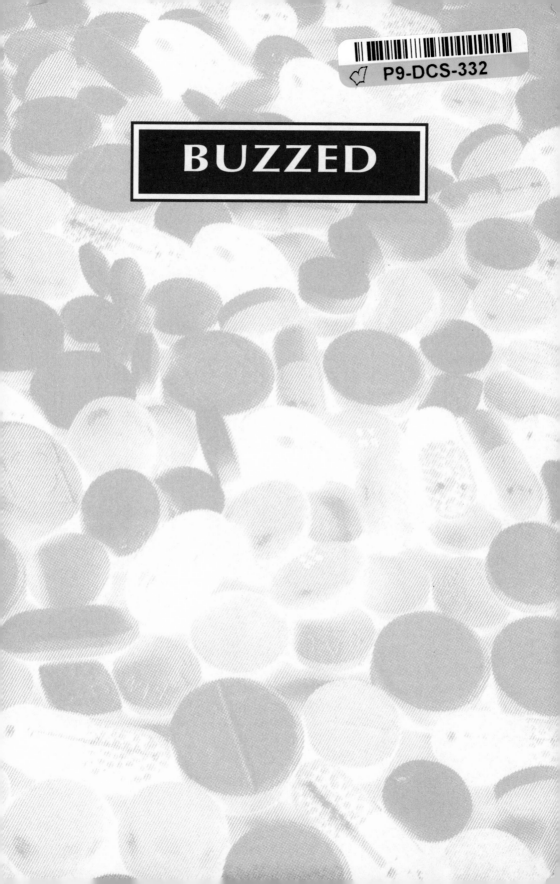

P9-DCS-332

BUZZED

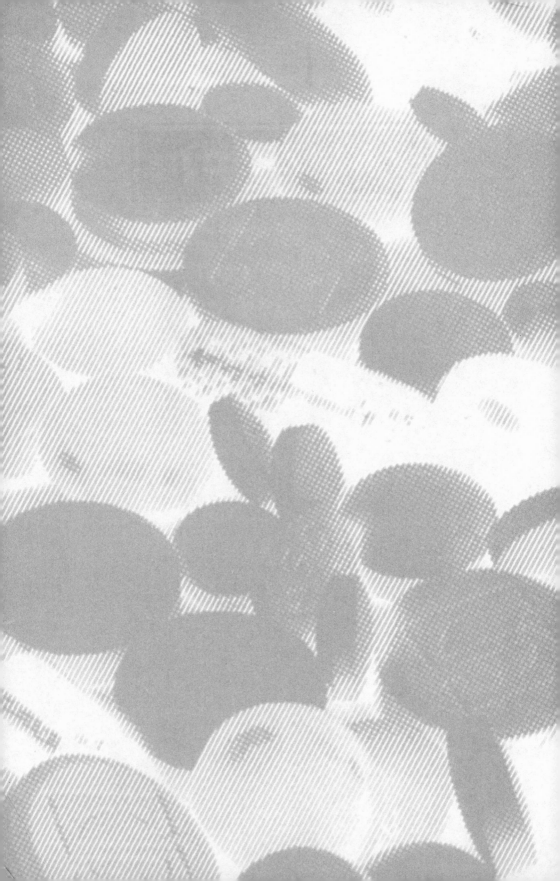

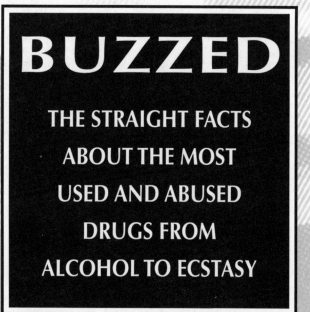

BUZZED

THE STRAIGHT FACTS ABOUT THE MOST USED AND ABUSED DRUGS FROM ALCOHOL TO ECSTASY

CYNTHIA KUHN, Ph.D.

SCOTT SWARTZWELDER, Ph.D.

WILKIE WILSON, Ph.D.

of the Duke University Medical Center

with Leigh Heather Wilson and Jeremy Foster

W. W. NORTON & COMPANY

NEW YORK • LONDON

For information about permission to reproduce selections from this book, write to Permissions, W. W. Norton & Company, Inc., 500 Fifth Avenue, New York, NY 10110.

The text of this book is composed in Electra with the display set in Optima
Composition and manufacturing by The Haddon Craftsmen, Inc.
Book design by JAM Design

Library of Congress Cataloging-in-Publication Data
Kuhn, Cynthia.
Buzzed : the straight facts about the most used and abused drugs from alcohol to ecstasy / Cynthia Kuhn, Scott Swartzwelder, Wilkie Wilson ; with Leigh Heather Wilson and Jeremy Foster.
p.   cm.
Includes index.
ISBN 0-393-31732-3 (pbk.)
1. Drugs of abuse—Popular works.   I. Swartzwelder, Scott.   II. Wilson, Wilkie.
III. Wilson, Leigh Heather.   IV. Foster, Jeremy.   V. Title.
RM316.K84   1998
615´.78—DC21   97-17914
CIP

W. W. Norton & Company, Inc., 500 Fifth Avenue, New York, N.Y. 10110
http://www.wwnorton.com

W. W. Norton & Company Ltd., 10 Coptic Street, London WC1A 1PU

1 2 3 4 5 6 7 8 9 0

Dedication

This is dedicated to my husband Mark, and my children Elena and Eric,
who have listened to every story in this book and
provided support and encouragement through
many evenings of writing.
—CMK

To my wife, Elizabeth, and my three children—
Sara, Nicholas, and Rita
—HSS

To Linda, Heather, Stephanie, and my father and mother,
Bill and Josephine Wilson, for their support and encouragement
in all the stages of my life.
—WAW

I would like to dedicate my efforts in creating *Buzzed* to my parents,
my sister, Stephanie, my grandparents, the administration and faculty of
Hollins College, and
Grey Magill, whose friendship I will always treasure.
—LHW

To my parents and my friends.
—JBF

Contents

Acknowledgments

This book arose from our recognition of how little most adolescents, parents, lawmakers, and even medical advisers know about drugs that we regularly use and abuse. Informal talks with Leigh Heather Wilson and Jeremy Foster (contributors to this book) about their college experiences, and our interactions with a large number of college students in our courses, led to our realization of the need for this book. These students asked hard questions, shared their experience honestly, and provided background research of their own. We thank each of them.

W. W. Norton representative Steve Hoge deserves our thanks for bringing the book to Norton's editors. Our agent, Reid Boates, was superb. He was recommended by Dr. Redford Williams, another Duke author. Thank you, Red. The editorial staff at Norton has seen us through the ups and downs of getting a book out, and we appreciate the good advice and editing from Alane Mason and Ashley Barnes. At Duke, we thank Dr. Barbara Markwiese for proofreading the text.

Two individuals were exceptional in helping us understand the rudimentary principles discussed in the "Legal Issues" chapter. Mr. Rick Glaser, First Assistant United States Attorney of the Northern Florida District, clearly and carefully explained some important parts of the federal laws that deal with illicit drugs as well as discussing the general nature of drug prosecutions at the federal level. He was remarkably insightful and helpful. (Mr. Glaser made it clear that his views do not necessarily represent the views of the Department of Justice, the Northern District of Florida, or the Middle District of North Carolina.) The Honorable James E. Hardin, Jr., the District Attorney for

Durham County, North Carolina, spoke extensively with us about drug prosecutions at the local and state levels. He was most patient with us nonlawyers, and quite helpful in explaining the basic laws regulating search and seizure as well as giving us an understanding of how local law enforcement is dealing with the drug issue. We are deeply grateful to both Mr. Hardin and Mr. Glaser.

Despite the fact that we received the best advice we could get, we want to be clear that the words written here are those of the authors, who are not lawyers, and should not be taken as legal advice.

In addition, Cindy thanks Dr. Anthony Means, Chairman of the Department of Pharmacology at Duke, for facilitating her undergraduate course, "Drugs and the Brain."

Scott thanks Jan Kaufman and Art Goldsmith for their encouragement and support throughout this project, Reynolds Smith for his interest and advice, and Drs. James Koury, Robert S. Dyer, Anthony L. Riley, and R. D. Myers for helping him learn how to think.

Wilkie thanks his daughter Heather, who, seeing her friends and acquaintances exposed to drugs in all sorts of social situations, was amazingly articulate in describing what she saw and absolutely relentless in pushing him to find some way to inform all of these people about the complexities of the drug issues in a user-friendly way. She became involved in this book as a research assistant, but she deserves enormous additional credit for her advice and counsel. He thanks her for her openness, her dedication to this project, and the grace she showed during some of the hard times. In addition, he thanks his wife, Linda, and his daughter Stephanie for support during some difficult moments when this was being written. Their love is beyond description.

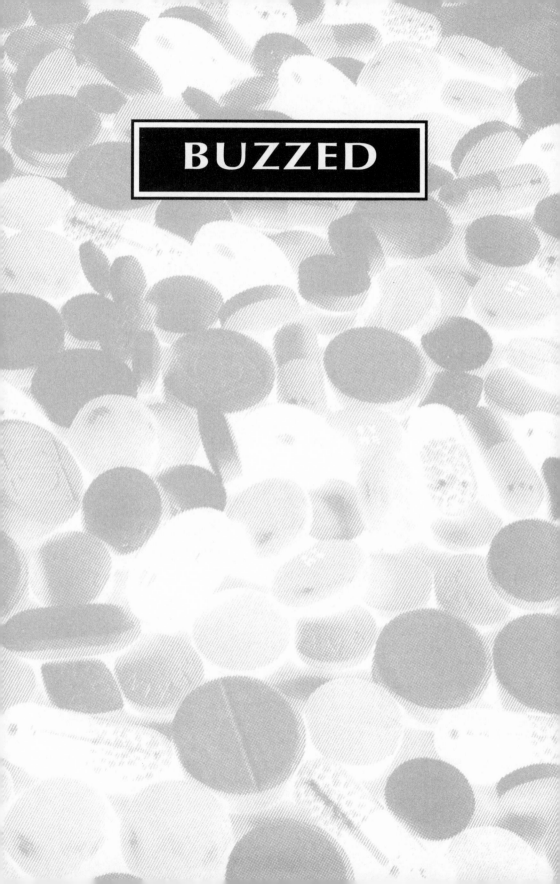

BUZZED

Introduction

For all of our history, we humans have believed that it is possible to reach beyond our simple consciousness. We hunger to expand ourselves into a universe that we feel but cannot touch. Chemicals that alter the way we perceive the world have played a large role in this search. In some instances, people have believed that the chemicals themselves had spiritual powers and mystical properties.

Others take a less spiritual view of drug use and choose chemicals that reduce a particularly painful state. They use drugs to reduce anxiety or suppress shyness, or they are prescribed drugs to treat serious illnesses like depression and schizophrenia. Some seek the stimulation and power they do not have in their social situations and choose drugs to help them attain this. As science has progressed, the laboratory has replaced nature as a source of chemicals, and the number of chemical choices has grown. There is every reason to believe that this will continue almost without bounds. So whether a person is seeking a way to expand his understanding or only trying to make normal life less painful, that person will have many, many choices of chemicals to use.

As scientists, we have devoted years to the study of the effects of drugs on the brain and behavior. We have seen the stunning advances in understanding the actions of the chemicals that have been with us for thousands of years. Yet surprisingly, little of this information is effectively translated for the public. We have become convinced that contemporary efforts to educate people about the effects of alcohol and other drugs are inadequate and misdirected. There is a lot of important information in the scientific literature about addiction and the effects of drugs, but it is not reaching the people who need to know it. The actions of drugs on the brain are complicated and vary tremendously from drug to drug and person to person, making it impossible to make blanket statements like "drugs kill" and have them believed by anyone who has any drug experience.

Imagine two trains headed at high speed in different directions, one being the scientific understanding of drug actions and addictions, the other being the public understanding of drug problems. The gap between scientific information and public information is growing hour by hour. This is the image portrayed in a recent speech by Dr. Alan Leshner, director of the National Institute of Drug Abuse. In his words, "There is a unique disconnect between the scientific facts and the public's perception about drug abuse and addiction. If we are going to make any progress, we need to overcome the 'great disconnect.' "

We agree that it is crucial to get these trains headed in the same direction. Each of us must understand what different drugs do to our brains and our consciousness, and what the physical consequences of their use might be. The number of consciousness-altering chemicals is increasing rapidly as medical scientists and pharmaceutical companies take advantage of new discoveries in neuroscience. Every time a new brain circuit or a new neurochemical is discovered, that discovery provides an opportunity to develop drugs that alter brain function in a new way. Some of these prove to be valuable treatments for mental illness, and many of the drugs that are currently abused, such as amphetamines, barbiturates, and "roofies," come directly from this same medical research.

Because of the incredible complexity of the brain, most drugs that affect it have actions in addition to those for which they were developed. Often dangerous drugs remain on the prescription market because they offer the only opportunity to treat a medical condition; their potential side effects seem worth the risk if they are used under medical supervision. Yet, recreational use may not be worth the risk of known and unknown effects on health. The fast-acting opiate fentanyl, which is used in the operating room, is a great example. This chemical is very safe and effective if there is a medical professional monitoring body functions such as heart rate, blood pressure, and the amount of oxygen getting to the brain. But with just a small error, it can turn dangerous and deadly. So imagine how risky it could be in some alley or dorm room, where it might be sold as "Apache" or "Jackpot."

It is easy to see how drug information can become subject to distortion. The public can be easily confused and manipulated. For example, some people (especially those in the drug culture) know individuals who consumed various drugs in various combinations in various settings over long periods of time and did not become permanently impaired, addicted, or involved with the legal system. Yet, they may not realize that many drug effects can be subtle enough to do a good deal of harm before the damage is recognized.

Conversely, others routinely carry out drug education by telling the worst horror stories they can recall, and often place any illegal substance in the category of "terribly dangerous." Not too long ago it was widely reported that a well-known basketball player, Len Bias, died after he used cocaine. This story has been used repeatedly to illustrate the dangers of cocaine use. However, most people who use cocaine do not die as a result of its use, and cocaine users and their friends certainly know it. Therefore, if horror stories are used as the principle tools in drug education, it does not take long for people to recognize that they do not represent the whole truth. The educator then loses credibility.

Good drug education will require a lot of effort. The scientific and medical literature is often difficult for most people to find and even more difficult to understand. Most interpretations of this literature to the general public are oversimplified, inaccurate, or disseminated by organizations that slant the research to further political and moral agendas.

The marijuana controversy is an excellent example. Some organizations have taken a hard line that this drug is devastating to anyone who uses it. Other organizations view it as harmless and support its legalization for totally unregulated consumption. In our opinion, the truth is somewhere in between. As you will read in the "Marijuana" chapter, marijuana causes memory problems and interacts with the immune system in unknown ways. It has effects many hours after it enters the body, even if the user is unaware of those effects. So it is not harmless. But people do not die from marijuana overdoses (as they do from overdoses of alcohol). Any truthful discussion of marijuana must include a range of topics and a realistic representation of risk. This cannot be accomplished by exchanging slogans.

Drugs should be viewed individually on a continuum of risk. Those we review in this book vary remarkably in their chemical structures, target systems in the brain, and in their pharmacological, behavioral, and psychological effects. Also, people vary markedly in their reactions to drugs. The rapidly expanding literature on genetic and hereditary predispositions toward addiction is just one example of our growing understanding of individual differences in drug reactivity.

The Internet is also making it difficult to carry out good drug education. An immense amount of easy-to-read information about drugs is accessible there, but, unfortunately, much of it is wrong. Anyone can create an Internet site and say whatever they please about drugs without anyone to weed out fact from fiction. A naïve reader could get into serious trouble following Web-site advice. The drug GHB, for instance, can be deadly at doses not far above those that produce a high. Yet some of the Internet literature would lead one to believe that the drug is not only safe but will treat alcoholism, insomnia, narcolepsy, sexual problems, and depression. One Internet site that we accessed in May 1997 provided directions for making GHB and stated that "GHB is the safest recreational drug ever used by humanity." Nothing could be further from the truth, and nothing could be more risky than believing this kind of misinformation. The counter on this Web site showed 300,270 visitor "hits" in the past eleven months. That's nearly 1,000 visitors per day getting dangerous information from just one Web page.

The primary goal of this book is to provide an unbiased, readable, and detailed presentation of the scientific facts about the drugs most commonly abused. We expect that this book will have its largest impact on people who are not addicted to drugs but are in a position to use drugs socially. During adolescence and young adulthood, most people—newly independent from parental control—will find themselves in situations in which drugs are available. College dorm rooms are often active, misguided psychopharmacology labs. We do not expect that this book will end drug abuse. However, it may prevent some bad experiences and some real tragedies.

We also hope that this book will begin a dialogue between scientists and legislators. The use of illegal drugs in the United States is rampant, and the social and legal reactions to that use have placed enormous stress on the resources of this country. President Clinton recently stated, "On the American side . . . we have less than five percent of the world's population and we consume about half the drugs." The debate about drug laws in the United States is raging and has been driven in part by this usage and the huge increase in the prison population. It is very costly to keep a person in prison, and during the last twenty years the number of sentenced prisoners in state and federal institutions has skyrocketed from about 200,000 to more than 1 million. About 30 percent of the current state prison population, and 60 percent of the people in federal prisons, are there for drug offenses.

The distinction between drugs that are considered legal or illegal in a given society is often based on much more than just scientific information. Traditions, economics, religion, and the popular media all influence the stance that a community takes on drugs. The religious rituals of some Native American communities include the use of hallucinogens, while many of those in Judeo-Christian traditions include the use of alcohol. Other cultures take very hardline stances against the use of any substance that is considered intoxicating. Even within a given culture, the legality of drugs can change over time. In the United States, the use of alcohol was legal for more than a century, was declared illegal during Prohibition, and is now legal again. Similarly, marijuana was legal until the 1930s, when its use was prohibited. Several recent state initiatives have permitted the use of marijuana for medical purposes and rekindled the debate about its legalization.

Again, in the words of Dr. Leshner, "Science must replace ideology as the foundation for drug abuse and addiction prevention, treatment, and policy strategies." The legislative authorities of developed societies must understand that no matter what legal efforts are taken, their citizens will have access to increasing numbers of chemicals that can cause addiction and impair human function. The only effective protection from the kind of societal disruption being experienced in the United States is good education that is accessible to everyone, and good scientific research that addresses the problems that drugs cause.

We hope that this book will be part of that process. The first twelve chapters in this book are devoted to particular drugs or classes of drugs. Each one starts with a quick-reference summary of the effects and dangers of the drugs. Next we present a detailed picture of how the drug works. We describe how the drug gets into and out of the body, its effects on physical and psychological functions, and its long-term effects. We've organized the drugs by class—even though some drug classes, like the enactogens, will be much less familiar to most readers than the specific drug names—because drugs in the same class generally have the same mechanisms of action, effects, and risks. However, the table of contents, the chapter of contents, and the index should make it easy to determine where to go for information on a specific drug, and the glossary provides translation for an impressive variety of street terms. In the second part of the book we've provided general chapters on the brain, how drugs work, addiction, and legal issues. We recommend that any reader using the book for a broad general understanding, rather than as a quick reference, read those chapters first, as they will provide an important background for all of the scientific information relating to specific drugs.

We believe that when provided with an unbiased and authoritative source of information about drugs and drug interactions, individuals will be empowered to make healthy decisions.

Just Say Know

(A College Student's Perspective by
Leigh Heather Wilson and Jeremy Foster)

"Just Say No." Well, no thanks. We would like a bit more information before making decisions about drug use. And when you say "Just Say No," does that mean you're telling us alcohol is as dangerous as cocaine? Before you start lumping everything from smoking cigarettes to shooting heroin together, could we have a little bit more information? "Just Say No" might not always be the right choice. Hasn't research shown that a glass of wine can be healthy? It is only natural that phrases like "Just Say No" are not sufficient to satisfy many young people. It is the very basis of our society to value proof, logic, and fact above all. Instead of asking us to respond blindly, convince us!

We have been friends all our lives. Because Heather's dad is a neuropharmacologist, we knew about psychoactive drugs early on. Since we can remember, drugs and how they do this or that to the something-or-another region of the brain has been a familiar topic of conversation.

Like many kids, in high school we became bored with the same-old, same-old that radio and MTV offered and wanted to broaden our musical horizons. This sparked an interest in some of the bands popular in the sixties and seventies. Consequently, we developed a fascination with the surrounding culture. It was clear that drugs, of one character or another, were cast in many roles during those times. The deaths of Janis Joplin, Jim Morrison, and Jimi Hendrix were all related to their drug use, and still, by way of their association with these and other musicians, drugs have an air of romance and intrigue.

Around the same time that we became aware of these issues, similar concerns about the nineties music culture became a trendy topic in the media. The flurry of publicity on the rising use of drugs again among young people, as well as the resurgence of heroin use, in particular, has led many to compare our times to the sixties and seventies. As one can imagine, all the hype made us quite curious about the subject. Not to mention the allure of the positive feelings people say they get from taking drugs. The rush from shooting heroin is commonly described as feeling even better than experiencing an orgasm.

We were both way past believing the slogans and hyperbole on the subject of drugs. Heather began nagging her dad with question after question about drugs in a struggle to understand their effects, and the questions evolved into a series of great conversations with him and some of his colleagues. We were so interested because finally we were getting straight, unbiased information about the actions of drugs in our bodies.

We learned a lot about heroin, which had seemed so attractively mysterious. We learned that its dangers included several major risks: addiction, overdose, and contracting HIV from needles. The risk of overdose, we learned, is unpredictable because of individual responses to the drug and varying degrees of purity of the compound sold by dealers. The particular compounds used to cut it can also be dangerous. So it became clear to us that with heroin, as with many other drugs, the safety issues are very complicated and often the danger is not limited to the specific effects of the drug but can include many other peripheral issues. For heroin, some of these issues arise from economic considerations because its high street value and relative scarcity leads dealers to cut it in unpredictable ways.

After all these conversations with Heather's dad and his colleagues, heroin seemed far less interesting and mysterious, and we avoided it. We felt lucky to have learned the truth, and with the new knowledge we felt armed. If someone offered heroin to one of us, we wouldn't be "just saying no," but defending an informed decision to stay away from the drug.

Nonetheless, there are people who will use drugs regardless of anything anyone says. And no amount of knowledge can save someone from a danger that is due to the drug's action in the body. Through learning about heroin we realized that not all the threats have direct causes and that by giving people good information, some of the dangers can be lessened. We know that a drug's effects can change in a novel environment, that the risk of overdose increases when the drug purity is not consistent, and that some drugs taken together become lethal. Making people aware of these kinds of issues could decrease some risks of using drugs.

Overall we were struck by the lack of unbiased and complete information available to people like us, and the contrast between the formal education we had received and the scientific facts we had learned.

By the time we were freshmen in college, we had both had experiences with alcohol, many of them positive. It wasn't until Heather went to college that she had her first really adverse experience with drugs. During Parents' Weekend, she, her roommate, and their parents went to her best friend's room and found her soaked in blood and tears on the dorm-room floor. Heather's friend had a history of depression, and the combination of this, a bottle of Jack Daniel's Black Label, and too much cold medicine left her ravaged and suicidal. Unfortunately, she didn't know that alcohol and antihistamines have a synergistic and depressing effect, and that at high levels the combination can even be lethal. They found her in time to save her, but she will always carry the scars where she cut her wrists.

Heather's friend wasn't the only girl left with scars. Everyone involved was affected. She and Heather were part of an unusually close-knit group of five. They had, unknowingly, become a family to each other. By doing almost everything together, they had become a source of strength and love for each other as they adjusted to college life. When Heather's friend went home she left a hole, a missing link in that safety net. An irresponsible act, taken without knowledge of drugs and their interactions, changed the lives of everyone who found her, all of her friends, and all of her family.

A second experience occurred on the same dormitory hall. Heather and her friends were invited to share some Ecstasy with boys from a nearby school. They were excited, having heard that Ecstasy was a lot of fun. Heather also remembered one of the strongest statements about drug use her dad had ever made. He had said, "Ecstasy permanently alters your brain, Heather. It is a bad drug and, frankly, this is one that I would like to ask you, as a personal favor because I'm your Dad and I love you, not to try. There are some kids who have used it and suffered problems with sleep, anxiety, and depression. These poor kids have changed their own brains and they will never be the same."

Cindy Kuhn had loaned Heather a neuropharmacology textbook the year before, the students used it to read about Ecstasy. With a clear view of what the drug could do to their brains, most of them chose not to try it, though others decided to take the risk.

With these experiences still vivid in our minds, the vast and cavernous difference between what we know from the most current research on drugs and what drug education and prevention programs teach was obvious. We realized that we are all being sold a bill of goods when it comes to recreational drugs. There are dangers involved in using drugs, but the issue is much more complicated than that. Each drug works differently in the brain, and there are very different issues to consider with each drug. Also, some drugs pose risks that are far greater than others. We do an injustice to ourselves when we try to make blanket statements like "Drugs Kill" or "Users Are Losers."

We realized that not everybody has a scientist to talk to and that the world needed a book that would not use scare tactics but would have reliable, in-depth information—a book that would not insult our intelligence. This book is about making the most current research on the pharmacological and psychological effects of drugs available to you in a friendly and useful way. We hope you enjoy reading it, but, most of all, we believe that with information that is both clearly presented and unbiased you will be qualified to make better decisions for yourself about drugs.

Test Your Drug Knowledge

1. The effects of smoking pot can last for two days. True or false?

2. Chocolate and marijuana stimulate the same receptors in the brain. How much chocolate would you have to eat to get the same effect as one joint?

3. Which cup of coffee has more caffeine—the one brewed in the office coffee maker from grocery-bought beans or the expensive cup from the new gourmet coffee bar?

4. Ecstasy was first popularized by Californian psychotherapists who tried to use it for "empathy training" in marriage counseling. True or false?

5. What popular recreational drug was originally developed as a treatment for asthma?

6. What popular nightclub drug is actually an animal tranquilizer—and the difference between a recreational dosage of it and an overdose is dangerously small?

7. What are the most dangerous drugs, and also the ones most often used by children under fourteen?

8. Which drug prescribed each year to millions of Americans impairs memory?

9. Put these drugs in the order of addictiveness: marijuana, nicotine, heroin.

10. Tonight you are at a club sipping on a soft drink, or still on your first beer, when suddenly you begin to feel very drunk and uncoordinated. What might have happened?

11. What was the drug misinformation promulgated by the movie *Pulp Fiction?*

12. What was the drug effect correctly portrayed by the movie *Trainspotting?*

13. Which drug carries a greater danger of fatal overdose, alcohol or LSD?

14. Right or wrong: alcohol before bed makes you sleep better.

15. Are the herbal remedies sold in health-food stores actually drugs?

16. Why do people inject a drug instead of just taking a pill?

17. What is the most popular illegal drug in America now?

18. If a child or an animal eats a cigarette, will it hurt?

19. Does marijuana kill brain cells?

20. Does alcohol?

21. Isn't it safe to drink a glass or two of wine with your dinner when you're pregnant?

22. Is caffeine addictive?

23. Are crack babies doomed to mental retardation and behavioral problems?

24. What drug that is popular on the club scene, and among high school students, causes definitive brain damage in rodents and monkeys?

ANSWERS

1. True. THC, the active ingredient in marijuana, is extremely fat soluble and can still enter the bloodstream from the fatty tissues and have effects on the brain for up to two days after smoking. Its by-products can turn up in the blood many months after the last use if the smoker suddenly loses a lot of weight. *(See Chapter 7.)*

2. About twenty-five pounds. *(See Chapter 2.)*

3. The office cup. The African robusta beans found in grocery stores can contain up to twice as much caffeine as the more expensive arabica beans found in specialty coffee shops. *(See Chapter 2.)*

4. True! *(See Chapter 3.)*

5. Amphetamine, which was originally synthesized as a derivative of ephedrine, the active ingredient of the Chinese herbal drug mahuang. *(See Chapter 12.)*

6. Ketamine, otherwise known as Special K (not the cereal!). *(See Chapter 4.)*

7. Chemical solvents such as toluene, benzene, propane, and those found in glue and paint. More than 20 percent of eighth graders have used such inhalants. *(See Chapter 6.)*

8. Valium and other drugs of its class. *(See Chapter 10.)*

9. Nicotine, heroin, marijuana (actually, there is little evidence that marijuana is addictive). *(See Chapter 7.)*

10. Someone probably slipped a sedative into your drink, like a roofie (Rohypnol) or GHB (gamma-hydroxybutyrate), also known as Easy Lay. These drugs can be fatal, and medical attention would be wise. *(See Chapter 10.)*

11. The movie shows a heroin overdose being treated by an injection of adrenaline into the heart. This is useless and dangerous: the opiate-blocking drug naloxone reverses heroin overdose after injection by more conventional routes. *(See Chapter 9.)*

12. The main character in the movie is overcome with diarrhea after coming down off heroin. Since heroin causes constipation, once it's eliminated from the body just the opposite effect kicks in. *(See Chapter 9.)*

13. Alcohol. Many deaths each year are caused by alcohol overdose. There is little danger of LSD overdose unless it is combined with or contaminated by other drugs. *(See Chapter 1.)*

14. Wrong. Alcohol might make you sleepy at first, but its by-products can cause sleeplessness, so after a night of drinking you might fall asleep quickly but wake up in the middle of the night feeling agitated. *(See Chapter 1.)*

15. Anything you take with the intention of changing how your body acts is a drug. Any drug that comes from a plant is herbal. This includes nicotine, ephedrine, and cocaine. "Herbal remedies" are completely unregulated and the amount and purity of what you buy is unknown. *(See Chapter 5.)*

16. For the speed with which the drug gets into the bloodstream, and into the brain. The faster it gets to the brain, the better the "rush." This faster delivery also means a greater chance of overdose because the amount of drug can reach fatal levels before the user can do anything about it. *(See Chapter 13.)*

17. Marijuana is used by far more people than any other illegal drug: 77 percent of all illegal drug users use marijuana, and almost 5 percent of the population used marijuana in the last month. *(See Chapter 7.)*

18. Yes. There is enough nicotine in a cigarette to make a small child or animal very sick, or even to kill one. *(See Chapter 8.)*

19. Probably not, but it does interfere with learning and memory. *(See Chapter 7.)*

20. It is unlikely that a single drink kills brain cells, but long-term chronic drinking can cause permanent memory loss and definite brain damage. *(See Chapter 1.)*

21. No. Studies have shown that even very moderate drinking during pregnancy can permanently hinder a child's ability to learn and to concentrate. *(See Chapter 1.)*

22. Not really. People who stop drinking coffee may experience mild withdrawal that includes drowsiness, headaches, and lethargy, but people very rarely engage in the compulsive, repetitive pattern of drinking coffee that typifies use of addictive substances. Addiction is not defined simply by the presence of withdrawal. *(See Chapter 2.)*

23. Not necessarily. In fact, the most common problems that crack babies experience are the same as those experienced by children of women who smoke cigarettes: small birth weight and the associated health risks, and subtle developmental delays in childhood. Cocaine can cause very severe problems, including premature separation of the placenta from the uterus, premature birth, and intrauterine stroke, but these are rare. *(See Chapter 12.)*

24. Ecstasy (MDMA). Studies show dramatic damage to nerves containing the neurotransmitter serotonin that is irreversible at doses approximating those consumed by humans. *(See Chapter 3.)*

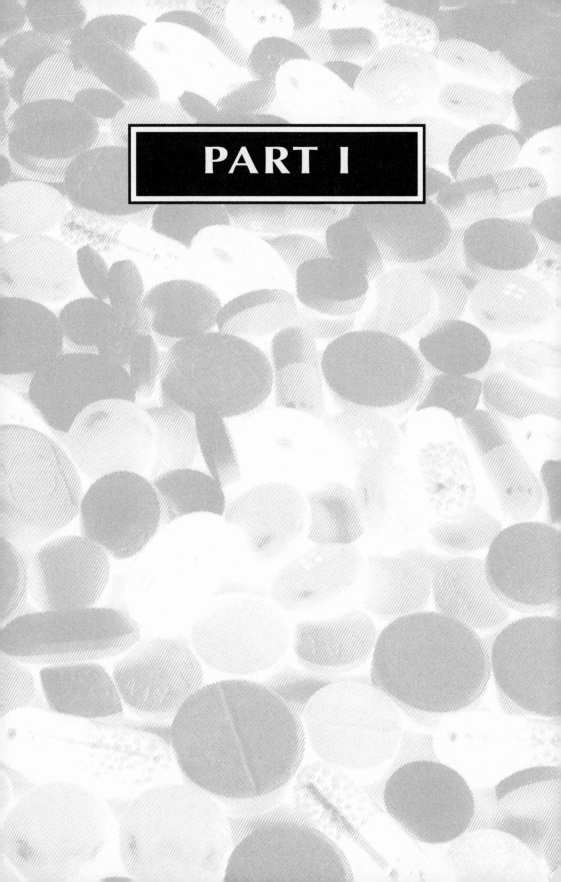

PART I

1

Alcohol

Drug Class: Sedative hypnotic

Individual Drugs: beer (5 percent or less alcohol); wine (9 to 12 percent alcohol); spirits, liquor, whiskey (40 percent or more alcohol)

Common Terms: liquor, whiskey, booze, hooch, wine, beer, ale, porter

The Buzz: When people drink alcohol, they feel pleasure and relaxation during the first half hour or so, often becoming talkative and socially outgoing, but these feelings are usually replaced by sedation (drowsiness) as the alcohol is eliminated from the body, so drinkers may become quiet and withdrawn later. This pattern often motivates them to drink more in order to keep the initial pleasant buzz going.

Overdose and Other Bad Effects: Under most circumstances, the chances of life-threatening overdose are low. However, people get into trouble when they drink a lot of alcohol very quickly—such as in a drinking game, on a dare, or when they can't taste the alcohol (as in punch or Jell-O shots). Drinking on an empty stomach is particularly risky. If a person becomes unconscious, is impossible to arouse, or seems to have trouble breathing, it is a medical emergency and immediate attention is necessary. Some very drunk people vomit, block their airway, suffocate, and die. Call for emergency medical assistance.

When drunk people pass out, their bodies continue to absorb the alcohol they just drank after they are asleep. The amount of alcohol in their blood can then reach dangerous levels and they can die in their sleep. Keep checking someone who has gone to sleep drunk. Do not leave him alone.

Binge drinking is particularly dangerous because it is during binges that most fatal overdoses occur.

Dangerous Combinations with Other Drugs: It is dangerous to combine alcohol with anything else that makes you sleepy. This includes other sedative drugs, such as opiates (e.g., heroin, morphine, or Demerol), barbiturates (e.g. phenobarbital), Quaaludes (methaqualone), Valium-like drugs (benzodiazepines), and even the antihistamines found in some cold medicines.

All sedative drugs share at least some of alcohol's effects and each increases the other's effects. Drugs can become deadly when combined. Even doses of drugs that do not cause unconsciousness or breathing problems alone can powerfully impair physical activities such as sports, driving a car, and operating machinery when taken together.

CHAPTER CONTENTS

INTRODUCTION

The use of chemicals to alter thinking and feeling is as old as humanity itself, and alcohol was probably one of the first substances used. Even the earliest historical writings make note of alcohol drinking, and breweries can be traced back some six thousand years to ancient Egypt and Babylonia. In the Middle Ages, Arab technology introduced distillation—a way to increase the alcohol content in beverages—to Europe. In those times alcohol was believed to remedy practically any disease. In fact, the Gaelic term *whiskey* is best translated as "water of life."

These days, beverage alcohol is clearly the drug of choice for much of Western culture, and one needs only to look closely at much of the advertising in this country to see that it is still sold as a magic elixir of sorts. We use alcohol to celebrate successes, to mourn failures and losses, and to celebrate holidays of cultural and religious significance. Implicit in these uses are the hope and promise that alcohol will amplify the good times and help us through the bad ones.

Nowhere is the alcohol advertising more targeted, or the peer pressure to drink more powerful, than on adolescents and young adults—particularly young men. Advertisements for alcoholic beverages take up eighteen times more space in college newspapers than do those related to books, and forty-eight times more space than those related to soft drinks. While young people do most of the drinking in American society, they are also the ones who need their brains to be functioning at their highest levels because of the intellectual demands of education and career preparation.

For most people alcohol is not a terribly dangerous drug—but it is a powerful drug, and must be treated accordingly. No one would take a powerful antibiotic or heart medication without the advice of a physician. But alcohol is available to virtually anyone who wants to have it, without a prescription. The vast majority of people in the United States face the decision of whether to use alcohol, and how much to use, during their high school or college years. The responsibility for making these decisions falls on each individual. This chapter will provide the latest information about alcohol and its effects.

TYPES OF "ALCOHOLS"

The alcohol that is used in beverages is called ethanol. It is actually only one of many different types. The alcohol a nurse rubs on the skin as a disinfectant before giving an injection or drawing a blood sample is not the same — it is isopropyl alcohol. The chemical structures of most alcohols make them quite toxic to the human body. Ethanol is the only one that should ever be consumed, but people regularly poison themselves with other alcohols. For example, methanol, produced in home-distilling operations, can cause blindness. A case of methanol poisoning requires immediate medical attention.

HOW ALCOHOL MOVES THROUGH THE BODY

The amount of alcohol a person consumes at any given time will influence these processes, but it's important to standardize the amount that we're talking about first, since beer, wine, and spirits contain significantly different concentrations of ethanol. A standard drink is often classified as the amount of alcohol consumed in one twelve-ounce beer, one four-ounce glass of wine, or a mixed drink containing one ounce of hard liquor.

GETTING IN

Ethanol is a relatively small molecule that is easily and quickly absorbed into the body. Once a drink is swallowed, it enters the stomach and small intestine, where a high concentration of small blood vessels gives the alcohol ready access to the blood. About 20 percent of a given dose of alcohol is absorbed through the stomach, and most of the remaining 80 percent is absorbed through the small intestine. Once they enter the bloodstream, the alcohol molecules are carried throughout the body and into direct contact with the cells of virtually all the organs.

Often a person who goes out for a drink in the early evening before dinner reports, "The alcohol went straight to my head." Actually, the alcohol went very rapidly throughout the whole body, and shortly after it was absorbed it became fairly evenly distributed. This process is called *equilibration*. But since a substantial proportion of the blood that the heart pumps at any given time goes to the brain, and since the fatty material of the brain absorbs alcohol (which dissolves in both fat and water) very well, that is where the effects are first and predominantly felt. However, as the alcohol is first entering the circulation (before equilibration), its concentration in the brain is actually higher than its concentration in the blood. Since it is alcohol's effects on the brain that lead to intoxication, soon after drinking a person may be more impaired than her blood alcohol level would indicate. So, there is some truth in the statement, "That drink went right to my head."

Indeed, the presence or absence of food in the stomach is perhaps the most powerful influence on the absorption of alcohol. When someone drinks on an empty stomach, the blood absorbs the alcohol very rapidly, reaching a peak concentration in about one hour. By contrast, the same amount of alcohol consumed with a meal would not be completely absorbed for nearly two hours. The food dilutes the alcohol and slows the emptying of the stomach into the small intestine, where alcohol is very rapidly absorbed. Peak blood alcohol concentration could be as much as three times greater in someone with an empty stomach than in someone who has just eaten.

The concentration of alcohol in the beverage consumed also significantly influences its absorption—in general, the higher the concentration, the faster it will be absorbed. So, relatively diluted solutions of alcohol, such as beer, enter the bloodstream more slowly than more highly concentrated solutions, such as mixed drinks or shots. Since more rapid absorption usually means higher peak blood alcohol concentrations, a person who drinks shots might have a higher blood alcohol level than a person who drinks the same amount of alcohol in the form of beer or wine.

The rapid absorption of high concentrations of alcohol can suppress the centers of the brain that control breathing and cause a person to pass out or even die. People who get into this kind of extreme medical emergency usually do so by accepting a challenge to drink a certain amount of alcohol in a short period of time, by playing drinking games that result in rapid consumption of multiple drinks, or by taking something like Jell-O shots, which get a lot of highly concentrated alcohol into the body in a short time. Often, young people, who cannot legally buy alcohol, "drink up" before going out to a mall or to a school dance. Some people do a lot of drinking before leaving for an event at a park or beach where alcohol is not permitted. Given the rapid accumulation of alcohol in the brain, under these circumstances the drinker may be very impaired in terms of her ability to drive or think clearly, though her blood alcohol level would not suggest this degree of impairment.

A person's body type also determines alcohol distribution. A particularly muscular or obese person may seem to be "really holding his booze," because he has more fat and muscle to absorb the alcohol. A heavy person would register a lower alcohol level in the blood than a lean individual after an identical dose. However, the extra weight also slows the elimination of alcohol, so he would retain it longer.

In pregnant women, alcohol is freely distributed to the fetus. In fact, because of the large blood supply to the uterus and developing fetus, some studies actually indicate that the tissues of the fetus may achieve a *higher* alcohol concentration than the mother. Later in this chapter, we will discuss the effects of alcohol on the fetus, and the lasting effects that prenatal exposure has on the child later in life. For now, it is important to recognize that when alcohol is distributed in the body, it does not discriminate between the tissues of the mother and those of the fetus.

GETTING OUT

The roadside Breathalyzer test is actually an excellent way of estimating the amount of alcohol consumed, even though 95 percent of the alcohol a person drinks is metabolized before the body excretes it. Only about 5 percent of the absorbed alcohol is eliminated unchanged, in the urine or through the lungs, but it is enough to result in "alcohol breath"—and the proportion exhaled stays constant enough to give a very accurate estimate of how much alcohol is in the blood.

Most alcohol is metabolized by the liver, where an enzyme called alcohol dehydrogenase, or ADH, breaks ethanol down into acetaldehyde, which in turn is broken down by another enzyme called acetaldehyde dehydrogenase into acetate, which is then excreted. The intermediate product, acetaldehyde, is a toxic chemical that can make a person feel sick. Although under normal conditions acetaldehyde is broken down quite rapidly, if it accumulates in the body, intense feelings of nausea and illness will result. One early drug therapy for alcoholism was a drug called disulfiram (or Antabuse), which allows the concentration of acetaldehyde to accumulate, making a person feel quite ill after drinking and less likely to drink again. While this strategy appeared promising initially, it has not resulted in consistent positive clinical outcomes with alcoholics.

The *rate* at which alcohol is metabolized and eliminated from the body is critical for understanding how long a person can expect to be affected by drinking. The rate of alcohol metabolism is constant across time. In general, an adult metabolizes the alcohol from one ounce of whiskey (which is about 40 percent alcohol) in about one hour. The liver handles this rate of metabolism efficiently. If the drinker consumes more than this amount, the system becomes saturated and the additional alcohol simply accumulates in the blood and body tissues and waits its turn for metabolism. The results are higher blood alcohol concentrations and more intoxication.

In addition, continued drinking increases the enzymes that metabolize alcohol. The increased level of these enzymes promotes metabolism of some other drugs and medications, harming the drinker in a variety of ways. For example, some medications used to prevent blood clotting and to treat diabetes are metabolized more rapidly in chronic drinkers, and are thus less effective. Similarly, these enzymes increase the breakdown of the painkiller acetaminophen (found in Tylenol), resulting in the production of substances that are toxic to the liver. Finally, metabolic tolerance to alcohol results in similar tolerance to other sedative drugs, such as barbiturates, even if the individual has never taken barbiturates. This is called *cross tolerance*, and may place the drinker at greater risk for the use or abuse of such drugs.

EFFECTS ON THE BRAIN AND BEHAVIOR

Once alcohol has been absorbed and distributed, it has many different effects on the brain and behavior. To a large extent these effects vary with the pattern of drinking. Therefore, it is useful to discuss the effects of *acute, chronic,* and *prenatal* alcohol exposure separately.

ACUTE EXPOSURE

Effects on Behavior and Physical State

Although the effects that a given dose of alcohol will have on an individual vary considerably, the following table shows the general effects of a range of alcohol doses:

Ethanol Dose (oz/hour)	Blood Ethanol (mg/100ml)	Function Impaired	Physical State
1–4	up to 100	Judgment fine motor coordination reaction time	happy talkative boastful
4–12	100–300	motor coordination reflexes	staggering slurred speech nausea, vomiting
12–16	300–400	voluntary responses to stimulation	hypothermia hyperthermia anesthesia
16–24	400–600	sensation movement self-protective reflexes	comatose
24–30	600–900	breathing heart function	dead

Still, there is often a substantial difference between *being* impaired and *appearing* impaired. In one study, trained observers were asked to rate whether or not a person was intoxicated after drinking. At low blood alcohol concentrations (about half the legal limit for intoxication) only about 10 percent of the drinkers appeared intoxicated, and at very high concentrations (greater than twice the legal limit) all the drinkers appeared intoxicated. However, only 64 percent of people who had blood alcohol concentrations of 100–150 mg/100ml (well above the legal limit in most states) were judged to be intoxicated. So, in casual social interactions, many people who actually would be quite impaired—and who would pose a real threat behind the wheel of a car—may not appear impaired even to trained observers.

Alcohol and Brain Cells

It is probably safe to say that many readers have heard some variation of the following statement: *"Every time you take a drink of alcohol you kill ten thousand brain cells."* Although it is highly unlikely that anyone would drink enough alcohol in a given sitting to kill brain cells directly, as with many such generalizations there is a grain of truth in the warning.

One way that researchers have tried to determine which brain regions control which behaviors in animals is by destroying, or *lesioning*, a specific brain region and then testing the animal on a particular behavioral task. Early in the use of this lesioning technique, some researchers found that if they injected a very high concentration of alcohol into the brain (far higher than would be achieved by a drinking person), the cells in that region would die. There is also another grain of truth in the warning about alcohol and brain cells: chronic, repeated drinking damages and sometimes kills the cells in specific brain areas. We will address this in the next section of this chapter: "Chronic Exposure."

There are fundamentally only two types of actions that a chemical can have on nerve cells—excitatory or inhibitory. That is, a drug can either increase or decrease the probability that a given cell will become active and communicate with the other cells to which it is connected. Alcohol generally depresses this type of communication, or synaptic activity, and thus its actions are similar to those of other sedative drugs, like barbiturates (such as phenobarbital) and benzodiazepines (such as Valium). Despite this general suppression of neuronal activity, however, many people report that alcohol activates or stimulates them, particularly soon after drinking, when the concentration of alcohol in the blood is increasing. Although we don't know exactly why alcohol produces feelings of stimulation, there are a couple of possibilities. First, there is the *biphasic* action of alcohol. This refers to the fact that at low concentrations alcohol actually activates some nerve cells. As the alcohol concentration increases, however, these same cells decrease their firing rates and their activity becomes suppressed. Or it might be that some nerve cells send excitatory signals to the other cells with which they communicate, prompting them to send inhibitory messages, actually suppressing the activity of the next cell in the circuit. So, if alcohol suppresses the activity of one of these "inhibitory" cells, the net effect in the circuit would be one of activation. Whatever the exact mechanism, it appears that there are several ways in which alcohol can have activating as well as suppressing effects on neural circuits.

Effects on Specific Neurotransmitters

GABA and Glutamate

Until recently it was generally thought that alcohol treated all nerve cells equally, simply inhibiting their activity by disturbing their membrane integrity. In this sense the effects of alcohol on the brain were thought to be very non-specific. However, recent research clearly shows that alcohol has specific and powerful effects on the function of at least two particular types of neuronal receptors: GABA receptors and glutamate receptors. GABA and glutamate are chemical neurotransmitters that account for much of the inhibitory and excitatory activity in the brain. When the terminals of one cell release GABA onto GABA receptors on the next cell, that cell becomes less active. When glutamate lands on a glutamate receptor, that cell becomes more active. It is in this way that many circuits in the brain maintain the delicate balance between excitation and inhibition. Small shifts in this balance can change the activity of the circuits and, ultimately, in the functioning of the brain.

Alcohol increases the inhibitory activity of GABA receptors and decreases the excitatory activity of glutamate receptors. These are the two primary ways alcohol suppresses brain activity. While the enhancement of GABA activity is probably responsible for many of the general sedating effects of alcohol, the suppression of glutamate activity may have a more specific effect: an impairment in the ability to form new memories while intoxicated. Recently it has become clear that the activity of a particular subtype of glutamate receptor, called the NMDA receptor, is very powerfully inhibited by alcohol—even in very low doses. The NMDA receptor is also known to be critical for the formation of new memory. Alcohol's powerful suppression of activity at the NMDA receptor may therefore account for the memory deficits that people experience after drinking.

Dopamine

The neurotransmitter dopamine is known to underlie the rewarding effects of such highly addictive drugs as cocaine and amphetamine. In fact, dopamine is thought to be the main chemical messenger in the reward centers of the brain, which promote the experience of pleasure. Alcohol drinking increases the release of dopamine in these reward centers, probably through the action of GABA neurons, which connect to the dopamine neurons. Very recent studies in animals show that the increase in dopamine activity occurs only while the concentration of alcohol in the blood is rising—not while it is falling. So, during the first minutes after drinking the pleasure circuits in the brain are activated, but this "dopamine rush" disappears after the alcohol level stops rising. This may motivate the drinker to consume more alcohol in order to start the pleasure sequence again. The problem is that although the dopamine rush is over, there is still plenty of alcohol in the body. Continued drinking in pursuit of the pleasure signals could push the blood alcohol concentration up to dangerous levels.

Effects on Memory

One of the most common experiences people report after drinking is a failure to remember accurately what happened "the night before." In more extreme cases, after heavy drinking, people often report that whole chunks of time simply appear to be blank, with no memory at all having been recorded. It is also clear that alcohol impairs the ability to form new memories even after relatively low doses. So, having a couple of beers while studying for an exam or preparing for a presentation at work is probably not a good strategy. The alcohol may promote relaxation, but it will also compromise learning and memory.

Hangover

One of the best known symptoms of a hangover is a pounding headache. The cause is not exactly clear, but probably relates to the effects of alcohol on blood vessels and fluid balances in the body. In any case, it is much easier to prevent the onset of pain than it is to relieve the pain once it has started. Therefore, the sooner a pain reliever is taken, the better. Some people take ibuprofen or Tylenol before going to bed after a night of drinking. This way the chemicals in the pain reliever can prevent the pain signals in the brain from getting started as the alcohol is eliminated from the body. Aspirin can serve the same purpose, but both aspirin and alcohol irritate the stomach and small intestine, and together they can result in uncomfortable gastric upset.

The upset stomach and nausea associated with hangover are harder to deal with. These may be caused by the toxic by-products of alcohol elimination, irritation to the stomach, or both. No medicines treat these effects specifically. Rather, the best strategy is to eat foods that are gentle on the stomach and to drink plenty of fluids. Morning coffee may help to start the day after a night on the town, but its irritating effects on the stomach may make it an unpleasant waking.

CHRONIC EXPOSURE

Everybody wants to know how much drinking is bad for them. Some want to know how much drinking they can get away with before they cause themselves health problems. This question always reminds us of a common response to the old warning that masturbation would cause blindness: Some people just wanted to know how much they could do it before suffering blurred vision.

The long-term effects of drinking depend on how much alcohol is consumed. Although there appear to be some health benefits associated with very moderate drinking in adults (see the section below), chronic heavy drinking creates very serious problems in a number of body systems, including the brain, liver, and digestive system. Between the extremes of heavy and light drinking lies a "gray area" that is not completely understood. Moreover, this gray area appears to be rather small. That is, while an average of one-half to one drink per day may be healthy for your heart, it is perfectly clear that an average of two drinks per day significantly increases your risk of dying from heart disease or cancer.

The Incredible Shrinking Brain

The brain-imaging techniques that have been developed during the past ten years create a window into the effects of alcohol on the brain. Using these techniques, researchers have observed shrinkage of brain tissue in people after long-term use of alcohol. The shrinkage is due primarily to the loss of nerve cells, not the loss of the "support cells" that surround them. So, it appears that chronic alcohol drinking does kill brain cells. Some studies indicate that certain parts of the brain may be more vulnerable to damage by alcohol than others, such as the cortex—the folded, lumpy surface of the brain (it gets its name because of its resemblance to the bark of a tree), which endows us with consciousness and controls most of our mental functions. Another vulnerable region is the mammillary bodies, which are very important for memory. (These small, round structures near the base of the brain got their name from the neuroanatomists who first noticed them and thought that they looked like breasts. Actually, their resemblance to breasts is quite remote, but neuroanatomists do have good imaginations!)

Most of the studies of brain shrinkage have been done with alcoholics. The shrinkage occurs while the person is still using alcohol. If she stops drinking for a prolonged period, her brain will recover somewhat—not because new nerve cells grow, but because support cells, or parts of the remaining nerve cells, grow. Therefore, the regrowth of brain size does not mean that the deficits in mental functioning that many alcoholics experience will be erased simply by abstaining from alcohol.

It is not known if there is a safe level of chronic drinking. Clearly many people who drink do not appear to suffer any damage to their mental functioning. Still, as with acute intoxication, the lack of any *obvious* impairment does not mean that there is none. Studies using animals instead of humans can look more closely at nerve-cell damage. Such studies have shown that more moderate alcohol exposure can damage and kill brain cells. A number of these studies have shown large areas of nerve-cell loss in a region of the brain called the hippocampus, which is known to be critical for the formation of new memories. This suggests that memory function could be damaged in someone who drinks chronically, though at a lower level than in someone who is clearly addicted to alcohol.

Effects on Mental Functioning

Four areas of mental ability are consistently compromised by chronic alcohol abuse: memory formation, abstract thinking, problem solving, and attention and concentration. As many as 70 percent of people who seek treatment for alcohol-related problems suffer significant impairment of these abilities.

Memory Formation
By memory formation we mean the ability to form new memories, not the ability to recall information that was learned in the past. That is, an individual with a chronic drinking habit might vividly and accurately recall what he learned early in life, but not be able to tell what he ate for lunch four hours ago. And the richness and detail of his memories during the past few years of drinking might be significantly less than in those earlier memories. On some tests of mental ability that assess different kinds of brain functions, chronic drinkers often perform just fine on most of the categories, but perform poorly on the memory sections. This selective and profound memory deficit may be a result of damage to specific brain areas, such as the hippocampus and the mammillary bodies.

Abstract Thinking
By *abstract* we mean being able to think in ways that are not directly tied to concrete things. We think abstractly when we interpret the meaning of stories, work on word puzzles, or solve geometry or algebra problems. Chronic drinkers often find these abilities compromised. One way to measure abstract thinking is to show someone a group of objects and ask her to group the objects according to the characteristics they share. Chronic drinkers will consistently group things based on their concrete characteristics (such as size, shape, and color) rather than on the basis of their abstract characteristics (such as what they are used for, or what kinds of things they are). It is as if abstract thoughts do not come to mind as easily for the chronic drinker.

Problem Solving
We all have to solve problems each day. Some are simple ones, like deter-mining whether to do the laundry or the grocery shopping first. Some are more complicated, like setting up a new personal computer, or deciding on what inventory to order for the next month's needs in a business. In either case, one of the abilities that is required is mental flexibility. We need to be able to switch strategies and approaches to problems (particularly the complicated ones) in order to solve them efficiently. People with a history of chronic drink-ing often have a lot of difficulty with this. Under testing conditions, it often ap-pears that they get stuck in a particular mode of problem solving and take a lot longer to get to a solution than someone who is better able to switch strate-gies and try new approaches.

Attention and Concentration
Chronic drinkers also develop difficulty in focusing their attention and main-taining concentration. This appears to be particularly difficult when related to tasks that require *visual* attention and concentration. Again, the deficits may not appear until the person is challenged. In casual conversation the sober chronic drinker may be able to concentrate perfectly well, but placed in a more challenging situation (like reading an instruction manual, driving a car, or operating a piece of equipment), she may be quite impaired.

Do These Deficits Go Away?
Heavy chronic drinkers who quit recover these functions partially during the first month or two after the last drink. However, once this time passes, they have gotten back all that they will recover. It is difficult to identify precisely how much recovery occurs, but clear deficits do appear to persist permanently in these individuals. In one study, people who had quit drinking completely after many years of alcohol abuse were examined for seven years. Even after this time they had significant memory deficits. This persistent pattern of mem-ory deficits in previous alcoholics is common enough to have a specific diag-nosis. It is generally called either *alcohol amnestic disorder* or *dementia associated with alcoholism*.

What About "Social Drinkers"?
It is important to define exactly what we mean when we say that someone is a social drinker. The most consistent definition, looking across the literature on alcohol use and treatment, would be this: someone who drinks regularly but does not get drunk when he drinks, nor has any of the clinical signs of ad-diction to alcohol. People who fit this pattern of drinking generally do not have deficits in mental functioning nearly as severe as those who drink heavily.

Among social drinkers the pattern of alcohol consumption plays a very important role in determining whether or not the person will develop deficits in mental functioning. The more alcohol he drinks during each drinking session, the higher the likelihood that mental deficits will develop. Consider two people who each drink five drinks per week, on average. The first person has one drink on each of five days of the week, and the second person has four drinks on each Saturday night and one in the middle of each week. The second person will be more likely to develop the kinds of deficits in the abilities described above for chronic alcoholics. This is a particularly important point for young people, since "binge drinking" on weekends is a typical pattern for many high school and college students as well as for young people in the work world.

Tolerance

Development Across Several Drinking Sessions
Tolerance means that after continued drinking, consuming an identical amount of alcohol produces a lesser effect, or more alcohol is necessary to produce the original effect. The development of tolerance means that alcohol exposure has changed the brain. *In some ways* it is less sensitive to the alcohol, but in other ways it may remain quite sensitive. The brain effects that produce the high may diminish, while the effects that are toxic to the brain cells themselves may remain the same. Another problem is that as tolerance develops, the drinker may drink more each time in order to get the high. As we just learned, such a drinking pattern is more likely to produce deficits in mental functioning over time. Also, since the brain is the organ of addiction, the tolerant person who increases her drinking runs a greater risk of addiction. Finally, although the brain may need more alcohol to produce the high, the liver and other internal organs are dealing with more and more alcohol, and they are at risk for permanent damage.

Development within One Drinking Session
Although tolerance to most alcohol effects develops gradually, and over several drinking sessions, it has also been observed even *within a single drinking session.* This is called *acute tolerance* and means that the intoxication is greatest soon after the beginning of drinking. Acute tolerance does not develop to all the effects of alcohol, but does develop to the feeling of being high. So, the drinker may drink more in order to maintain the feeling of being high, while the other intoxicating effects of alcohol (those which interfere with driving, mental function, and judgment) continue to build, placing the drinker at greater and greater risk.

Dependence

It is important to distinguish between alcohol dependence and alcohol abuse. Generally, alcohol abuse refers to patterns of drinking that give rise to health problems, social problems, or both. Alcohol dependence (often called alco-holism) refers to a disease that is characterized by abnormal seeking and con-sumption of alcohol that leads to a *lack of control over drinking*. Dependent individuals often appear to crave alcohol. They seem driven to drink even though they know that their drinking is causing problems for them. The signs of physical dependence begin within hours after an individual stops drinking. They include profound anxiety, tremors (shaking), sleep disturbances, and, in more extreme cases, hallucinations and seizures. Therefore, until a chronic drinker actually stops drinking, it is quite difficult to make a definitive assess-ment of alcohol dependence. However, for most practical purposes this formal diagnosis is unnecessary, since the social and medical problems that most al-coholics experience should be recognizable to health professionals. See the section on "How to Spot a Problem Drinker" (below) for some general guide-lines.

PRENATAL EXPOSURE

The dangers of prenatal alcohol exposure have been noted since the time of Aristotle in ancient Greece. However, it was not until 1968 that formal reports began to emerge. The early studies of *fetal alcohol syndrome* (FAS) described gross physical deformities and profound mental retardation among children of heavy-drinking alcoholic mothers. Although this was a very important set of findings, at first there was no evidence that women who drank more mod-erately were placing their children at risk. In fact, until quite recently, pregnant women were often encouraged to have a glass of wine with dinner or take a drink now and then during pregnancy to help them fall asleep or just to relax.

It took a while for the effects of moderate prenatal drinking to be noticed, since the children have none of the very obvious defects associated with the full-blown fetal alcohol syndrome. However, it is now clear that there is a less severe, but very clear, pattern of deficits associated with more moderate pre-natal drinking—a pattern described as *fetal alcohol effects* (FAE). School-age children with FAS or FAE are frequently described as hyperactive, distractible, and impulsive with short attention spans—behaviors similar to those observed in children with attention deficit disorder (ADD). However, the FAS and FAE children differ from ADD children in that they are *more intellectually im-paired*.

The impairments of intelligence and behavior in people with FAS and FAE appear to persist at least into adulthood, resulting in IQ scores markedly below average, often well into the moderately retarded range. Those with FAS scored worse than those with FAE, but both were significantly below normal, ham-pered in reading and spelling, and most profoundly deficient in mathemati-cal skills. More important, the FAE patients did not perform any better than the FAS patients on academic achievement tests, though their IQs were some-what higher. What all this means is that even moderate drinking during preg-nancy can create permanent intellectual disabilities. Some studies using animal models of FAE even suggest that just one drink per day impairs the function of brain areas related to learning in the adult offspring.

The bottom line is that there is no identified safe level of drinking during pregnancy. The smart decision for a woman is simply not to drink if she is pregnant or thinks that she might be.

RISK FACTORS FOR ALCOHOL ADDICTION

Anyone can become dependent on alcohol. Continued exposure to alcohol changes the brain in ways that produce dependence. Although there are large differences in individuals' risk for dependency and addiction, any person who puts enough alcohol into his brain over a long enough time will become physically dependent on the drug. Putting aside for a moment the risk factors that have been identified for alcohol dependence, the numbers generally show that the chances of a man becoming addicted to alcohol increase markedly if he drinks more than about three to four drinks per day. For women, the number of drinks is about three. Another consistent finding is that people who become addicted to alcohol are often those who report that they drink to relieve their emotional or social difficulties. In other words, if some-one drinks in order to self-medicate—to block out emotional or social prob-lems—he is especially likely to become addicted. But self-medication simply cannot account for all of the alcohol addiction in the world, and the big ques-tion remains: Why do some people choose to drink enough to get addicted?

GENETIC FACTORS

Much of the evidence that genetic factors may lead to alcohol dependence has come from studies on twins and children of alcoholics who were adopted at birth and raised by nonalcoholic adoptive parents. Studies like these allow re-searchers to begin to tease apart the separate influences of nature and nurture in the development of alcohol addiction. At present it seems clear that the basis of alcoholism is partly genetic, but that genetic factors alone cannot ac-count for the development of the disease. The real value of the nature versus nurture studies so far is that they have identified certain traits, or *markers*, that run in families and predispose people to alcohol dependence. Thus, they help to identify individuals who may be at risk for developing alcohol problems. If a person knows that he is at more risk than normal for this disease, then he can make better decisions about drinking.

It is very clear that alcoholism, like diabetes, runs in families. First-degree relatives (children, siblings, or parents) of alcoholics have been estimated to have a seven times greater chance of developing alcoholism. More important, male relatives of male alcoholics appear to be at particular risk. So, the son, brother, or father of an alcoholic should take special care in deciding about the use of alcohol. Although the general lifetime expectancy for a man becoming an alcoholic is 3 to 5 percent, for sons of alcoholics the percentage estimates can range between 20 and 50 percent. This is a huge difference in risk for alcoholism among these men. The general chances of a woman becoming an alcoholic are between 0.1 percent (1 in 1,000) and 1 percent. Among daughters of alcoholics the percentage increases to between 3 and 8 percent. So, being the child of an alcoholic increases the risk of becoming an alcoholic regardless of sex, but boys are at considerably more risk than girls.

It is important to know that these family studies do not conclusively demonstrate a genetic basis for alcoholism. It is likely that factors other than biological ones, such as being raised by an alcoholic parent, also contribute to drinking behavior. A number of studies show that being raised in a family in which alcohol is abused increases a child's chances of becoming alcohol-dependent.

This problem is effectively controlled in studies of adopted children of alcoholics. In general, these studies indicate that persons with an alcoholic biological parent are approximately two to three times more likely to develop alcoholism *regardless of their home environment*. Studies of twins are even more powerful indicators that genetic factors contribute to alcoholism.

A SPECIAL RISK FOR MEN

Although genetic influences significantly affect the risk of alcoholism in both men and women, these influences appear to be more powerful in men. A number of studies compare the sons of alcoholic fathers with sons of nonalcoholic fathers. In general, it appears that the sons of alcoholic fathers are less impaired by alcohol than other men. However, early in the drinking session (when the pleasurable effects of alcohol prevail), the sons of alcoholics appear to be more affected by alcohol. This suggests that sons of alcoholic fathers may have a more powerful experience of the pleasurable effects of alcohol and a less powerful experience of the impairing effects of alcohol than other men, creating a setup for these men to continue drinking over time and making them more susceptible to addiction.

In addition, a specific type of alcoholism seems to occur only in men. This is called Type II alcoholism and is characterized by an onset of drinking problems in adolescence, aggressive behavior, trouble with the law, and the use of other drugs. Type II alcoholism is considered to be very strongly influenced by genetics. Type I alcoholism is more common and less severe than Type II alcoholism, occurs in both men and women, and begins in adulthood. Men with fathers or brothers who show signs of Type II alcoholism should be particularly careful about alcohol use.

How to Spot a Problem Drinker

Health-care practitioners use several simple screening tests to assess whether an individual may have an alcohol problem. Before describing them, though, we must make two cautionary notes. First, a diagnosis of alcohol abuse, alcohol dependency, or alcoholism can only truly be made by a health professional trained specifically in addiction. These are very complex medical and psychological states, and no simple screening tool is adequate to make a foolproof assessment. Second, it sometimes does considerably more harm than good to confront a friend or relative with the impression that she may have a drinking problem. Although a concerned person may have the best of intentions, and may be acting out of true concern, the other person may simply feel accused and withdraw from the very help being offered. The screening tests we describe below are often used in doctor's offices and clinics as a *first indication* that there might be a problem.

The most widely used screening test is called the **CAGE:**

- Have you ever felt the need to Cut down on your drinking?
- Have you ever felt Annoyed by someone criticizing your drinking?
- Have you ever felt Guilty about your drinking?
- Have you ever felt the need for an Eye opener (a drink at the beginning of the day)?

If the person gives two or more positive responses to these questions, there is a good chance that she has some degree of an alcohol problem. But remember that screening tests are, by their nature, imperfect. For example, it is easy to imagine that a person with a history of heavy drinking might answer yes to all the questions, even if she hadn't had a drink for years.

Another screening test, which has proven particularly useful with women, is called the **TWEAK:**

- Tolerance: How many drinks does it take to make you high?
- Worried: Have close friends or relatives worried or complained about your drinking?
- Eye opener: Do you sometimes take a drink in the morning to wake up?

- Amnesia (memory loss): Has a friend or family member ever told you things you said or did while you were drinking that you could not remember?
- (**K**)Cut: Do you sometimes feel the need to cut down on your drinking?

This test is scored differently than the CAGE, but a positive score of three or more is considered to indicate that the person likely has a drinking problem.

One final word of caution regarding these screening techniques: they all rely on one critical component (which is not always so reliable)—the person's own responses. There are any number of reasons why a person might not respond fully accurately. Therefore, while these screening tools may be useful as a first-pass indicator of a possible problem, they must not be used in isolation to form impressions about a person.

SPECIAL CONSIDERATIONS FOR WOMEN

DIFFERENT SENSITIVITY

Alcohol does not treat all people equally, and there are some big differences between the effects of alcohol on women and on men. As women have taken a more visible role in our society, they have found more freedom (and perhaps more encouragement) to drink. Consequently, drinking is on the rise among women in general. Surveys indicate that the percentage of women who drink alcohol has increased from 45 to 66 percent over the past forty years, and that as many as 5 percent of women are heavy drinkers.

Women's bodies differ from men's bodies in a number of ways that make them react differently to alcohol. For one, women are generally smaller than men, and their bodies have a larger percentage of fat, which causes them to develop higher blood alcohol concentrations than men after drinking similar amounts of alcohol. In fact, after a given dose of alcohol, a woman may achieve a blood alcohol level 25 to 30 percent higher than a man. Women should know that they will likely be considerably more impaired than their male companions if they drink comparable amounts of alcohol.

BIRTH CONTROL PILLS

Another specific issue for women is that oral contraceptives (birth control pills) slow down the rate at which alcohol is eliminated from the body. A woman who is on the pill can, therefore, expect to feel the sedating effects of alcohol for a longer period of time than a woman who is not.

Health Effects

Women who drink are at significantly greater risk for liver damage than men *even if they drink less alcohol or drink for a shorter period of time.* This increased risk has been reported for women who drink between one and a half to three drinks of alcohol per day, and may be due to the differences in the way a woman's body eliminates alcohol.

The pancreas, too, is more likely to be damaged by alcohol in women. The cells of the pancreas make chemicals that are used for digestion. When alcohol damages the pancreas cells, the digestive chemicals begin to leak out and can actually begin to digest the pancreas itself. Although this happens in both women and men, women tend to develop the disease sooner.

Women are also more likely than men to develop *high blood pressure* due to alcohol drinking. High blood pressure is one of the major causes of heart attack and stroke. Women who drink two to three drinks per day have a 40 percent greater risk of developing high blood pressure. The good news is that this additional risk diminishes when the woman stops drinking. Still, for women who drink even moderate amounts of alcohol, the increased risk of high blood pressure is substantial.

Social and Psychological Issues

Despite the increased acceptance of drinking by women during the past several decades, recent studies have shown that women who drink a lot meet with more disapproval of their drinking than do men. In addition, the divorce rate for alcoholic women is higher than for alcoholic men. This suggests that women are less likely to leave relationships with alcoholic men than the reverse.

It is also clear that women who drink heavily are at a much higher risk for domestic violence and sexual assault than other women. One particularly compelling study of more than three thousand college women found that the more alcohol a woman consumed, the higher her chances were of being sexually victimized. This might occur because a woman impaired by alcohol may have more trouble accurately interpreting a man's behavior as threatening and resisting unwanted sexual advances.

ALCOHOL AND SEX

Anyone who has ever watched a commercial for beer can tell you that your sex life will improve considerably with drinking. The truth of the matter is that most of the effects of alcohol on sexual functioning are bad. Of course, a person may *feel* more suave and sexy after drinking, and he may more easily convince himself that his sexual prowess is unparalleled. But all too often the mind makes a promise that the body can't keep after a night of heavy drinking. Men, in particular, should consider the meaning of the term "brewer's droop."

As many as 40 to 90 percent of chronic male drinkers (depending on the study) report reduced sex drive. Chronic drinkers show reduced capacity for penile erection, decreased semen production, and lower sperm counts. In fact, in alcoholic men the testes may actually shrink (a fact generally not presented in beer commercials). In extreme cases of chronic heavy alcohol abuse among men, a *feminization syndrome* can develop, which involves a loss of body hair and the development of breast tissue. Although these effects are most often seen in men who drink heavily over a prolonged period, some sexual and reproductive functions are impaired even by lesser intake. For example, evidence is accumulating that consuming two to three drinks per day may decrease sperm counts.

CHILDREN AND ADOLESCENTS

By far, alcohol is the drug used most often by high school seniors. Although most seniors cannot buy alcohol legally, 90 percent of them have tried alcohol and nearly a third report that they have drunk heavily (more than five drinks in a row) in the past two weeks. More than 40 percent of college students report recent heavy drinking. In fact, one study shows that colleges in the northeastern United States and those with fraternities, sororities, and big sports programs may pose a real hazard for freshmen. On these "high risk" campuses it was found that of freshmen who come to school without a history of binge drinking, 46 percent become binge drinkers. Even on "low risk" campuses, 17 percent of freshmen with little or no drinking experience become binge drinkers.

However, the use of alcohol by much younger people (children as young as second grade are known to use alcohol regularly) is in some ways a more frightening problem. Though the problems associated with underage drinking are well known, we know very little about how alcohol affects the brains of younger people. We do know some interesting things about the young brain, though. For example, we now know that the brain does not finish developing until a person is around twenty years old, and one of the last regions to mature is intimately involved with the ability to plan and make complex judgments. Young brains also have rich resources for acquiring new memories, and seem to be "built to learn." It is no accident that people are educated in our society during their early years, when they have more capacity for memory and learning. However, with this added memory capacity may come additional risks associated with the use of alcohol. Recent studies using animals have shown that when the brain is young it is more vulnerable to some of the dangerous effects of alcohol, especially on learning and memory function. If this turns out to be true in humans, then children and adolescents who drink may be powerfully impairing the brain functions on which they rely so heavily for learning.

DANGEROUS INTERACTIONS WITH OTHER DRUGS

Sedatives

Clearly the most dangerous drugs to mix with alcohol are other sedatives, or "downers," such as phenobarbital and pentobarbital. The depressing effects of alcohol on brain function combined with the effects of the barbiturates can cause extreme impairment, unconsciousness, or even death. One of the most famous recent cases in medical ethics was that of a young woman, Karen Ann Quinlan, who drank alcohol in combination with Quaaludes (methaqualone—a powerful sedative drug) and went into a coma from which she never recovered. This tragic case gained national attention because it raised the issue of whether a person should be removed from life-support machines after it becomes clear that he or she will never recover from a vegetative state.

Although few people take alcohol-sedative combinations severe enough to cause coma or death, the combination of even relatively low doses of alcohol and sedatives can be dangerous, powerfully impairing the ability to think clearly, make good decisions, or drive a car. A person who is normally able to perform these tasks perfectly well at the end of an evening after having had three or four beers over the course of several hours might find that he is totally unable to perform them if even a small dose of sedatives is added to the mix. The effects of the alcohol may be totally unexpected in the presence of the other sedative drug.

Antianxiety Medications (Valium, Librium, etc.)

These drugs fall into the general category called benzodiazepines and are used to treat anxiety, sleep disturbances, and seizures. They are also used to treat alcohol-withdrawal symptoms in detoxification clinics. These drugs are sedating and may cause severe drowsiness in the presence of alcohol, increasing the risk of household and automobile accidents.

Antibiotics

In combination with acute doses of alcohol, some antibiotics can cause nausea, vomiting, headache, or even convulsions (seizures). Among the potentially dangerous ones are Furoxone (furazolidone), Grisactin (griseofulvin), Flagyl (metronidazole), and Atabrine (quinacrine).

Anticoagulants (blood thinners)

Warfarin (Coumadin) is prescribed to decrease the blood's ability to clot. Alcohol increases the availability of warfarin in the body and increases the risk of dangerous bleeding. But in chronic drinkers, warfarin's action is *decreased*, lessening these patients' protection from the consequences of blood-clotting disorders.

Antidepressants

Many people who are depressed use alcohol, and many alcoholics are also depressed. So, it is quite common for people to use alcohol with antidepressant drugs. Alcohol increases the sedative effects of the tricyclic antidepressants such as Elavil (amitriptyline). This impairs both mental and physical skills such as those necessary for driving. Chronic drinking appears to increase the action of some tricyclic antidepressants and decrease the action of others. Anyone who is on antidepressants should consult closely with her doctor about how her medication reacts with alcohol.

Antidiabetic Medications

Orinase (tolbutamide) is given orally to help lower blood sugar in diabetic patients. Acute alcohol drinking prolongs the action of this drug, and chronic drinking decreases its availability in the body. Alcohol can also cause nausea and headache when taken with some drugs of this class.

Antihistamines (diphenhydramine—Benadryl and others)

These drugs are available without a prescription and are used to treat allergic symptoms and sometimes insomnia. They have sedative effects that may be intensified by alcohol, increasing the probability of accidents. In older persons these drugs can cause excessive dizziness and sedation, and their combination with alcohol may be particularly dangerous.

Antipsychotic Medications

Drugs such as Thorazine (chlorpromazine) are used to treat psychotic symptoms such as delusions and hallucinations. Acute alcohol drinking can increase the sedative effects of these drugs, resulting in impaired coordination and potentially fatal suppression of breathing.

Antiseizure Medications

One of the most widely used drugs prescribed to treat epilepsy (seizures) is Dilantin (phenytoin). Acute alcohol drinking increases the availability of Dilantin in the body, and increases the probability of side effects. Chronic drinking may decrease the availability of Dilantin, dangerously hampering its effectiveness and increasing the patient's risk of seizures.

Heart Medications

There are many medications used to treat disease of the heart or circulatory system. Acute alcohol drinking can interact with some of these to cause dizziness or fainting upon standing up. These drugs include the angina medicine nitroglycerin and the following blood pressure medications: reserpine, Aldomet, Apresoline, and guanethidine. In addition, chronic alcohol drinking reduces the effectiveness of the blood pressure medication Inderal (propranolol).

Narcotic Pain Relievers (morphine, Darvon, codeine, Demerol, etc.)

These drugs are prescribed for moderate to severe pain, such as after surgery or dental work. The combination of any of these drugs with alcohol magnifies the sedative effects of both. This increases the risk of death from overdose. Even a single drink can significantly increase the sedative effects of Darvon.

Nonnarcotic Pain Relievers (aspirin and other nonprescription pain relievers)

Some of these drugs can cause stomach bleeding and prevent the blood from clotting normally. Alcohol can worsen these side effects. In addition, aspirin may increase the availability of alcohol within the body, thereby increasing the intoxicating effect of a given drink. In chronic drinkers, certain enzymes are formed that transform acetaminophen (used in Tylenol and others) into chemicals that can cause liver damage. This can occur even when the pain reliever is used in recommended doses.

HEALTH BENEFITS OF MODERATE ALCOHOL USE

RELAXATION AND STRESS REDUCTION

It is perfectly clear that heavy drinking, either in one session or across decades, carries with it significant risks to health and safety. However, alcohol is not all bad. Used in an informed and moderate way, alcohol can convey some health benefits. For example, the similarity of its actions to those of antianxiety medications such as Valium make alcohol a good antianxiety agent. The feeling of relaxation that accompanies an occasional drink of alcohol can help to reduce stress, and stress reduction is healthy. But remember: people who use alcohol heavily or too regularly as a way of coping with the difficulties in their lives are at considerable risk for becoming addicted. Ultimately, the use of alcohol for relaxation and stress reduction is a personal choice that must be made in as informed a way as possible.

PROTECTION AGAINST HEART DISEASE

There is no doubt that chronic heavy drinking damages the heart. However, recent studies show that light (and perhaps moderate) drinkers have a reduced risk for coronary artery disease—a principle cause of heart attacks. Remember, though, that this is a relatively recent area of study, and it is not possible to arrive at an exact "prescription" of alcohol use for cardiovascular protection. Still, a growing number of studies suggest that an average of a half to one and a half drinks per day may significantly lower a person's risk for coronary artery disease.

A recent study from Harvard Medical School further supports these early findings—at least in men. A group of more than twenty-two thousand men who ranged in age from forty to eighty-four were studied over a ten-year period. Compared to men who drank less than one alcoholic beverage per week on average, those who drank two to four alcoholic beverages *per week* were significantly less likely to die of a heart or circulatory disorder. These light-drinking men also suffered fewer cancers over the ten-year period. However, among men who drank two or more drinks *per day*, the death rate was 51 percent higher. This means that there is a narrow window for the possible health benefits of alcohol for men. Two drinks per week seems to be good; two drinks per day seems to be bad.

For women, however, these findings present a double-edged sword. Studies have shown that women who drink an average of three to nine drinks *per week* are significantly more likely to develop breast cancer than women who do not drink. Still, the causes of breast cancer are quite complex, and much work remains to determine the exact relationship of alcohol drinking to breast cancer. Women who choose to drink moderately, for whatever reasons, should keep in close touch with the latest information related to breast cancer risks.

DEATH RISK

There have now been several large-scale studies, in both Eastern and Western countries, indicating that light to moderate drinking may diminish the risk of death in middle-aged men. A recent study in China showed that men who drank one to two drinks per day over a six-and-a-half-year period reduced their risk of death by about 20 percent—a finding that is consistent with studies in European countries. The protective effect was not limited to death from heart disease (the drinkers were also less likely to die from cancer or other causes) nor to any particular type of alcoholic beverage. Beer drinkers, wine drinkers, and drinkers of hard liquor shared equally in the benefits, as long as their consumption was not more than an average of two drinks per day. Beyond that level the risk of death was increased by about 30 percent. Unfortunately, such studies have not yet been undertaken with women, so it's unknown whether they share the same benefits and risks associated with men.

2

■

Caffeine

Drug Class: Stimulant

Individual Drugs: coffee (75–150 mg per 8-oz cup), tea (30–60 mg per 8-oz cup); soft drinks (30–70 mg per 12-oz serving), over-the-counter pain relievers (30–70 mg), over-the-counter stimulants (100–200 mg), some prescription medications (concentrations vary)

The Buzz: At low to moderate doses, many people report increased alertness and ability to concentrate, and even euphoria. Higher doses can result in nervousness and agitation.

Overdose and Other Bad Effects: Fatal overdose with caffeine is extremely rare, but it is possible. Some symptoms of caffeine poisoning include tremors (involuntary shaking), nausea, vomiting, irregular or rapid heart rate, and confusion. In extreme cases, individuals may become delirious or have seizures (convulsions). In these cases, death may be caused by seizures that result in an inability to breathe. In less severe cases, high doses have been associated with panic attacks.

In small children toxic effects may be observed with doses of around 35 milligrams per kilogram (about 800 milligrams in a fifty-pound child). This level could be achieved by taking four Vivarin tablets or drinking about seven cups of strong coffee.

Dangerous Combinations with Other Drugs: Caffeine can raise blood pressure, so some physicians caution hypertensive patients to limit their use of caffeine. In addition, it should be used cautiously by people who are taking other drugs that can raise blood pressure. These drugs include antidepressants that are MAO inhibitors, such as Marplan, Nardil, and Parnate; as well as high doses of cold medicines that contain phenylpropanolamine. Since caffeine is a stimulant, it can add to the effects of stronger stimulants such as cocaine, amphetamine, or methamphetamine.

CHAPTER CONTENTS

A BRIEF HISTORY

It is difficult to write a "brief" history of caffeine because its history of use in human culture is very old and very detailed. Today, caffeine is found in a variety of sodas, pain relievers, and other medications, but historically, coffee, tea, and chocolate were the caffeine-containing products consumed by people. The origins of tea use can be traced back to China in the fourth century, when it was thought to have significant medicinal properties. In the 1500s medical uses also fueled interest in tea in Europe, but soon its stimulant actions came to be appreciated as well. Some ancient legends suggest that the effects of coffee beans on their early users were so powerful that they were thought to have powers given by divine intervention. These legends also indicate that the stimulant properties of these beans were appreciated and sought after from the very beginning. One often-cited story describes how a goat herder began chewing coffee beans after he observed the stimulating effects of the beans on his herd. Soon he and others began chewing the beans regularly in order to maintain their stamina and concentration through long, isolated hours of work.

Coffee began to be cultivated in Yemen in the sixth century. However, many religious leaders of the time thought poorly of coffee, contending that it gave rise to personal (and political) treachery. On the other hand, users enjoyed its ability to combat fatigue and enhance physical endurance. Among some it gained a reputation for stimulating thought and intellectual conversation.

By the 1600s, trade merchants had introduced coffee to Europe, and "coffeehouses" spread rapidly. One of the hallmarks of these establishments was intellectual conversation. Not all of this conversation was viewed as politically correct, however, and coffeehouses were outlawed in England. That ban was very brief, and the growth of coffeehouses and the use of coffee spread even more rapidly thereafter. In fact, coffeehouses came to be known as places where one could go to learn from notable academic and political figures of the day. The environment created in coffeehouses turned out to be one that gave rise to creative thinking in the entrepreneurial and business realms as well. As an example, the giant insurance firm Lloyd's of London actually began as a coffeehouse in the early 1700s.

Coffee and the United States have a strong relationship. Although tea was the caffeinated drink of choice in the English colonies for quite a while, the British Stamp Act of 1765 and the Trade Revenue Act of 1767 levied high taxes on the importation of tea to the colonies. This, of course, gave rise to the tide of rebellion that was symbolized so powerfully at the Boston Tea Party, ushering in the Revolutionary War. In protest of the tea taxes, coffee became our caffeinated drink of choice. By the 1940s, coffee consumption in the United States reached a high of around twenty pounds per person per year. Though by the early 1990s that level had dropped to ten pounds per person per year, this did not mean that Americans were cutting their caffeine consumption in half. While the consumption of coffee was falling off, the consumption of caffeinated soft drinks was growing rapidly. In recent years coffee has been making a comeback. Specialty coffee shops and cafés began to spring up on the West Coast in the 1980s, and they have spread over much of the nation. Americans are now consuming more varieties of coffee and more types of coffee drinks than ever before. It is estimated that more than half of the American population drinks at least two cups of coffee per day, and that among coffee drinkers, nearly 50 percent drink five or more cups per day.

Finally, we cannot leave the history of caffeine without mention of another caffeine-containing delight—chocolate. Chocolate was actually introduced to Europe before either coffee or tea, but it did not become popular as rapidly because it was presented mostly as a thick preparation made from processed and ground cacao kernels. In the 1800s the Dutch developed a process that removed much of the fat from this crude preparation, and the result was a more refined chocolate powder. The fat that was removed was then combined with sugar and the chocolate powder, and the result was the birth of the chocolate bar in the 1840s. As the technology for producing chocolate became better known in Europe, its use spread rapidly. Dark chocolate contains about 20 milligrams of caffeine per ounce. That means that a four-ounce bar of chocolate would contain approximately 80 milligrams of caffeine—about the same as in a cup of percolator-brewed coffee.

HOW CAFFEINE MOVES THROUGH THE BODY

Caffeine is almost always taken by mouth, and so it is absorbed into the blood primarily through the linings of the stomach, small intestine, and large intestine. It is only slowly absorbed through the stomach, and so most absorption occurs at the next step along the gastrointestinal tract, the small intestine. However, once it reaches the intestines, virtually all of the caffeine that was ingested is absorbed. A given oral dose of caffeine takes effect within thirty to sixty minutes, depending upon how much food is in the stomach and intestines and how concentrated the caffeine is in the substance that contains it.

Caffeine is evenly distributed throughout the body, metabolized by the liver, and its breakdown products are excreted through the kidneys. The body eliminates it rather slowly, with the half-life of a given dose of caffeine being approximately three hours. Thus, some of the caffeine that one consumes in the morning is still around well into the afternoon. A person who drinks several cups of coffee or caffeinated sodas across a morning or afternoon is adding onto an existing load of caffeine with each subsequent drink, and may end up feeling rather jittery by the end of the day.

HOW CAFFEINE WORKS

Caffeine is the most well known of a class of compounds called xanthines (pronounced "zan-theenes"). Theophylline, another xanthine found in tea, is prescribed for breathing problems because it relaxes and opens breathing passages. However, there is so little of it in brewed tea that it exerts no significant stimulant effects in that form. Chocolate contains theobromine, another xanthine, but one with far less potency than caffeine.

All the xanthines, including caffeine, have multiple actions. The major action is to block the action of a neurotransmitter/neuromodulator called adenosine, which is in the brain (more on this below). There are also adenosine receptors throughout the body, including those in blood vessels, fat cells, the heart, the kidneys, and many types of smooth muscle. These multiple actions create a confusing picture because the direct effects of caffeine on a system can be enhanced or suppressed by indirect effects on other systems.

EFFECTS ON THE BRAIN

Adenosine receptors, the main site of caffeine action, cause sedation when adenosine binds to them. Adenosine, a by-product of cellular metabolism, leaks out of cells. So, as neurons become more active, they produce more adenosine, and this provides a "brake" on all the neural activity—an ingenious self-regulation by the brain. Caffeine thus produces activation of brain activity by reducing the ability of adenosine to do this job. This is a good example of how a drug can produce an effect (in this case, CNS stimulation) by *inhibiting* the action of a neurotransmitter that produces an inhibiting effect (a positive coming from two negatives). At moderate doses of around 200 milligrams (about what one gets from one to two strong cups of coffee), electroencephalograph (EEG) studies indicate that the brain is aroused. Higher doses, in the range of 500 milligrams, increase heart rate and breathing. Activation of these centers also causes a constriction, or narrowing, of blood vessels in the brain (though outside the brain caffeine has a direct effect on blood vessels that does just the opposite—it dilates, or widens, them).

Mild tolerance develops to the repeated use of caffeine, but most tolerant people can achieve an arousing effect by increasing their dose by two to three times. The tolerance that develops to the brain-arousing effects of caffeine is less severe than the tolerance that develops to some of its effects on other parts of the body (see below).

Dependence on caffeine can develop as well. As discussed in earlier chapters, one of the principle indicators of dependence is the occurrence of withdrawal symptoms when a drug is abruptly stopped. When caffeine users stop, they generally experience headaches and fatigue. These signs usually begin about twenty hours after the last dose of caffeine and may persist for several days to a week. Generally, they are at their worst during the first two days after quitting. Nonprescription pain relievers such as acetaminophen (Tylenol) or ibuprofen relieve the headaches, and moderate doses can be taken through-out the withdrawal period. If one decides to stop using caffeine entirely, one should avoid pain medications that include it (see table, Over-the-Counter Drugs, page 67.

Many people have found that they enjoy, and indeed rely on, the psycho-logical effects of caffeine. While this wouldn't meet our definition of addic-tion, most caffeine users find the effects pleasant enough to continue using this drug. Therefore, those who decide to quit should also be prepared to give up those caffeine-aided feelings of alertness and mild euphoria, which may have become a very regular and important part of each day. A related issue is that people who drink caffeinated beverages often do so at the same or similar times of day. In that way the drinking itself may become a part of important daily rituals. It is important to anticipate that changing those rituals may be dif-ficult as well.

EFFECTS ON OTHER BODY PARTS

The Heart

Caffeine affects the heart in two ways: it acts on brain centers that regulate the cardiovascular system, and it acts directly on the heart. In people who are not tolerant to caffeine, a high dose (generally above 500 milligrams—about four cups of strong coffee) can increase the heart rate by as much as ten to twenty beats per minute (from a baseline of eighty to ninety). In some, this dosage can result in brief periods of irregular heartbeat. However, in general, the morning cup of coffee does not have much effect on heart function in a healthy person.

There is controversy over the issue of caffeine and the gradual develop-ment of heart disease. At present, the scientific literature is inconsistent in its findings on the question of whether continued caffeine use increases the risk of heart disease or heart attack. One very large study of men found no rela-tionship between coffee drinking (up to six cups per day) and heart disease, while others have found an increased risk of heart attacks in coffee drinkers. Moderate caffeine consumption (up to 500 milligrams per day) probably does not place the user at significant risk for heart problems. Above that level, how-ever, the risk of heart attack appears to increase. This would be particularly true for individuals with other risk factors for heart attack, such as smoking, being overweight, or a family history of heart disease.

Cholesterol

Coffee can increase the amount of cholesterol and fat in the blood, but only when it is brewed in particular ways. A recent study has shown that five to six cups of coffee per day can increase LDL cholesterol levels (this is the "bad" type of cholesterol as far as risk of heart disease is concerned) by 10 percent or more. This is not the case, however, if the coffee is prepared using a paper filter. While it is not clear exactly why filtered coffee fails to raise cholesterol levels, some researchers think that it is because oils from the coffee beans and other substances that promote fat buildup in the blood are trapped by the paper filter as the water passes over the coffee grounds.

THE KIDNEYS

The well-known bathroom break that follows the morning coffee is probably caused both by a direct effect on the kidneys and by effects in the brain. There are adenosine receptors in the kidneys, and caffeine acts on these, causing effects similar to those of diuretics, which increase urine production. Caffeine may also slow the release of a hormone from the brain (an antidiuretic hormone) that normally slows urine production.

THE DIGESTIVE SYSTEM

In coffee drinkers, the acids, oils, and caffeine can all irritate the stomach lining and promote secretion of acid, leading to gastritis (inflammation of the stomach). However, caffeine may not be the major villain, as decaffeinated coffee has effects almost as great as caffeine-containing coffee. Although coffee was once blamed for ulcers, the primary cause of ulcers is now thought to be a bacteria *(Helicobacter pylori)*. Irritating agents like coffee and aspirin can contribute to the process by damaging the protective mucous lining of the stomach walls, but they probably don't cause ulcers on their own. In some individuals, caffeine in coffee can promote the reflux of stomach acid into the throat, resulting in painful heartburn.

THE RESPIRATORY SYSTEM

Caffeine and similar drugs have two quite separate effects on breathing. The first was mentioned above: they stimulate the rate of breathing. Theophylline is sometimes used in treating premature infants with breathing problems. Xanthines also relax the smooth muscle in the bronchioles that take air into the lungs. This is very helpful in treating asthma, a disease in which breathing difficulties arise because these tubes constrict. Theophylline was used widely in the past to treat asthma, and is still sometimes used today. However, concerns about side effects (restlessness, stomach upset) and the development of more effective treatments have diminished its use.

THE REPRODUCTIVE SYSTEM

Although studies in humans have not confirmed a link between caffeine consumption and birth defects, some studies report that babies born to women who used caffeine during pregnancy have lower birth weights. There is some evidence, furthermore, that caffeine consumption (equivalent to more than one cup of coffee per day) can significantly reduce the chances of a woman becoming pregnant. There have also been contradictory findings about the association between caffeine use, fibrocystic breast disease, and eventual development of breast cancer. All of these associations are questionable, and most studies do not support an association with the development of breast cancer.

THE EYES

Caffeine causes the tiny blood vessels in the eyes to constrict (become narrower), and thus decreases the flow of nutrients to the cells within the eyes and the clearing of waste products.

CAFFEINE AND STRESS

Caffeine increases some of the normal stress responses because it increases the amount of adrenaline that is active in the body under stressful circumstances. Thus, it seems that caffeine users who find themselves under stress (or who use caffeine even more during stressful periods to work more effectively) may experience more of the effects that stress can produce. Adrenaline release increases blood pressure during stress, and the caffeine-induced rise adds to this. Thus, caffeine and stress together lead to greater bodily stress responses than either does alone.

CAFFEINE AND PANIC ATTACKS

In some people, caffeine can contribute to the experience of panic attacks, which generally come on suddenly and involve powerful feelings of threat and fear. The experience can be very debilitating for a brief period of time. It seems that caffeine is more likely to bring on panic attacks in people who have had them previously. However, relatively high doses of caffeine (greater than 700 milligrams) have been reported to lead to panic attacks in people who have never experienced them.

ENHANCEMENT OF PHYSICAL PERFORMANCE

Caffeine can slightly enhance physical endurance and delay fatigue associated with vigorous exercise in some people. One way that caffeine might accomplish this is by releasing fats into the blood for use as energy, enabling the body to conserve its other energy stores (in the form of stored sugars), thus allowing the athlete to sustain physical activity for a longer period of time. Caffeine may also help muscle performance during physical exercise, although the way this happens is not clear.

Two words of caution, though, for those who use caffeine for this purpose. Since caffeine causes increased loss of water through urine production, a person exercising on caffeine may become dehydrated more rapidly during long periods of exercise such as distance running or cycling. This caution is particularly important for hot-weather exercisers. The other concern is the effects of caffeine on heart rate and heart rhythms. Since strenuous exercise obviously stresses the heart, a person with cardiovascular disease could experience problems while using caffeine to promote physical performance.

People who worry about their weight might be interested in the issue of fat metabolism. Products based on the supposed ability of caffeine and theophylline to "burn fat" include a theophylline cream placed on the market a couple of years ago that was supposed to melt fat away. Just rub it on the offending fat pad! Unfortunately, the effectiveness of this treatment hasn't been established (one big problem is probably getting the theophylline through the skin and into the fat cells).

Likewise, there is tremendous interest in whether a combination of caffeine and exercise can help to promote the burning of fat as fuel for weight loss. Since fat cells really do have adenosine receptors, and xanthines really can cause a small release of stored fat, some foods that include caffeine have been sold as fat burners. However, the scholarly research on these products has demonstrated only small weight-loss effects. Coffee and its cousins may prove to be a useful part of weight-loss programs in the future, but at this point nothing "melts" fat except old-fashioned exercise and a good diet.

TREATMENT OF HEADACHES

Caffeine causes constriction of blood vessels, and this is likely the reason that it can be an effective treatment for migraine headaches, especially if it is taken at the first sign of the headache. In general, it is easier to head off growing pain than to remove pain once it is strong, so a strong cup of coffee at the first sign of a migraine can help stop the problem before it really gets started. Caffeine also increases the effectiveness of ergotamine tartrate, a medication that is used to treat migraines, if taken at the first sign of the headache. Caffeine has also been touted as an effective treatment for nonmigraine headaches in some individuals. It is easy to see why some over-the-counter pain relievers (such as Anacin, Excedrin, and Goody's Powders) contain caffeine. However, its effectiveness in this regard really hasn't been proven.

HOW WE TAKE CAFFEINE

COFFEES

The amount of caffeine in a cup of coffee varies tremendously and depends on several factors.

Types of Coffee Beans

Robusta beans are often grown in Africa and may have as much as twice the caffeine as arabica beans, which are grown in South America and the Middle East, among other places. Robusta coffees are generally cheaper and are often used in the mass-produced canned coffees sold in grocery stores. Arabica coffees are considered to be of higher grade and to yield a better-tasting cup. Although generally available, they are predominant at specialty coffee retailers and through the rapidly growing mail-order coffee businesses. Arabicas are also much more often sold in whole-bean form than are robustas. For purposes of comparison, a typical cup of coffee brewed from arabica beans generally has 70 to 100 milligrams of caffeine, whereas the comparable amount of robusta coffee may have closer to 150 milligrams.

Roasting

Dark-roasted coffee beans contain less caffeine and less acid than lighter-roasted ones. Many people think that dark-roasted coffees contain more caffeine because they often have a more powerful taste than the lighter roasts. In fact, the additional roasting associated with the darker product allows more time for caffeine to be broken down in the beans.

Brewing

The method of brewing and the size of the granules of ground coffee interact to have a significant influence on the amount of caffeine per ounce of coffee produced. The more fine the grind, the more surface area of ground coffee comes into contact with the brewing water. This creates more opportunity for caffeine to be extracted from the ground beans. As for brewing method, a cup of coffee made using a drip-type coffee maker generally has about 20 percent more caffeine than a cup made in a percolator. "Plunger pots" can also extract maximal caffeine levels from ground coffee because the grounds are actually soaked continuously in water prior to the plunger being lowered to separate the water from them.

Espresso

Espresso is really a different drink from brewed coffee. It is made by passing water rapidly through relatively tightly packed coffee grounds under high pressure. The result is that the oils and other products in the coffee are more fully extracted than under other coffee brewing conditions, and the taste is considerably richer than that of other coffee brews. A typical "cup" of espresso contains about 1.5 to 2.0 fluid ounces, much less than a cup of coffee. But espresso contains more caffeine per fluid ounce than coffee does. Thus, the amounts of caffeine in a cup of coffee and a cup of espresso are about the same. While an average cup of coffee brewed from arabica beans will contain in the range of 70 to 100 milligrams of caffeine, the average cup of espresso usually contains about 60 to 90 milligrams.

This seems contradictory to the impression that many people have that espresso creates more of a "caffeine buzz" than coffee does. This could be because of the higher *concentration* of caffeine in the espresso. When a drug is more concentrated in a certain solution, it will tend to be absorbed more rapidly across the membranes of the stomach and small intestine. So, even though a single espresso *(espresso solo)* may have the same or less caffeine than a cup of coffee, its more rapid absorption can result in a more rapid onset of the caffeine effects and a greater feeling of "rush." Of course, a double espresso (or *espresso dóppio*) will contain twice as much caffeine.

Other drinks, such as cappuccino, *caffè latte,* and café mocha, are each generally made by adding one single shot of espresso to other ingredients. So, the caffeine content of these drinks should be roughly equal to that of a single espresso, though less concentrated.

Based on the above information, it is obviously impossible to present a simple table describing the amount of caffeine in coffee drinks. Remember that these are broad averages based on a survey of the pharmacological and dietary literatures.

AVERAGE CAFFEINE CONCENTRATION

Drink	*Milligrams*
Dripped robusta coffee (8 oz)	150
Dripped arabica coffee (8 oz)	100
Percolated robusta coffee (8 oz)	110
Percolated arabica coffee (8 oz)	75
Instant coffee (8 oz)	65
Decaffeinated Coffee (8 oz)	3
Espresso (and espresso-based drinks) made from arabica beans (1.5–2 oz)	90

Teas

Tea leaves are harvested from bushes that are grown mostly in India, Indonesia, and Sri Lanka. Leaves are of differing qualities, depending upon how far out on the stalk of the bush they grow. Generally, the bud leaves, which are closest to the stalk, are considered to be of the highest quality. The leaves are dried and allowed to ferment, which turns them to an orange hue. However, some tea leaves are not fermented in this way and remain green. Green teas are the type found in most Chinese restaurants in the United States.

In general, a cup of tea will contain less caffeine than a cup of coffee. Although there is more caffeine in a pound of fermented tea than in a pound of coffee, that pound of tea might be used to brew three to four times as many cups as a pound of coffee would. In addition, the amount of tea in a "cup" is often less than the amount of coffee, by tradition. As with coffees, the amount of caffeine in a given cup may vary considerably, depending on several factors.

AVERAGE CAFFEINE CONTENT

Drink	*Milligrams*	
Brewed tea, domestic brand		
5-minute brew time	40	(20–90)*
1-minute brew time	30	
Brewed tea, imported brand		
5-minute brew time	60	(25–110)*
1-minute brew time	45	
Iced tea (12-oz glass)	70	

*depending upon the particular brand tested

Sodas

The consumption of caffeinated sodas in the United States has been on the rise for a number of years. Some people are bothered by the gastric upset that is sometimes associated with the acids in coffees and prefer to drink caffeine-containing soft drinks. In general, the concentration of caffeine per ounce in sodas is considerably lower than in coffees, but the typical serving of soda is 12 ounces, compared to 6 to 8 ounces for coffee. The general range of caffeine doses in soft drinks is about 30 to 60 milligrams. The diet drinks contain the same amount of caffeine as their nondiet equivalents. However, there are some products, such as Jolt cola, that contain 100 milligrams or more per serving. Some examples are as follows:

AVERAGE CAFFEINE CONCENTRATION

Drink	Milligrams
Canada Dry Jamaica cola	30
Coca-Cola	46
Dr Pepper	46
Mello Yello	53
Mountain Dew	54
Pepsi-Cola	38

OVER-THE-COUNTER DRUGS

There are quite a few preparations that contain caffeine, some in very high amounts. The chart below lists some of these.

CAFFEINE CONCENTRATION

Brand Name	Milligrams
Cold Remedies	
Coryban-D	30
Dristan	16
Triaminicin	30
Diuretics	
Aqua-Ban	100
Pain Relievers	
Anacin	32
Excedrin	65
Goody's Powders	33
Midol	32
Vanquish	33
Stimulants	
Caffedrine	200
No Doz	100
Vivarin	200

CHOCOLATE

Chocolate is made from the bean of the *Theobroma cacao* bush, which contains a unique xanthine called theobromine. An average cup of cocoa may contain as much as 200 milligrams of theobromine, but this compound is much less potent than caffeine as a stimulant. However, chocolate also contains caffeine. For example, a 1-oz bar of baker's chocolate contains about 25 milligrams of caffeine, and a 5-oz cup of cocoa may contain 15 to 20 milligrams. On the other hand, a typical 8-oz glass of chocolate milk generally contains under 10 milligrams of caffeine.

One final note about chocolate. Caffeine and theobromine may not be the only psychoactive compounds in it. A recent report has indicated that one component of chocolate is very similar to the natural chemical in the brain that interacts with our THC receptors—the receptors to which the psychoactive compound in marijuana binds. Although the concentration of this compound is quite low in chocolate (it was estimated that one would have to eat twenty-five pounds of chocolate to stimulate the receptors as much as a typical dose of marijuana), it is possible that its presence could supplement the natural THC-like compound in the brain enough to produce a subtle effect. These results have led some to speculate that the vague sense of well-being and happiness that some people report in response to chocolate may be related to the interaction of two subtle drug effects—those of low-dose caffeine, and those associated with activating the natural THC receptors in the brain.

TOXICITY OF CAFFEINE

Overall, caffeine is fairly safe, *if* a healthy person takes it in moderate amounts. The undesirable side effects that most people experience are gastric upset and nervousness or jitteriness. As people age, they tend to have more problems with sleeplessness, and often will limit their caffeine consumption in the afternoon and evening. Pills containing fairly hefty amounts of caffeine, however, can result in severe side effects in people who load up on them to stave off sleep (procrastinating students and sleepy truck drivers, for example). It is also important to note that while caffeine may allow one to keep sleep at bay, sleeping is a very important biological need that should not be ignored for long.

Children who take theophylline for treatment of asthma can also experience toxicity if their blood levels get too high. The major symptoms are severe gastrointestinal upset and vomiting, extreme nervousness, and nervous sys-

tem excitability that eventually leads to seizures if blood levels get high enough. Remember, too, that people who have other conditions that impair their cardiovascular system (obesity, hypertension, etc.) are more vulnerable to anything that affects heart function.

3

Enactogens

Drug Class: Enactogens

Individual Drugs: methylenedioxymethamphetamine (MDMA), methylenedioxyamphetamine (MDA), methylenedioxyethylamphetamine (MDEA)

Common Terms: Ecstasy, X, XTC, Adam (MDMA); Eve (MDEA)

The Buzz: MDMA and MDA increase heart rate, blood pressure, and body temperature and produce a sense of energy and alertness like that observed after amphetamine. (See "Stimulants" chapter.) These drugs also suppress appetite. However, the effects of MDMA on mood are quite different from those caused by amphetamine. Instead of an energizing euphoria, MDMA users experience a warm state of "empathy" and good feelings for all those around them.

Overdose and Other Bad Effects: At high doses of MDMA, users often describe a jitteriness and teeth clenching that is unpleasant. MDMA has caused a number of deaths when it was used in conjunction with high levels of physical activity (at rave dance parties). Death is usually typical of stimulant overdose, with greatly increased body temperature, hypertension, and kidney failure. Long-term damage to serotonin neurons is suggested by animal studies.

Dangerous Combinations with Other Drugs: These drugs can be dangerous if taken in conjunction with antidepressants that are monoamine oxidase

(MAO) inhibitors. They can cause a dangerous or lethal increase in heart rate and blood pressure.

A BRIEF HISTORY

MDMA was originally made in the 1930s as an experimental amphetamine. It was patented as an appetite suppressant but was never used clinically and never tested on humans. It languished, mainly unstudied, for many years. It returned to the scene in the 1980s when a group of enterprising psychotherapists decided that the empathic state produced by Ecstasy could be useful in couples therapy by producing at least a temporary state of openness during the therapy session that could help patients achieve insight and mutual understanding. This hope proved short-lived, as the drug experience was not easily controlled, and concerns about neurotoxicity led to its classification as a Schedule I drug by the DEA (a drug with no valid clinical use). Ecstasy moved quickly into the underground "rave" scene. Its most popular use today is at all-night dance parties, where users take Ecstasy and other drugs and dance for hours.

HOW MDMA GETS INTO AND OUT OF THE BODY

MDMA is usually taken orally in the form of pills, synthesized by bootleg labs which make them in several different colors (white, yellow, and beige), although sometimes pure powder is dissolved in water and injected, or inserted into the anus. The actual composition of pills can vary from 50 mg up to 200 to 300 mg. A number of other substances have been identified in pills sold as Ecstasy, including amphetamine, ephedrine, caffeine, and ketamine. The drug is well absorbed from the gastrointestinal tract, and peak levels are reached in about an hour. The effects last for three to six hours.

WHAT MDMA DOES TO THE BRAIN AND BODY

MDMA users provide very consistent reports of the feelings that result from taking it. Almost all users say that it causes a feeling of empathy, openness, and caring. The enhancement of positive emotions has been described as a decrease in defensiveness, fear, the sense of separation from others, aggression, and obsessiveness.

One first-time user reported the effects in this way: "What happens is, the drug takes away all your neuroses. It takes away your fear response. You feel open, clear, loving. I can't imagine anyone being angry under its influence, or feeling selfish, or mean, or even defensive. You have a lot of insights into yourself, real insights, that stay with you after the experience is over. It doesn't give you anything that isn't already there. It's not a trip. You don't lose touch with the world. You could pick up the phone, call your mother, and she'd never know."*

In both animals and humans, MDMA seems to cause a combination of amphetamine- and hallucinogen-like effects. While MDMA does not cause overt hallucinations, many people have reported distorted time perception while under the influence of the drug. It causes an amphetamine-like hyperactivity in people and animals, as well as the classic signs of stimulation of the flight-or fight response. For instance, heart rate and blood pressure are increased, and the smooth muscles of the breathing tubes (bronchioles) dilate. The pupils dilate, and blood flow to muscles increases.

One way to test the qualities of an unknown drug is to give it to an animal that is trained to recognize a certain class of drugs and see if it recognizes this one. This is called a *drug discrimination test*. When such tests are done with MDMA, some animals trained to recognize amphetamine also recognize MDMA, while other animals trained to recognize LSD or other hallucinogens also recognize MDMA. This confusion almost never happens with other drugs. Amphetamine-like drugs are almost never confused with hallucinogens.

People report that MDMA decreases feelings of aggression, and animal studies confirm this impression. MDMA also usually decreases sexual behavior in both humans and animals. There is mixed information about whether MDMA is pleasurable (and addictive) the way cocaine is. Small-scale studies have shown that primates will take this drug voluntarily, and the general profile of the way the drug acts on the brain indicates that it has this potential. However, the typical pattern of human use is quite different from those of cocaine and amphetamine. While people clearly use it repeatedly, it is used

*From Nicholas Saunder Londson, *Ecstasy and the Dance Culture*, 1995. (This is a self-published book.)

most frequently in a specific environment, like rave dance parties. There are no reports of people self-administering MDMA in a compulsive, repetitive manner, which occurs with many addictive drugs.

Overall, MDMA creates a very unusual behavioral profile. The positive feelings that people report are most similar to the effects of fluoxetine (Prozac) and fenfluramine (the main component of the recently withdrawn diet pill Pondimin). This makes sense, as we will see below, because these three drugs share some biochemical actions. Overall, MDMA doesn't fit into any other drug category, and the term *enactogen* has been coined to describe drugs such as this.

MDA is very closely related to MDMA in chemical structure, and though it shares the amphetamine-like effects, its effects on mood are different. MDA acts more like a typical hallucinogen. MDEA effects more closely resemble those of MDMA, but this drug also lacks the unusual empathic qualities of MDMA.

HOW MDMA WORKS IN THE BRAIN

Much of what MDMA does is explained by its ability to increase the levels of the monoamine neurotransmitters in the synapase. MDMA increases levels of dopamine, norepinephrine, (see "Stimulants" chapter) and serotonin (see "Hallucinogens" chapter). Like amphetamine, MDMA actively "dumps" them into the synapse, and the amount of these neurotransmitters that is released is much larger than is usually seen with cocaine. Unlike amphetamine, MDMA does a very good job of increasing the levels of serotonin. While amphetamine is ten to one hundred times better at releasing dopamine and norepinephrine than serotonin, MDMA is the opposite: it releases serotonin far more effectively than it does dopamine.

Some of the things MDMA does makes sense, given its biochemical profile. The big increase in body temperature, the relatively low addiction potential, and the decrease in aggressiveness are typical of drugs that produce a big increase in serotonin levels in the synapse. The serotonin-specific uptake inhibitors (SSRI), such as fluoxetine (Prozac), do this is in a *much* more limited but important way. While MDMA actively dumps serotonin into the synapse and produces very large increases this way, Prozac and drugs like it prevent serotonin recapture but do not actively release it. This means that the neuron has to release serotonin first before antidepressants can do anything. MDMA can make much more serotonin available because it doesn't have to wait for the neuron to fire.

We don't know if its effects on serotonin alone are enough to explain the unique effects of MDMA on mood, or whether some undescribed effect is responsible for the sense of empathy and positive feelings. While similar trends are apparent with Prozac and similar drugs, they never create a state just like this. Additionally, fenfluramine, an amphetamine derivative that has a similar ability to dump serotonin, shares some of these actions (like its ability to decrease aggression) but has not been reported to cause the same emotional changes. The actions of MDMA really are a mystery, because no other drug produces an identical state, and because the neurochemical effects we have observed so far don't really explain all of these effects.

This drug raises an ethical question: What is the benefit and harm caused by a drug that can apparently treat "personality" rather than disease? The effects seem overwhelmingly positive. While this particular drug has dangerous side effects that would limit its clinical use, would a "safer" enactogen be a valid clinical drug or a "tonic" for treating the ills of normal life? Can insights and positive feelings aroused during a drug-induced state carry over into normal life? The same issue has arisen with the incredible popularity of Prozac (as addressed in the book *Understanding Prozac*). We can't answer that question here, but we will raise a cautionary note. Sometimes there is a good reason for bad feelings: they are caused by bad experiences, and they often motivate personal change for the better. Furthermore, discontent is part of human diversity. Our world would seem so much blander in the absence of negative emotions.

MDMA TOXICITY

MDMA can be extremely dangerous when used in high doses (two to three times greater than a usual single dose). The bad effects are typical of an overdose of amphetamine. People report jitteriness and teeth clenching as the dose moves up, as well as all the classic signs of overstimulation of the sympathetic nervous system. Hunger is suppressed (remember, MDMA was first tested as an appetite suppressant), and people typically experience dry mouth, muscle cramping, and sometimes nausea. At higher doses, MDMA causes a large increase in body temperature, and that is one reason for its toxicity: the high temperature may be responsible for the muscle breakdown and kidney failure that have been seen in lethal cases reported from raves. When people dance for long period of time in close quarters, the physical activity and tendency to dehydration can synergize in an especially dangerous way with the effects of the drug. MDMA has also caused lethal cardiovascular effects in people with underlying heart disease. It has caused heart attacks and strokes in a few people. Unfortunately, it is hard to know how much causes dangerous effects in humans based on these reports, because the drugs were usually taken at a party, often with other drugs, and later the patient had little recall of how much drug they took. Like most amphetamine-like drugs, MDMA can cause seizures at extremely high doses.

MDMA use, especially repeated use of high doses, has been responsible for a number of psychiatric/psychological problems. Some patients have complained of panic attacks after repeated use of MDMA. These usually resolve eventually, but have continued for months in a few people. Similarly, hallucinations and amphetamine-like paranoid psychotic symptoms have occurred in chronic, high-dose users. Again, these symptoms waned when drug was discontinued. These may represent the development of tolerance to MDMA, or the development of irreversible changes in the brain.

IS MDMA REALLY NEUROTOXIC?

There is a raging controversy about whether MDMA causes long-term damage to serotonin neurons, a concern that arose from previous experience with similar amphetamine-like serotonin-releasing drugs. Most of the drugs that release both dopamine and serotonin have been shown definitively in laboratory studies to cause *permanent destruction* or long-term damage of either (or both) dopamine or serotonin neurons in the brain. The ends of the serotonin neurons that normally release serotonin onto its receptors (nerve terminals) are simply gone. Not only is the neurotransmitter gone, but all the other components of the terminal are gone. The transport molecules that accumulate serotonin, and the vesicles that store serotonin, have disappeared. With almost all these drugs, the amount of damage is dose- and time-related. Small doses produce little or no damage, moderate doses produce damage but leave the serotonin system still functional, while large doses can destroy it completely and eliminate the ability of these neurons to release serotonin.

MDMA acts like other drugs that are neurotoxic to serotonin neurons in every animal model that has been used. In rats as well as primates, MDMA not only produces the temporary loss of serotonin (which doesn't present any real long-term problem) but also produces the same kind of damage that the other amphetamine-like drugs produce. With some dose regimens, a limited amount of recovery occurred, while with higher dose regimens, no recovery occurred.

How much MDMA is necessary to produce significant long-term damage? The dose range that produced permanent damage in experiments with squirrel monkeys was about the equivalent of a 150-pound person taking 350 milligrams spaced over four days. The drug was administered by injection in the monkeys, which very likely produced higher tissue levels of drugs. An average human dose of Ecstasy is about 100 milligrams. Does the same type of damage happen in people who take high doses of MDMA for a long time?

There is one very disturbing scientific study that suggests that the answer is yes. In a study of about thirty MDMA users and thirty nonusers, scientists found that the levels of the major serotonin marker in the nervous system were decreased in the users, especially in the women users who probably experienced higher levels of drug in the bloodstream. This is a preliminary report involving only a few patients who had used the drug between eighty and one hundred times, but the news is quite troublesome given the well-documented effects in animal models. We'll know more in a few years, but for now caution is well advised.

What are the long-term effects of this type of serotonin loss? Are some of the anxiety disorders that we discussed above due to this type of damage? Again, we don't know for sure. Since increased levels of serotonin have been associated with improved mood (see "Hallucinogens" chapter), and its loss with depression in some cases, it is not far-fetched to speculate that mood disorders might be in the future for heavy Ecstasy users.

There is currently a similar controversy raging about recently withdrawn diet pills containing the drug fenfluramine, which is also an amphetamine derivative that releases serotonin and causes definite neurotoxicity in animal models. While thousands of people in Europe have taken very low doses of this drug without overt signs of toxicity, recent findings of serious heart valve changes in U.S. studies have caused fenfluramine to be taken off the market. Since we don't really know how to assess the behavioral effects of serotonin neurotoxicity, the only test involves imaging studies of the brain to measure whether or not the serotonin neurons are present. We don't yet have such definitive tests, and until we do it is appropriate to approach these drugs with considerable caution.

4

Hallucinogens

Drug Class: Hallucinogens

Individual Drugs: lysergic acid diethylamide (LSD), psilocybin, mescaline (peyote), Jimsonweed (belladonna alkaloids), phencyclidine (PCP), ketamine, dimethyltryptamine

Common Terms: acid, blotter, California sunshine, microdot, trip, yellow sunshine, and many others (LSD); boomers, magic mushrooms, shrooms (psilocybin); buttons, mesc, mescal, topi, peyote (mescaline); atropine, scopolamine, belladonna, deadly nightshade, Jimsonweed, stink weed, mandrake (belladonna alkaloids); PCP, angel dust, T, PeaCe pill, Special K, K (Phencyclidine; ketamine); DET (Diethyltryptamine), DMT, businessman's special (dimethyltryptamine)

The Buzz: Hallucinogen experiences vary incredibly. Even the same person can have dramatically different experiences with the same drug on different occasions. The experience is strongly shaped by the user's previous drug experience, her expectations, and the setting in which she takes the drug.

Mild effects produced by low doses can include feelings of detachment from the surroundings, emotional swings, and an altered sense of space and time. With higher doses, visual disturbances and illusions (hallucinations) occur. A hallmark of the hallucinogen experience is a sensation of separation from one's body. Some users experience intense feelings of insight with mystical or religious significance. These effects can last for minutes (with DMT) or for hours (with LSD).

Physical effects vary from drug to drug, but with LSD and similar drugs, users report jitteriness, racing (or slowed) heartbeat, nausea, chills, numbness (especially of the face and lips), and sometimes changes in coordination. In some cases these effects are caused by other drugs added to the LSD.

Overdose and Other Bad Effects: The hallucinogens should be divided into two groups: the drugs that usually produce psychological problems—the LSD-like drugs, and the much more physically dangerous belladonna and PCP-like compounds. The belladonna drugs, such as atropine and scopolamine, can be lethal in the usual amounts that people ingest for intoxication. These drugs can stimulate the heart and increase body temperature dangerously. At the point where a user is experiencing hallucinations from these drugs, he is at or very near the life-threatening level. PCP can also be lethal at high doses, causing seizures, coma, or a psychosis-like state that can last for some days.

The greatest danger of other hallucinogens, like LSD, is a bad trip, which can be physical or psychological in nature. The most common of these is a frightening experience that results in acute anxiety and the physical effects of that anxiety. In addition, users can accidentally injure or kill themselves because they are not thinking clearly about their environment. They may try to fly, for example, and jump from a high place. Actual psychotic reactions are much more unusual, happening in about 1 to 3 percent of cases, but they can require hospitalization. Another problem can be flashbacks, which are visual disturbances or other recalled events of the drug experience that emerge long after the drug is out of the body. Flashbacks are fairly common in heavy hallucinogen users. Surveys have shown that up to 30 to 60 percent of heavy users experience these in one form or another. Finally, as with any street drug, unknown contaminants can be present, and some, like strychnine, can be dangerous. Remember that most of these compounds are manufactured and packaged by illegal and uncontrolled laboratories and distributed in a completely unregulated fashion. The old phrase "let the buyer beware" could not be more appropriate.

Dangerous Combinations with Other Drugs: The dangers of these drugs vary by class. The most dangerous combination is the combination of PCP-like drugs with alcohol or other sedatives. This combination can kill you. Taking atropine-like drugs with anything that stimulates the cardiovascular system or raises body temperature (like ecstasy) can lead to dangerous disturbance of heart rhythms or increased body temperature. Hallucinogens with amphetamine-like actions (like mescaline) can be dangerous when taken in combination with stimulants. Any drug that increases blood pressure as it begins to take effect can be dangerous in people with heart disease if they combine it with other drugs that can raise blood pressure (like nasal decongestants). The physical risks of drug combinations with serotonin-like hallucinogens (like LSD) is much less, although an already unpredictable experience becomes even more unpredictable if combined with marijuana, a common practice.

HALLUCINOGEN HISTORY

This class of drugs boasts a longer history; a greater mystique; and more botanical, cultural, and historical diversity than almost any other. The use of hallucinogens is evident in plant remains from cultures on every continent. Each student of hallucinogens has his favorite "oldest story." One of ours explains how Siberian hunters discovered the fly agaric mushroom (*Amanita mus-*

caria). As the story is usually told, hunters noticed the abnormal behavior of reindeer grazing on these mushrooms, so they experimented with them. They found that not only did the mushrooms have a profound hallucinatory effect, but they were so potent that the urine of those who had ingested the drug still contained active drug, and so the drug could be recycled among tribe members. We can only imagine how they figured that out. It has been suggested that the same mushroom provides the drug Soma described in the Rig-Veda, the book of religious writings from India that has been dated to at least thirty-five hundred years ago. Hallucinogens were used in early Greece, and the plant riches of the New World provided a wealth of hallucinogenic agents that were known to the earliest migrants into South America from Eurasia. Archeological evidence suggests that the use of the peyote cactus goes back thousands of years.

WHAT IS A HALLUCINOGEN?

Hallucinogens are drugs that change one's thought processes, mood, and perceptions. The word itself is derived from the Latin word *alucinare*, which means "to wander in mind, talk idly, or prate." At high doses, these drugs cause people to perceive an experience as actually happening when, in fact, it is not. At lower dose levels, they cause milder disturbances of perception, thought, and emotion, but not the complete fabrication of unreal events.

Hallucinogens have often been called psychotomimetics, psychedelics, and illusinogens. All of these names suggest that these drugs induce or mimic mental illness, and they are wrong to varying degrees. Hallucinogens do not really mimic psychosis or mental illness. Although they can trigger a psychotic experience in a vulnerable person, the drug experience itself is probably quite different. For one example, the hallucinations caused by most of these drugs are usually seen, while the hallucinations of schizophrenia are usually heard.

The term *psychedelic* developed in the late 1950s to describe drugs that were "mind-expanding," a vague term that was popular at the time but not very descriptive. A similar term used to describe these drugs is *entheogenic,* which conveys the idea of finding "the god within." None of these terms is really adequate. The lack of good terminology to describe these drugs almost certainly results from the tremendous variation in the experiences that people have had with them.

In this chapter, we are going to talk about three broad categories of hallucinogens. The most familiar is the LSD, or serotonin-like, group. The prototype of this group is lysergic acid diethylamide (LSD). Dealers most often package LSD by placing drops of solution onto a piece of absorbent paper

(blotter paper) or a sugar cube, although it can also appear in pill form. Psilocybin mushrooms contain the active compounds psilocin and psilocybin, which roughly resemble LSD in the effects they produce. The peyote cactus contains mescaline. Mushrooms containing psilocybin and cactus buttons containing mescaline are usually consumed as the dried plant and look like it. There are many other "designer" hallucinogens that resemble LSD in their actions, including dimethyltryptamine (DMT) and bufotenine. There is also a group of amphetamine derivatives, including DOM (2,5 dimethoxy-4-methylphenylisopropylamine), also known as STP; TMA (trimethoxyamphetamine); and DMA (dimethoxyamphetamine), which resemble mescaline in their actions. Many of these hallucinogens appear in pill form, and the actual content of the pills often differs from what the dealer has described.

The belladonna alkaloids are the second major group of hallucinogens we will discuss. These have been used medically for thousands of years, and have been used ritually for even longer. However, their recreational abuse is just now becoming popular. Belladonna alkaloids in the United States are most often obtained either through prescription medication that contains them or from tea prepared from the leaves of the wild growing Jimsonweed (*Datura stramonium*).

Finally, there are the dissociative anesthetics, or "horse tranquilizers," phencyclidine (PCP) and ketamine. PCP appears in several different forms: pills, a powder for snorting, or "rocks" that can be smoked or, more rarely, dissolved for injection. Sometimes tobacco, marijuana, or parsley leaves are coated with PCP solution. These produce a bizarre, dissociative state that comes closer to resembling psychosis than the other hallucinogens do.

GETTING IN AND GETTING OUT: MOVEMENT OF HALLUCINOGENS IN THE BODY

Ritual use of hallucinogens by primitive peoples involves many routes of administration, ranging from herbal teas to application to the skin in potions to hallucinogenic snuffs. However, the major hallucinogens used in Western civilization are almost always taken by mouth. All the drugs listed above can be absorbed easily from the stomach or intestines. PCP is an exception because users also smoke or inject it. Only LSD is potent enough to appear in effective doses on paper. Users most often simply chew and swallow plant-derived hallucinogens such as cactus buttons or dried mushrooms. All the designer hallucinogens, and frequently LSD or various drugs that are supposed to be LSD, are ingested in pill form.

The lag time between taking drug and beginning the drug experience, and the duration of the experience itself, depends upon the drug. A typical LSD

experience begins between thirty and sixty minutes after a user takes the drug. LSD is absorbed efficiently from the stomach and intestines and enters the brain fairly quickly. It is unique among the hallucinogens in acting for an extremely long time: often the drug effects last up to twelve hours for a typical single dose. The reason for this is simple: the liver degrades LSD slowly, so active drug remains in the body for hours.

Despite many rumors to the contrary, LSD is not stored in the spinal fluid for months, nor does it remain hidden in any organ. It is eliminated just like other drugs, but more slowly. LSD flashbacks do not occur because hidden drug in the body suddenly reappears. We do not understand the neurobiology underlying flashbacks, but it would be reasonable to speculate that they represent a plastic change, or a memory, in the brain that is retained after the drug experience. As we will see later, in the "Brain Basics" chapter, the central nervous system has the capacity to recall all sorts of experiences, and flashbacks may be just that.

Peyote trips can last almost as long as LSD trips. In contrast, psilocybin experiences usually last two to four hours. Dimethyltryptamine (DMT) is the shortest-acting of the commonly used hallucinogens, producing noticeable effects within ten minutes, peaking at about thirty minutes, and ending within an hour. This drug is often described as a "businessman's special" for that reason. The differences from drug to drug are caused by differences in two properties. First, the more fat-soluble a drug is, the more quickly it enters the brain (this explains the rapid onset of DMT action). Second, the more slowly the drug gets degraded, the longer the trip. Again, this varies according to the particular chemical structure of the drug. Some drugs, like LSD and mescaline, produce particularly long-lived effects because they are not quickly metabolized by the liver.

PCP deserves some special notice because of the problems its chemical characteristics often cause. PCP is well absorbed when taken by mouth, and peak blood levels are reached even faster (within fifteen to thirty minutes) if it is smoked. However, it is broken down quite slowly, so the effects last a long time. The main drug experience lasts four to six hours, but significant amounts of the drug are present for twenty-four to forty-eight hours. The body's slow metabolism of PCP, along with some users' tendency to use it repeatedly over a day's time, leads to overdose and very persistent drug effects for days after ingestion.

Myths about how to stop a trip abound; drinking milk is the most unlikely we have heard. Most of these stories are just that: *myths*. There is no simple way to speed up removal of most hallucinogens from the body. One must simply wait for the liver and kidneys to do their job. PCP is the only exception. In critical situations, emergency room personnel can use a drug that makes the urine more acidic, speeding up the removal of PCP by the kidneys. Some drug

treatments (see below) can help with the symptoms of acute panic, and a drug is being tested that should be useful in the future in blocking the action of LSD. However, at the moment there is no quick fix, like there is for opiate overdose.

So it's important to remember that, once begun, the trip on some of these drugs can last for hours. If the trip is unpleasant, there is not much to do except receive support from unimpaired companions. If someone is going to experiment with any of these drugs, it is crucial that he or she do so in a safe and supportive environment. Doing even the least dangerous of these drugs alone invites trouble.

THE HALLUCINOGEN EXPERIENCE: WHAT HALLUCINOGENS DO TO THE BRAIN

It is very difficult to describe what a person experiences under the influence of these drugs because each experience is so individualized. The identity and amount of the drug, how it is taken, the user's expectations, and the user's previous experience all play a role. However, there are some effects that are commonly reported. Often, a trip begins with nausea, a feeling of jitteriness, and mild increases in blood pressure, heart rate, and breathing. After that, the first effect is usually a slight distortion of sensory perception. Visual effects predominate, with wavering images and distortion of size (things may seem much larger or smaller than they are).

At high doses, users experience frank hallucinations that are highly individual and profoundly influenced by the setting. They can range from simple color patterns to complex scenes, often with the drug taker watching his or her own actions from outside the body. The confusion of senses, or synesthesia, such as seeing sounds and hearing colors, is commonly reported. The sense of time is distorted, so that minutes can seem like hours. At the peak of the drug experience, the user will frequently describe a sense of profound understanding or enlightenment. Perhaps there will be a sense of oneness with the world, which is rarely maintained after the drug experience is over. Profound euphoria or anxiety can occur. As the drug effect wanes, the user usually feels a sort of otherworldly sense and fatigue.

Although eloquent, fantastic, and entertaining reports abound in the literature, one of the best descriptions of the hallucinogenic experience was written by Dr. Albert Hoffman, the chemist who first synthesized LSD. The report is especially believable because Dr. Hoffman wrote it at a time when the effects of the drug had never before been described, so he could not have been influenced by expectations.

This was in the era when scientific self-experimentation was more common than it is today, so after an accidental experience in the laboratory that alerted him to the profound effect of the drug, he took some of it intentionally and recorded what happened.

"After 40 minutes, I noted the following symptoms in my laboratory journal: slight giddiness, restlessness, difficulty in concentration, visual disturbances, laughing . . . Later, I lost all count of time. I noticed with distress that my environment was undergoing progressive changes. My visual field wavered, and everything appeared deformed, as in a faulty mirror. Space and time became more and more disorganized and I was overcome by a fear that I was going out of my mind. The worst part of it being that I was clearly aware of my condition. My power of observation was unimpaired. Occasionally, I felt as if I were out of my body. I thought I had died. My ego seemed suspended somewhere in space, from where I saw my dead body lying on the sofa. It was particularly striking how acoustic perceptions such as the noise of water gushing from a tap or the spoken word were transformed into optical illusions. I then fell asleep and awakened the next morning somewhat tired but otherwise feeling perfectly well."*

INDIVIDUAL HALLUCINOGENS

LSD

Lysergic acid diethylamide (LSD) is probably the best known and most commonly used hallucinogen in the United States. It is also the most potent of commonly used hallucinogens. Typical doses today are between 10 and 80 micrograms, lower than the typical doses of the sixties (100 to 200 micrograms). These levels are still enough to produce full-blown hallucinations in nontolerant individuals, although some experienced users take multiple "hits."

Because LSD is so potent and so easily dissolved, it is often diluted and dissolved in liquid, and then absorbed into a piece of paper. This is the common dosage form of blotter paper, and no other drug is potent enough to be used in this form. However, LSD also appears in other guises, including pills. Many a drug dealer will market a pill as LSD that actually contains other adulterants, including the poison strychnine, phencyclidine (PCP, or angel dust), or methamphetamine.

Although LSD itself was originally synthesized in a laboratory in the 1940s, the hallucinogenic (and the toxic) effects of lysergic acid derivatives (the ergot alkaloids) have been recognized for thousands of years. Certain species

*From *Interim Drug Report of the Commission of Inquiry into the Nonmedical Use of Drugs* (Ottawa: Information Canada, 1970), pp. 58–59.

of morning glory seeds that provided a drug called *ololiuqui* in ancient Mexico contain a related chemical, lysergic acid amide. Some people have used these seeds in search of a drug experience, but this is quite risky since many seed suppliers intentionally adulterate these seeds with toxic chemicals, and since native seeds contain many other chemicals that can cause nausea, vomiting, and other unpleasant side effects. Even worse, a fungus that commonly grows on rye *(Claviceps purpurea)* also produces poisonous LSD-related ergot alkaloids and amino acids that cause hallucinations, gangrene, loss of limbs, spontaneous abortion, and sometimes death. The disease caused by eating ergot-infected rye became known as St. Anthony's fire, after the burning sensation caused by the intense constriction of blood vessels, and after the patron saint of the order of monks founded to care for the victims of these poisonings.

What physical changes accompany the LSD experience? As the experience begins, many people report unusual sensations, including numbness, muscle weakness, or trembling. A mild flight-or-fight response occurs: heart rate and blood pressure increase a little, and pupils dilate. Nausea is quite common. These changes are rarely large enough to be dangerous, although they can be in individuals with underlying heart disease. Many users report phantom pains. Internet discussions of hallucinogen experiences usually reveal several conversation threads about particular pains. A recent look at these found complaints ranging from chest pain to testicular pain.

PATTERNS OF CLINICAL EFFECTS FOR HALLUCINOGENS OF THE LSD
GROUP*

Time	Clinical Effect
0–30 min.	Dizziness, nausea, weakness, twitches, anxiety
30–60 min.	Blurred vision, increased contrasts, visual patterns, feelings of unreality, incoordination, tremulous speech
1–2 hr.	Increased visual effects, wavelike motions, impaired distance perception, euphoria, slow passage of time
2–4 hr.	Waning of above effects
4–12 hr.	Returning to normal
Late effects	Headache, fatigue, contemplative state

*Adapted from R. M. Julien, *A Primer of Drug Action* (New York: W. H. Freeman and Company, 1995).

The effects of LSD depend upon the dose. Many experienced users have compensated for the decreased dose in contemporary LSD by taking multiple doses up to amounts equaling doses that were present in LSD in the 1960s. While this practice is usually not physically dangerous, it increases the risk of a particularly intense bad trip. Obviously, any contaminant present will be taken in increased levels with double dosing.

Rapid tolerance develops to LSD. Probably this effect, as well as the lingering exhaustion from a drug experience that lasts so long, is the reason why most users take LSD at fairly widely spaced intervals (once a week to once a month). The tolerance diminishes quickly, so that a week's abstinence is usually enough to restore sensitivity to the drug.

PSILOCYBIN MUSHROOMS

Hallucinogenic mushrooms are probably the most frequently used hallucinogen after LSD in the United States. The popular cottage industry that has arisen promoting sales of home-growing kits has increased public awareness of these agents. However, there is probably almost as much misinformation about "shrooms" as there is about LSD.

The shrooms to which most users refer belong to several genera of mushroom (*Psilocybe, Panaeolus,* and *Conocybe*). The most commonly used species in the United States are *Psilocybe mexicana* and *Psilocybe cyanescens*. These mushrooms contain two related compounds: psilocin (4-hydroxy-N,N-dimethyltryptamine) and psilocybin (4-phosphoryloxy-N,N-dimethyltryptamine). Although many people think that psilocybin is the active agent, this is probably not the case. Only after the liver has removed the extra chemical group (a phosphate group) can the remainder of the molecule (psilocin) enter the brain. Although there are rumors that phosphorylated serotonin, or phosphorylated DMT, provide a unique new high, these groups actually prevent rather than promote psychoactivity, because they slow the entry of drug into the brain. Psilocybin is distributed both in the dried mushroom form and as a white powder of purified crystalline compound. A typical dose is 4 to 10 milligrams (two to four mushrooms of the genus *Psilocybe cyanescens*).

Use of these mushrooms is very ancient. Statues of mushrooms dating from A.D. 100 to 1400 have been found throughout Mexico and Central America, and a group of statues from central Guatemala that are even older (about 500 B.C.) are widely interpreted as mushroom stalks associated with mushroom worship. Use of *teonanactl*, or "flesh of the gods," persisted in Mexico until the Spanish, who attempted to extinguish its use, arrived. Ethnobotanists, including R. Gordon Wasson, Richard Schultes, and others, worked in central Mexico in the 1930s to identify almost twenty species of mushrooms belonging to the general *Psilocybe* (the majority), *Conocybe, Paneolus,* and *Stropharia* that were used for healing and religious purposes.

Psilocybin's careful ritual use by native peoples has evolved into college students' recreational shroom use during spring break and at weekend parties. This experience is generally viewed as a milder and shorter LSD-like experience. At low doses, psilocybin causes simple feelings of relaxation, physical heaviness or lightness, and some perceptual distortions (especially visual). At higher doses, more physical sensations occur, including lightheadedness, numbness of the tongue, lips, or mouth, shivering or sweating, nausea, and anxiety.

The psychological effects mirror those of LSD. The records of a group of scientists who gave LSD, psilocybin, and PCP to college students during the mid-1960s provide a good description of the effects in contemporary terms. They published the verbatim transcripts of the experiences of three students. The following is an excerpt from a transcript of a female college senior (who previously had never taken hallucinogens) that was recorded during a psilocybin experiment.

About an hour after the drug: "When I close my eyes, then I have all these funny sensations. Funny pictures, they're all in beautiful colors. Greens and reds and browns and they all look like Picasso's pictures. Doors opening up at triangular angles and there are all these colors . . . an unreal world. It must be my subconscious or something. If I open my eyes, now the screen is, the dome gets darker. Looks like something is moving on the outside. Right along the edge. Some writhing. There's a figure—isn't exactly a figure, huge wings like a hawk, head of a hawk, but legs of a man beneath a bed. Now it's gone."

About two hours after the drug: "Ho, ho, I wonder if, I know I can sing as I sang before, but there's some flower vines running up. They start at one point, like at the bulb, and then they go up over an archway or something. And they have flower on them: the vines are green . . . I have the feeling that someone is sticking their high-heeled shoe into the cotton in my right hand. But I can't feel it, it's not there. When I move my hand, my hands are very wet. And the lower part of my body, body, well, my body's bent. Freud. I think he went too far. Ohh. I'm moving. I look like I'm just moving. I just looked down at my body. I wish I had a mirror. I suppose that wouldn't help my seeing. . . . Now I can see a fire. It looks like a key and there's the crackling again. There's a cage and someone is opening the door of the cage. And there's a spider inside. But I'm not going in. I could stay here forever. It's so pleasant. Move slowly up and down, up and down, back and forth, ripple and wave. I keep my eyes closed now and I see a purple flower . . ."*

---

*From J. C. Pollard, *Drugs and Phantasy: The Effects of LSD, Psilocybin and Sernyl on College Students* (New York: Little, Brown and Co., 1965).

Trips are not always so benign as this one, and in some cases they can be terribly frightening. The following are descriptions of two very unpleasant trips experienced by friends of the authors. The first indicates the depth of fear that can be experienced.

"It was late in the evening and I had been hanging out with two friends since the afternoon. We were all pretty tired, but decided to take some mushrooms. I remember as the trip began that every time I closed my eyes huge, vividly colored plants would seem to grow really rapidly in the darkness behind my eyelids. I found this pretty interesting and entertaining. It happened every time I closed my eyes—as though the process and the images were completely beyond my control." Later that night, after a botched attempt to go to a party and a brief spell of unconsciousness, our friend "lay there looking up into the darkness and perceived the darkness to begin to move ever so slightly in a circular motion. It was not a dizzy feeling that happens sometimes to people who are really drunk and think that the room is moving. I had not been drinking heavily at all. In my mind it was the darkness that was moving. I already felt pretty unsettled because of having passed out, and the sense of moving darkness was quite frightening. As I stared into the darkness it began to swirl slightly faster, and I had the feeling that it was moving toward me—bearing down on me. Lightly at first, but the force seemed to increase as the swirling gained speed. Before long I was consciously fighting with that swirling dark force, having to push hard against it with my mind to keep it at bay. The process continued. The swirling got faster, and the darkness now seemed bent on overtaking me. I was overcome with the thought that if I let it get all the way to me that I would be dead. So, I mustered all the concentration and focus I could to continue holding it off. I struggled for some time, but very slowly it seemed to wear me down.

"I remember thinking that it was going to win, and I was going to die. I held it off with all the will I could muster, and finally, feeling quite exhausted, gave up with the thought that fighting that force was useless and I should just let it take me. So I did. I relaxed and felt that at least I was facing my death calmly. The swirling malevolence seemed to enter into my body in the middle of my belly. Then everything was calm and quiet again. I really thought I was dead. After a brief moment, I remember suddenly feeling that an intense white light was bursting from within me, moving outward. It was as if single, white laser beams were shining out through each and every pore of my skin. Later I remember interpreting the experience in terms of my fear of, and struggle with, my image of my own death. But while it was going on, I was more afraid than I can ever remember having been."

The second trip illustrates another death theme that produced extreme fear.

"When the trip started, I was scared. It was the first time I had ever tripped.

I sat Indian-style on my bed and let the waves of thought bombard me. I waited to see rainbows where the walls should have been or angel fish swimming in the sky. I didn't. I just felt fragments of a hundred emotions fly in and out of my mind in a frenzy and life began to feel tragic. I was confused and felt out of control. In an effort to gain control over my mind I tried focusing. I became fascinated with my hands, and I tried to let everything else go and just look at the moonstone on my ring finger. I watched and my hand slowly began to change. The variation in color around my knuckles became more extreme, and I could see the lines around them were getting deeper. The smooth brown skin was aging, and I could see sunspots develop on it. The hand grew thinner and the fingers bony with little meat left between the joints. A blue vein bulged near the surface on the back of my hand. My skin no longer had a healthy glow but took on a green tint. My fingers began to curl and were contorted from arthritis. The slight inward bend in the top joint of my pinky was now a crook, and just like my grandmother's, my index finger had also curved inward. The wrinkles were deep now and the skin was just a thin layer of crumpled tissue paper. Soon even the skin was gone and all that was left was an X-ray image of the arthritic old bones."

These stories illustrate the wide variation in experiences one can have. The fear inspired in some can be so profound that the memory of it stays with an individual for life, and should be considered a risk of taking these drugs.

Cautionary Note on Mushrooms

Psilocybin mushrooms are not the only ones that produce discernible mental effects. However, they are the only mushrooms in wide use in North America. The other well-described hallucinogenic mushrooms are extremely dangerous and can kill you. *Amanita muscaria*, which we discussed at the beginning of this chapter, contains a number of compounds that produce hallucinations, including muscimol and ibotenic acid. This mushroom also contains muscarine, which stimulates acetylcholine receptors in the body and can be lethal. This compound mimics stimulation of the parasympathetic nervous system, causing intense salivation, nausea, vomiting, spasm of the bronchioles (breathing tubes), slowed heart rate, and extremely low blood pressure. These last two effects can lead to shock and death.

OTHER LSD-LIKE HALLUCINOGENS

DMT

Dimethyltryptamine (businessman's special) is one of the other serotonin-like hallucinogens that appear on the drug scene in North America. The compound originally derives from a vine *(Piptadenia peregrina)*, and has been used by South American tribes as a hallucinogenic snuff called *yopa* or *co-*

hoba. However, it is most often available today as the pure compound, which users prepare as a tea or in conjunction with marijuana, by first soaking the leaves in a solution of DMT and then drying and smoking them. The drug takes effect very rapidly: the entire experience develops and finishes within a hour. Probably because the onset of action is so fast, DMT causes anxiety attacks much more frequently than LSD, although the basic experience is similar.

Some serotonin-derived compounds, such as 5-methoxy dimethyltryptamine (5-MeO-DMT) and bufotenine, are found in the skins of some toads, including the Colorado River toad. Milking the glands on the back of the toad to obtain the hallucinogens, which are then smoked or ingested, was an old Native American trick that has recently been repopularized to the extent that *The Wall Street Journal* reported it. The high that is produced is extremely brief and accompanied by much worse side effects than most hallucinogens, including increased blood pressure and heart rate, blurred vision, cramped muscles, and temporary paralysis. These are due mainly to the bufotenine. The same compounds also appear in the seeds of a number of trees that grow in Haiti, Central America, and South America *(Piptadenia peregrina).* The powdered seeds provide the basis for hallucinogenic snuffs used by indigenous peoples, and have been identified as a component of voodoo powders.

Peyote Cactus (mescaline)

The peyote cactus has likely been used as a hallucinogen by native tribes in Mexico for thousands of years, and its use by North American tribes is an accepted part of their histories. A cactus that grows in northwest Mexico produces mescaline, the active hallucinogen, as well as many other compounds. The dried "button" of the cactus is the usual form in which the drug is sold, although it also appears in other dried forms (powders, etc.), as well as in a tea made from buttons. It can be smoked, but this is unusual. The button is usually swallowed without chewing, and the active agent is absorbed from the stomach and intestine.

Mescaline's chemical structure does not resemble LSD or psilocybin and the other serotonin-like hallucinogens. Instead, it looks more like amphetamine. While the physical effects resemble those of amphetamine—dilated pupils, increased heart rate, and increased blood pressure—the mental effects as described by ritual and recreational users are surprisingly similar to LSD. Nausea and vomiting are common, especially soon after ingestion of the cactus buttons. After a user ingests a number of cactus buttons, he often feels an increase in sensitivity to sensory images and sees flashes of color followed by geometric patterns and sometimes images of people and animals. Time and space perception are distorted, as with LSD, and people often feel that they are outside of themselves. It should be emphasized that the effects of ingestion of pure mescaline used in some experiments and the cactus button are similar but not identical, as there are at least thirty other compounds in the cactus.

The ritual use of this cactus by the shamans of native tribes, like the Huichol in Mexico, persisted into recent times, and North American tribes adopted it in the late nineteenth century. The ritual use by North American tribes was integrated with a number of Christian practices in the form of the Native American Church. The use of peyote as a part of this church's religious rituals has been protected by the First Amendment, though certain states have attempted to restrict use of peyote, which is otherwise banned by the DEA. However, the Religious Freedom Restoration Act, passed in 1993, will likely provide new protection for its use. It requires that the government can limit a person's exercise of religious freedom only if "it is in furtherance of a compelling government interest, and is the least restrictive means of furthering that compelling interest." Recent court cases have upheld peyote use, for example that of *The United States* v. *Boyll* in 1991, when the government argued that Robert Boyll was not entitled to possess peyote because he was not a Native American. The court ruled that this rationale imposed racial discrimination in the practice of religion, since no one can practice in the Native American Church without using peyote.

"Designer" Mescaline-like Drugs

A large number of these drugs were first made during the original chemical studies of mescaline. The names sound like an alphabet soup: DOM (2,5 dimethoxy-4-methylphenylisopropylamine, also known as STP), MDA (methylenedioxyamphetamine), DMA (dimethoxy amphetamine), MDMA (methylenedioxymethamphetamine, or Ecstasy). All these drugs are less specific than mescaline, and produce strong amphetamine-like effects in addition to hallucinations. As a result, all are more toxic than mescaline, and appear much more rarely on the street today. Ecstasy provides a unique profile of effects, discussed in the "Enactogens" chapter.

The spices nutmeg and mace deserve a final note as we discuss the mescaline-like hallucinogens. Someone who takes several teaspoons of nutmeg (if he can figure out how to avoid the overwhelming taste) can experience a very mild hallucinogenic state that includes perceptual distortions, euphoria, and sometimes mild visual hallucinations and feelings of unreality. The active compounds in nutmeg and mace are myristicin and elemicin, compounds with structures somewhat like mescaline. The drawback (besides the taste) is that these compounds are very weak hallucinogens, and the dose required to evoke changes in perception causes a number of unpleasant side effects, including vomiting, nausea, and tremors. Furthermore, an aftereffect of sleepiness or a feeling of unreality can persist into the next day.

BELLADONNA ALKALOIDS

The "Jimsonweed" nickname comes from records of a famous poisoning that left the settlers of the Virginia colony of Jamestown deathly ill. Someone unfamiliar with the edible plants of the New World included the leaves of this plant in a salad, resulting in severe intoxication in the diners. Teas prepared from any part of the plant, or the chewed seeds alone, produce a bizarre dream state at extremely high doses. Most users do not remember the experience because the drug causes amnesia. Ingesting doses large enough to produce this mental state causes severe and dangerous effects on heart rate, breathing, and body temperature.

The belladonna alkaloids atropine and scopolamine are the active agents in Jimsonweed. Atropine is responsible for many of the effects outside of the brain. At low doses, this compound or similar drugs are effective in the treatment of asthma and some stomach problems, as well as in the diagnosis of eye problems. However, at higher doses atropine can be lethal. The dramatic effects on thought and perception are caused by the scopolamine. Scopolamine, unlike atropine, enters the brain easily and is responsible for all of the behavioral effects of this plant.

The belladonna alkaloids mimic the complete shutdown of the parasympathetic nervous system—the mouth is extremely dry, the pupils are dilated, the heart speeds up, the bronchioles (breathing passages in the lung) dilate, and digestion slows. These drugs also affect regions of the brain involved in control of body temperature, which can rise to dangerous levels. Finally, they block a neurotransmitter receptor that is important for memory, so amnesia for some of the experience can occur.

These compounds and related ones also exist in other plants, including the deadly nightshade (*Atropa belladonna*) and the mandrake root (*Mandragora officinarum*). Used properly, they are important and effective medicines. However, recent recreational use, mainly by teenagers, has resulted in an increasing number of hospitalizations and deaths. The mandrake root is showing up in herbal remedies and has caused accidental poisonings in this form.

Belladonna alkaloids have very different actions from the serotonin-related hallucinogens. They induce a bizarre delirium that users remember only as strange dreams. These dreams often include the sensation of flying, which may have contributed to modern stories of witches flying (the broomstick image may derive from the use of vaginal applicators to permit absorption of the drug from the mucous membrane of the vagina).

These compounds have been used throughout history, as often for poisoning as for hallucinations. The term "belladonna," or beautiful woman, refers to their use during the Middle Ages to dilate the pupils of the eyes for enhancement of beauty. These drugs also were supposedly used by practitioners of female-deity worship in Europe and Eurasia during the rise of Christianity, when those using these drugs were depicted as "witches" by the early Church.

Phencyclidine (PCP) and Ketamine (Special K): Hallucinogenic Anesthetics

Phencyclidine (PCP, angel dust, etc.) has a bad reputation and deserves it. Both PCP and ketamine were initially marketed as general anesthetics under the names Sernyl and Ketalar. However, so many patients experienced hallucinations and delirium as they were waking up that doctors stopped using it in humans unless they received a Valium-like drug to minimize the hallucinations. Currently, ketamine is used mainly as a veterinary anesthetic. This is a drug that is frequently taken intentionally for recreation, but it is also often part of mixtures sold as LSD, amphetamine, or Ecstasy. It is sold in many different forms: as rocks that are smoked like crack, as PCP-impregnated marijuana joints, as white powder, or as pills. It is taken orally, snorted, or injected intravenously. The main effects of a single dose last four to six hours, although the lingering effects can last for up to two days.

PCP and ketamine are the most complicated drugs we discuss in this book, because they have so many different effects on brain activity. Put simply, taking PCP can produce a state similar to getting drunk, taking amphetamine, and taking a hallucinogen simultaneously. It is most frequently taken for the amphetamine-like euphoria and stimulation it produces. Many of PCP's bad side effects also resemble those of amphetamine, such as increased blood pressure and body temperature. However, at the same time it causes a "drunken" state characterized by poor coordination, slurred speech, and drowsiness. People under the influence of PCP are also less sensitive to pain. Finally, at higher doses it causes a dissociative state in which people seem very out of touch with their environment. Observers frequently report that a PCP-intoxicated person has a blank stare and seems very detached from what is going on around her.

So, in total, you have someone running around drunk, insensitive to pain, and very uninhibited. Is it any wonder that PCP-intoxicated people frequently find themselves in trouble with the law? Their driving skills are poor, their judgment worse, they are not attending to their environment, and they are insensitive to pain. This condition indeed can resemble the "drug-crazed," sometimes violent state that many misinformed people attribute to any drug of abuse. In the case of PCP, the stereotype has some truth. Few drugs create a person more difficult to treat in an emergency room situation because he or she can be so out of touch, belligerent, and agitated. At high doses, muscle rigidity and general anesthesia occurs. Extremely high doses can result in coma, seizures, respiratory depression, dangerously high body temperature, and extremely high blood pressure.

HOW HALLUCINOGENS WORK

This section must begin by clearly stating that neuroscientists know little about hallucinations. In part, this is because hallucinations can be studied only in humans. No one would volunteer for the kinds of careful brain-lesion studies that are used to answer such questions, although imaging studies in intact, living humans are becoming feasible. However, we do have a lot of information about the neurotransmitter systems involved. Since there are so many hallucinogenic drugs, it will come as no surprise that there are several different neurochemical routes to hallucinatory states, and that each drug produces a somewhat distinct state that overlaps but does not coincide with the state produced by other drugs.

LSD, PSILOCIN, AND MESCALINE

The suspicion that drugs like LSD have something to do with the neurotransmitter serotonin (5HT) has been prevalent since scientists first described the similarity of the chemical structures of LSD and psilocin to serotonin in the 1940s. It has been a long and torturous road from this initial suspicion to a molecular understanding of what these drugs do. Serotonin is an important neurotransmitter that is necessary to permit sleep, regulate eating behavior, maintain a normal body temperature and hormonal state, and perhaps limit vulnerability to seizures. Drugs that enhance all of the actions of serotonin are useful for treating depression and suppressing overeating. How, then, can drugs that affect serotonin produce such bizarre effects on perception without disrupting many of these other actions of serotonin?

Part of the difficulty in understanding hallucinogens came from using LSD as a test hallucinogen. All of the early test systems involved organs other than the brain. For example, serotonin can make the heart of a clam beat faster, so these hearts were an early favorite test system. The clam heart would be suspended on a wire attached to a pen that would move if the heart muscle contracted. When serotonin was dripped on the heart, it contracted. LSD prevented the effects of serotonin on clam hearts and other test systems, and for years it was thought that hallucinogens acted by preventing the actions of serotonin. When more sophisticated tests of serotonin action in the brain became available, they seemed to support this idea. Scientists measuring the rate at which serotonin neurons were firing showed that LSD inhibited their firing. However, this didn't make a lot of sense, because shutting down the serotonin neurons so dramatically should have affected all of the other processes of such drugs be tightly restricted, as native societies seem to have decided as well.

Although many people use hallucinogens for recreation, and some use them for spiritual experiences, many also use them as a tool to find new ways of thinking and feeling. Since the nature of these experiences is so subjective and individual, it is impossible to gauge the real value of these drugs for people seeking personal enhancement. Still, many people do report that after using hallucinogens, they have a slightly new viewpoint on the world and possibly on themselves.

For example, some people report a sense of "dissolving boundaries" while under the influence. A user might be sitting on the ground and feel that the boundary between the ground and his body no longer exists. This feeling can then go in a number of directions. It could lead to the very unsettling feeling of being sucked into the earth, or it could lead to a calming sense of "oneness" with mother earth. After the trip the memories of such experiences move some people to reconsider some of their ideas about who they are and how they fit into the world. Some report that such reflections have led them to more healthy perspectives. Enlightening or not, though, it is very important to emphasize that everyone reacts differently to these complicated drugs, and one person's enlightenment can be another person's hell.

DANGERS AND MYTHS

IDENTIFICATION

First and foremost: one can never really be sure which hallucinogen one is taking. Blotter paper–like preparations are most likely to be actual LSD because other hallucinogens are not potent enough for an effective dose to be delivered in this way. However, a pill/capsule/powder could be anything, or any combination of things. Laboratory analyses of blood from people admitted to emergency rooms for LSD toxicity indicate that in some urban settings, only about 50 percent of the drug samples that were thought to be LSD by their possessors actually were LSD. Strychnine, PCP, and amphetamine are common, potentially dangerous contaminants. Strychnine is a poison favored by snake handlers and pest-control agents (it has been used historically as rat poison). It's a convulsant (a drug that causes seizures). It does so by preventing the action of a neuromodulator (glycine) that normally slows neural activity. In the small doses in which it usually appears when mixed with LSD, it simply causes jitteriness and some muscle cramps. However, with multiple dosing or higher single doses, worse effects can emerge, including convulsions.

Finally, LSD or any drug that has been synthesized in an underground laboratory can contain various by-products that arise from poor chemical synthesis.

that rely on serotonin, but LSD did not produce such effects. Furthermore, mescaline did not have the same effect as LSD in these types of experiments, but since the structure of mescaline, unlike the other drugs, did not resemble serotonin, scientists were willing to assume that mescaline was working in some different way.

The answer to the question of what hallucinogens have to do with serotonin had to wait for the era of molecular biology, when scientists discovered that the neurotransmitter serotonin acts on a number of different receptors. It turns out that there are two major groups of serotonin receptors (serotonin 1 and serotonin 2 receptors). This is where the problem with LSD was explained. LSD acted on both classes of receptors, but it blocked one while stimulating the other. It turns out that receptors stimulated by serotonin (serotonin 2 receptors) were the important ones for hallucinogenic activity. So far, every experimental drug tested that stimulates the serotonin-2 receptors causes hallucinations. We don't know how this happens, but we are pretty sure that stimulating these receptors can do it. Most of these receptors are in the cerebral cortex, where we think hallucinogens have their major action.

The true marvel of serotonin neurons lies in their receptors. We mentioned two groups of serotonin receptors above, but this was a bit of a simplification. At least eight types of serotonin receptors are now recognized, and we know that some seem to have very specific effects on behavior. Only one of these (as we described above) can trigger hallucinations.

The serotonin-3 receptors offer the best example of how specific the actions of these receptors can be. They exist only in a very restricted place in the brain, where they serve a very specific purpose: they seem to be involved in triggering vomiting when a person ingests toxic substances. The fact that so few of these receptors exist anywhere else in the brain has allowed the development of near "miracle drugs" that block the actions of serotonin at this receptor to prevent vomiting, an incredible boon to cancer treatment. Many cancer medications are very toxic, and induce such strong vomiting that people will stop their therapy rather than experience it. The serotonin-3 antagonists prevent this vomiting with very little effect on any other part of the brain.

The recent technical innovation of being able to knock out a specific gene in animals has given us additional insight about another serotonin receptor, the 5HT1b. Mice without this receptor have a number of problems, but one more striking than all the others: they are incredibly aggressive and do not survive if housed together because they kill each other. This was quite unexpected, as no one would think that simply changing one gene would have such a big impact on behavior, but it certainly is consistent with the research associating low serotonin levels with increased aggressiveness.

Given how many receptors for serotonin there are, and how particular their actions are, it seems less surprising that drugs that stimulate 5HT2 receptors would stimulate hallucinations so specifically. However, even these receptors have other jobs, and hallucinogens can actually stimulate all the additional things that these receptors do. Animals in which the 5HT2c receptor (the one that LSD probably activates) has been eliminated genetically seem fairly normal most of the time. But they occasionally have seizures that kill them, and they become very overweight because they cannot control their eating. These findings implicate the hallucination receptor in important controls on feeding behavior and the general excitability of the central nervous system. However, LSD is unlikely to be the diet drug of the future!

One mystery that remains about serotonin drugs is why the antidepressant drugs that increase the amount of serotonin in the synapse (see "Brain Basics" chapter) *do not* usually cause hallucinations. These drugs increase serotonin everywhere in the brain, including sites that have 5HT2c receptors, but although a rare patient taking one of these drugs will experience hallucinations, when the 5HT2c receptors are stimulated in balance with all the other serotonin systems, there are generally no hallucinogenic effects.

BELLADONNA ALKALOIDS

The belladonna alkaloids work by a completely different mechanism, which might explain the different state that they cause. They act by preventing the actions of the neurotransmitter acetylcholine at one of its receptors. Acetylcholine is the neurotransmitter that nerves use to stimulate muscle and allow movement, and it is also the neurotransmitter mimicked by nicotine. It has two types of receptors: one is stimulated by nicotine, and the other (called the muscarinic receptor, because researchers discovered that it was stimulated by the compound muscarine from the *Amanita muscaria* mushroom) slows the heart and probably helps to form memories. We'll describe this in more detail below.

PCP AND KETAMINE

Both PCP and ketamine block the actions of the neurotransmitter glutamate at one of its receptors. This blockade can, on its own, produce a feeling of disconnection from one's body or environment. This is extremely unfortunate, because similar glutamate-blocking drugs had great promise a few years ago for medical use—in experimental studies they protected against the nerve death that results from stroke. However, in clinical trials of these drugs, patients hallucinated. As you can imagine, it was terrifying for patients to wake up in the hospital, seriously ill, afraid that the stroke rather than the treatment was causing hallucinations.

If PCP were just a glutamate blocker, it would be a hallucinogen and would pose a tremendous overdose hazard, but it would not cause the excitation

and loss of pain sensation that cause people to behave unpredictabl[y] themselves. However, PCP also acts like amphetamine to release [the] transmitter dopamine. This accounts for the running around [that] intoxicated people can experience.

PCP also acts on another neurotransmitter system to relieve p[ain sensa]tions. There are a group of opiate-like drug receptors that, when [stimulated,] cause a spectrum of effects, including loss of pain sensations as we[ll as hallu]cinations. We know little except that these receptors (the sigma op[iate recep]tors) are unlike any others yet defined. Interest in this system h[as grown in] recent years since researchers found that drugs that specifically [stimulate] this receptor system produced hallucinations without affecting the [opi]ate systems. Dextromethorphan, the active ingredient in many [over-the-]counter cough remedies, is a very weak stimulant of this recep[tor. This] explains the slightly hallucinogenic state that results from this drug[, but it] takes a lot (at least a four-ounce bottle) to create even a mild effe[ct. Taking] a whole bottle of cough syrup can be quite dangerous not because [of dex]tromethorphan but because some cough syrup preparations con[tain a de]congestant that could raise blood pressure dangerously in such exce[ss.]

PCP clearly is a complicated drug. Ketamine probably is more s[imple, as] it lacks the effect on dopamine and sigma opiate receptors. The la[tter is still] used in particular situations in surgery, but it is used with a benz[odiazepine] (a Valium-like drug) to prevent the adverse effects.

ENLIGHTENMENT OR ENTERTAINMENT?

The use of hallucinogens by many indigenous peoples is tightly co[nnected to] their cultures. These cultures restrict such drugs to ritual use for p[urposes of] healing, enlightenment, or prophecy. In many cases, only particu[lar individ]uals in a society are permitted to use the drugs at all.

Has the use of hallucinogens evolved from this spiritual purpo[se to recre]ational use/abuse in contemporary society? If you talk to college stu[dents,] the reasons they give for using these drugs vary tremendously. So[me are curious] and simply aim for a novel and exciting experience. However, inter[views with] regular and heavy users will reveal a substantial percentage who u[se them] for the sense of enlightenment they feel they gain by separating f[rom them]selves. The sensation of dissociation resembles that reported by [some reli]gious practitioners. Many such users are well informed, artic[ulate, and] persuasive. Dr. Timothy Leary abandoned a successful tradition[al academic] career for exactly this reason. Unfortunately for such advocates, the[ir views] conflict directly with the illegal status of these drugs. Both sides car[ry on the] issue persuasively, but the fact is that the majority of Americans pre[fer]

Hallucinogenic mushrooms represent another identification problem. It takes an educated and practiced eye to identify any mushrooms in the field, and this is always a dangerous proposition. Many mushroom species, including the *Amanita muscaria* described above, contain psychoactive compounds that are extremely dangerous or lethal. Other species *(Amanita phalloides)* contain toxins that produce fatal damage to the liver and kidneys. While simple "home" tests are much touted ("if the stem turns blue, it is psilocybin"), none of these are foolproof. A number of mail-order operations exist that claim to send out psilocybin-containing mushrooms, but the identity of the dried mushrooms can be very difficult to establish.

PHYSICAL AND PSYCHOLOGICAL PROBLEMS

LSD, psilocybin, and mescaline do not generally cause dangerous physical reactions, and blood pressure, body temperature, and other vital signs remain reasonably stable unless there are acute anxiety reactions. A user is in little danger of seizures or coma. Furthermore, there is little evidence that these drugs activate the pleasure centers, and addiction and physical dependence do not really occur. In this sense, they are remarkably safe. However, the psychological consequences for some users can be extreme. The bad trip, in which the drug user feels acute anxiety and perhaps fears that he will not be able to return, is the most common. Fortunately, this reaction ends as the drug is eliminated from the body. Furthermore, the acute anxiety can usually be treated with a dose of a benzodiazepine (a Valium-like drug). "Talking down" can be helpful, but it is not always practical. While antipsychotic medications like Thorazine (chlorpromazine) were once popular, they are not always effective on bad trips, and in fact can make things worse. Now that we understand that hallucinogens act on serotonin-2 receptors, it's possible that an antagonist (blocking) treatment will become available that would terminate the trip immediately. Such drugs exist but have not yet been investigated or approved for this purpose in the United States.

What about the myth that taking LSD will make you crazy? As with many myths, it is an exaggeration, but it still has a grain of truth in it. Hallucinogens definitely can worsen the symptoms of people who are already psychotic. But can they cause psychosis? We don't know. They certainly don't very often. However, a number of studies have shown that hallucinogen users are disproportionately represented among psychiatric inpatients, and that one to five people out of one thousand who take hallucinogens experience an acute psychotic reaction.

There is a chicken-and-egg problem in understanding this statistic. Most people who are hospitalized for a psychotic reaction to hallucinogens have never before been seen by a psychiatrist. So, it is impossible to know whether they were completely healthy before the drug experience. However, we do know that a small number of people have very serious reactions to LSD and similar drugs, including prolonged psychotic states. Also, people with a family history of, or other predisposition toward, mental illness should be particularly careful. Sometimes a hallucinogenic experience can reveal symptoms in such individuals.

FLASHBACKS

The issue of flashbacks, or posthallucinogen perceptual disorder (PHPD), is much clearer. Flashbacks are the reemergence of some aspect of the hallucinogen experience in the absence of drug. The most common form includes altered visual images, wavering, altered borders to visual images, or trails of light. While this can occur after a single use of the drug, flashbacks become increasingly common as the number of hallucinogen experiences increases. Use of other drugs, like marijuana and alcohol, and even extreme fatigue, can trigger this phenomenon. A recent survey of college students showed that up to 60 percent of heavy users (people who admitted to having taken LSD between twenty and eighty times or more) have experienced some form of PHPD. People's reactions to these experiences vary widely. For some, they trigger anxiety and depression. Others view them as an acceptable side effect of an otherwise positive experience. In many cases, they diminish with abstinence, although symptoms that persist for years have been reported.

These symptoms might actually reflect long-term changes in how the brain processes sensory images. Studies of vision of habitual LSD users (when they are not under the influence of the drug) show that their brains may continue to respond to visual stimuli after the stimuli are removed. This suggests that the repeated LSD usage may cause some neuroplastic changes that persist. In the "Brain Basics" chapter we discuss the brain's capacity to remember all sorts of experiences, including repeated drug applications.

CHROMOSOMAL DAMAGE

We have one final myth to discuss: the idea that LSD will break chromosomes. This concern was raised during the 1960s, based on scanty research. While women who used LSD during pregnancy have given birth to children with birth defects, it has been difficult to show that this rate is higher than that of the general population. Furthermore, most of these women used other drugs during pregnancy. Most animal research has not shown remarkable effects of LSD on the developing fetus. Some concern about the effects of LSD goes back historically to the widespread use of related ergot alkaloids to induce abortion. However, LSD itself does not have this effect. Nevertheless, women who are pregnant, or who might be, should avoid drugs in general.

DEATH

While the LSD-like hallucinogens are fairly unlikely to produce terrible physical effects, the other drugs discussed in this chapter may. The belladonna alkaloids represent a particular danger. These drugs prevent the action of one of the major neurotransmitters in the body (acetylcholine) at many of its synapses. At doses that cause hallucinations, they increase heart rate and body temperature to dangerous levels: death can result. It is important to understand that there is *not* a dose that produces significant behavioral effects that is not toxic: the behavioral effects, like delirium, are signs of overdose. These effects are easily treated by medical personnel *if they know what the intoxicating drug is.* Therefore, it is extremely important to seek medical attention.

PCP also can cause dangerous side effects or death from overdose (two to five times a single recreational dose). As the user increases the dose, general anesthesia can result (remember, this was the reason the drug was invented). However, a number of dangerous effects occur after high doses, any one of which can be lethal. Body temperature can rise to 108 degrees, blood pressure can rise so much that a stroke occurs, breathing can cease, or a prolonged period of seizure activity can result. PCP can also cause a prolonged state resembling paranoid schizophrenia. This most often happens in people who use PCP for long time. However, an abnormal psychiatric state that persists for days can result from a single use. The acute delirium caused by PCP or ketamine can be alleviated with benzodiazepine drugs, like Valium.

INTERACTIONS WITH OTHER DRUGS

Many people who experiment with hallucinogens are known to combine drugs. For example, it is not uncommon for people to take LSD or mushrooms and smoke marijuana at the same time. The effect of these combinations is highly individual, and depends on the previous drug experience of the user, the doses, and the particular drugs involved. For example, smoking marijuana often triggers PHPD (flashbacks) in heavy LSD users. Many of these combinations produce bizarre, anxiety-provoking, but not dangerous states.

The most troublesome reactions are those that are caused by the user taking something without knowing it. PCP is a frequent culprit in this regard. Marijuana can be adulterated with PCP without the user's knowledge, and can induce a terrifying or dangerous state in the unsuspecting users.

What about interactions with prescription drugs? Not surprisingly, other drugs that influence serotonin systems have been involved in reported interactions. There are several reports of Prozac (fluoxetine) triggering flashbacks in heavy LSD users. There is much curiosity but not much credible information about how LSD affects patients who are taking Prozac for depression.

5

Herbal Drugs

Drug Class: Herbal drugs

Individual Drugs (just a few examples): Herbal X-tacy, smart drugs, melatonin

The Buzz: Most of these drugs are either members of other classes we have discussed or don't have a buzz because they are ineffective.

Overdose and Other Bad Effects: The biggest danger of these drugs is that many are untested and unregulated. For some, there may be anecdotal support for effectiveness and safety, or even evidence of traditional use by other cultures for centuries. For most, however, effectiveness of the drugs has not been tested in controlled scientific studies. Even for effective medicines like ephedrine, the actual contents of herbal preparations are unknown. Furthermore, the user cannot rely on the instructions to be a reliable guide for safe use. In the worst cases, instructions suggest use of dangerous amounts of the drug.

Dangerous Combinations with Other Drugs: Ephedrine can be quite dangerous when taken in combination with monoamine oxidase inhibitors, which are used to treat depression. The combination of these two drugs can lead to fatal increases in blood pressure or heart rate. The combination of ephedrine with caffeine is much more likely to lead to symptoms of cardiovascular activation, jitteriness, anxiety, and arousal than either drug alone.

CHAPTER CONTENTS

WHAT IS AN HERBAL DRUG?

Herbal drugs are simply drugs from plant matter that appear in plant form rather than as "synthetic"-looking capsules or tablets. Often they are touted as safe and effective because they are "natural," or a normal constituent of the body. This drug classification is simply a marketing device, not a uniquely new or rediscovered form of traditional medicine. Marketing drugs as "herbal" makes them sound safe: nontraditional and milder. The herbal strategy has been effective: the current market in herbal drugs in this country amounts to millions of dollars. Since most of these preparations are sold as nutritional supplements rather than as drugs, they are not subject to FDA requirements. Therefore, neither their safety nor their effectiveness has been established in controlled scientific studies. This doesn't mean that none of the drugs are effective: some certainly are. Furthermore, one should never discount the placebo effect: the promise of a remedy can have a powerful healing effect. However, the manufacturer is not responsible for effectiveness or safety. It is up to the buyer to decide what risk to take (if only wasting his money on something useless). Also, just because a substance is herbal and one does not need a prescription does not mean that one can safely increase the recommended doses.

Many of the drugs discussed in this book are herbal drugs. Many of the commonest intoxicants are ultimately derived from plant products. Nicotine comes from tobacco plants, and many forms of alcohol are prepared by fermentation of yeast in the presence of grain products. Most of the hallucinogens, ranging from psilocybin mushrooms to belladonna alkaloids, could be described as herbal drugs, along with many natural stimulants, including caffeine, ephedrine, and cocaine. There are also herbal sedatives: hypnotics, like kava, that act very much like alcohol.

HERBAL DRUGS ARE NOT SUBJECT TO TESTING AND RESTRICTIONS

Herbal drugs are not all dangerous, or ineffective. However, the buyer should consider several issues. First, what is the source of claims for effectiveness? Some herbal drugs have been tested by credible, well-controlled scientific studies. Others have been used by other cultures for centuries in a carefully documented way. Unfortunately, there is little evidence to back up claims by many other drugs. Furthermore, there is a growing romanticism about Eastern medicine and uncritical acceptance of herbal healing techniques. While many effective medicines derive from these sources, many ineffective ones do as well.

The second consideration is the safety and reliability of formulation. A frightening example occurred several years ago in the marketing of the amino acid tryptophan. Tryptophan, a normal constituent of the body, is used by some as a "smart drug" to improve mental functioning and facilitate sleep. It is a component of many foods, and has no known hazards when taken as a nutritional supplement. However, a contaminant in a tryptophan preparation from one particular supplier caused a serious and fatal disease—eosinophilia-myalgia syndrome. As these drugs are not regulated by the FDA, there is no guarantee of safety. In addition, there is no guarantee of product identity. A recent survey of melatonin products showed that the melatonin content of some preparations was half or double the amount listed on the label.

Finally, most people who use these drugs must rely upon self-experimentation to establish effective doses that lack side effects. There are few professionals in the United States who are qualified to give knowledgeable advice about their use. For example, we know of an elderly man who was given an herbal preparation for his flu by his pharmacist of many years. Fortunately, the man read the label, which strongly warned against use of the drug by people with immune disorders like one he had suffered from for years (a condition known to his pharmacist!). The situation in Europe is quite different, where use of herbal and patent medications is broader and pharmacists are more informed. So, for now, users in the United States are dependent upon an informal (and often uninformed) network of advocates—often those marketing the compounds.

EPHEDRINE (HERBAL X-TACY AND OTHER NAMES)

We have discussed ephedrine in detail elsewhere, in the "Stimulants" chapter. We are also visiting it here, because it is sometimes sold as an herbal (and safer) substitute for Ecstasy (methylenedioxymethamphetamine—MDMA) rather than as ephedrine itself. It is also marketed as a safe drug to enhance athletic performance. It is sold in pill form, as a loose herb, and as an herbal preparation for a tea used for asthma. All of these guises are the same compound. Ephedrine is an effective medicine for treating asthma, and has been used medically as such in appropriate doses for thousands of years because it acts as a mild stimulant on the sympathetic nerve endings to dilate bronchioles, increase heart rate and blood pressure, and raise blood glucose. However, this drug does not enter the brain well, and at best causes a jitteriness that most people find discomfitting even when used in appropriate amounts for the treatment of asthma. At higher doses, ephedrine causes an arousal and anxiety state that most people find unpleasant, although some report positive feelings with the arousal. Relative to other stimulants, these effects are mild.

These characteristics explain why ephedrine, especially at excessive doses, can be mistaken for MDMA, or can be used to improve athletic performance. Ephedrine can mimic some of the signs of MDMA intoxication or increased athletic performance, including the increased heart rate, blood pressure, etc. It can give the feeling of greater physical activation, which can be mistaken for improving athletic performance. If high enough doses are taken, these effects are associated with some increase in arousal and anxiety, so the users can "feel" a drug effect. But, in fact, ephedrine does nothing to improve muscle development.

There may be some truth to claims that ephedrine can help contribute to weight loss due mainly to its effects on the body to facilitate fat breakdown and increase energy production, but the effects are minor. Ephedrine and ephedrine/caffeine preparations have been tested on obese humans, and have been found to have a modest benefit (one well-controlled study reported a five-pound weight loss in two months, and a total of ten pounds of weight lost in five months).

So what is the harm in taking ephedrine? *Taking too much can lead to high blood pressure and stroke.* There have been reports of at least eight deaths due to excessive ephedrine use. Usually, the cause of death was heart attack or stroke. There are many more reports of milder side effects, including tremors, headache, insomnia, nausea, vomiting, fatigue, and dizziness, all of which are common. Chest pain, palpitations, and seizures have occurred in people taking doses in excess of therapeutic levels or those recommended on the package.

Ephedrine interactions with other drugs can also be dangerous. Ephedrine/caffeine/aspirin combinations are often "stacked" by weight lifters, and used for weight loss. Combinations of ephedrine with caffeine are much more likely to lead to effects on the heart and circulation, jitteriness, anxiety, and arousal than either drug does alone. Furthermore, the potential for overdosing is high given the free availability of both drugs. Since ephedrine releases monoamines, in patients taking monoamine oxidase inhibitors for treatment of depression (Marplan, Nardil, Parnate) its effect can be lethal.

Finally, since the content of these products is unregulated, there is no guarantee about their identity. At least one case of hepatitis associated with herbal ephedrine use has been reported. It was attributed to unknown constituents in the herbal preparation, since ephedrine is not known to cause liver injury.

COMMON SOURCES OF EPHEDRINE

Product	Serving Size	Ephedrine Dose
Ephedrine herb capsules	500 mg	1–15 mg
Ephedra herb tea	2 g dried herbs	10–50 mg
Over-the counter asthma drugs	2 tablets	48 mg

MELATONIN

Melatonin is widely sold in capsule form in health-food stores as the new cure for jet lag and other sleep disorders, as well as a cure-all that can prevent aging and such diseases as cancer. It could be called the prototype herbal drug. On the positive side, melatonin is the product released by the pineal gland, so it is a normal part of the human body. It has been the object of at least some scientific study, and some of the claims of substantial effects have been borne out in these studies. Therefore, melatonin is not a completely fraudulent product. On the negative side, however, no safe and effective dose has been determined in clinical studies, the safety of long-term use has never been established, and the content of preparations marketed as melatonin is unregulated and varies widely.

WHAT IS MELATONIN?

Melatonin is a neurotransmitter that is released from the pineal gland, which is a tiny gland that sits on top of the brain. Structurally it is very similar to serotonin, but it is made only in this one place in the body. Melatonin is released only at night. Visual signals travel from the eye to an area in the brain that sets the circadian rhythm, and then to the nerves that travel to the pineal gland and cause it to release melatonin into the bloodstream, where perhaps it has some of its actions. Eventually, it crosses the blood brain barrier to enter the brain and acts on receptors at certain places in the brain. The very marked day-night rhythm in melatonin release is one reason why it is thought to be involved in sleep. Normally, when darkness falls, the nerves that stimulate melatonin release become active. A number of different receptors for melatonin have recently been discovered.

MELATONIN AND SLEEP

The claim most often made for melatonin is that it restores normal sleep in people experiencing jet lag or switching work schedules. The reason for this speculation is the marked day-night differences in melatonin levels in the blood, which are so consistent that they can be used to test whether such rhythms are normal.

The nighttime release of melatonin suggests that it is involved in sleep. The next step is to prove that giving melatonin to people can cause sleep. The answer is only a qualified yes. Some studies show that if melatonin is given at a time earlier than normal bedtime (such as in the early evening or late afternoon), it does seem to help people sleep. However, giving melatonin at normal bedtime does not make people fall asleep faster or sleep longer.

Does melatonin actually create day-night rhythms in other aspects of body function? It may contribute to the fall in body temperature that occurs at night. In species other than humans, melatonin may be very important in allowing animals to breed at appropriate times of the year. The shorter days and longer nights of winter cause an increasing release of melatonin. For some species, like sheep, which are triggered to breed during the short days of winter, this increasing release of melatonin improves fertility, while it decreases fertility in animals like hamsters, which breed in the summer, when days are long. Melatonin has a much less certain role in human reproduction. Humans are not "seasonal breeders": they maintain fertility throughout the year. This fits nicely with the fact that the nightly rises in melatonin are not so great in humans as they are in other animals. Can human reproduction be affected by causing a larger nighttime rise in melatonin? Some scientific studies suggest that melatonin decreases fertility in humans, although there is little research in this area. Melatonin (in doses that exceed usual doses by tenfold) has even been tested as a contraceptive, but given the possible side effects on sleep, it has some real disadvantages in comparison to more completely tested medications.

MELATONIN AND AGING

Melatonin might also have a slight antioxidant action. Much of aging-related tissue damage and disease may result from by-products of oxygen metabolism (oxygen radicals) that damage tissue. Certain compounds, such as vitamin E, are known to "scavenge" and eliminate these products before they interact with proteins and DNA and thus produce tissue damage. There are some reports that melatonin can function in this way. The most persuasive are findings that giving melatonin to experimental animals can prevent the DNA damage caused by compounds known to produce such oxygen radicals. However, this research is in its early stages, and effectiveness in lower primates or humans has not even been tested. Again, taking a psychoactive compound that might suppress fertility for years to delay aging seems like a strategy that offers more risks than rewards.

MELATONIN AND IMMUNE FUNCTION

Melatonin is also claimed to improve immune function, but scientific proof of these claims is even scantier than it is for its antioxidant properties.

CAUTIONS ABOUT MELATONIN

Melatonin may be effective in some situations, but is it safe? The first caution relates to the dose. Doses in scientific studies range from to 0.1 to 5 milligrams. In most health-food stores, it is sold in amounts ranging from 1 to 5 milligrams, which is in the appropriate range. However, there is no control over how much a user takes because it is available over-the-counter rather than by prescription, and excessive doses might affect reproduction or other aspects of body function. The second caution relates to the lack of testing of long-term effects. It isn't even known whether melatonin is effective if given for a long period of time. Most sleep medications lose their effectiveness with time, and it wouldn't be surprising if melatonin did as well. If so, a dangerous situation could develop if a person started increasing his dose to compensate for the loss of effect.

GINSENG

The ginseng root has been used in Chinese medicine for thousands of years for a variety of ailments ranging from fatigue and stress to high blood pressure and even cancer. It is used traditionally and is available here in the United States in a wide variety of forms, from teas to chewing the root itself. It is used as a tonic to increase resistance to stress. It is being used widely in the United

States for reasons that vary from improvement of athletic performance to decrease in anxiety to curing disease.

Does ginseng have real biologic activity? Testimonials by happy users have provided much of the support for this drug. And in a few small-animal studies, the active ingredients in ginseng (the ginsenosides) have proved to have activities in the brain. One study showed that giving a rat a large dose of active ginsenosides decreased anxiety as much as diazepam (Valium) does. Other studies have shown them to decrease the response of the adrenal gland to stress. There are even a couple of studies that indicate that extracts of ginseng showed some effectiveness in improving the ability of rats to learn a maze. Unfortunately, we don't have any controlled studies showing effects on human memory, anxiety level, or response to stress, although mild effects on blood pressure were seen in one study when it was given (in combination with gingko) to humans.

Reassuringly, the recommended dose on preparations sold in a local health-food store came in the same range as doses used in the experimental studies (about 700 milligrams for a normal adult male). However, the exact content of these formulations is unknown and not controlled by any agency, so potency can vary wildly. In addition, the effectiveness of a single dose is not clear. Some studies fail to show significant effects except with repeated dosing. Fortunately, no dangerous side effects of high doses are known with single doses, although the safety of repeated doses is not documented in the Western scientific literature. As with many ancient herbal cures, there is active research ongoing to test the efficacy of ginseng in treating disease.

GINGKO

An extract of the leaves of the *Ginkgo Biloba* tree is a popular herbal cure that is supposed to improve circulation in small blood vessels in the brain, and so improve memory and alertness. Like ginseng, it has many advocates. Unfortunately, it has even less in the way of research to back up the claims of satisfied users. However, as with many herbal drugs, serious research is just beginning, and a recent study in Alzheimer's patients suggests that gingko provided some help. It is often marketed in combination with ginseng for similar conditions, such as stress. Its effectiveness as a stress cure remains to be proved.

HERBAL "SMART DRUGS"

The so-called smart drugs may win the contest for popularity due to the ingenious marketing of marginally effective agents. Their popularity has been fueled in part by the general enthusiasm for cleansing and lack of intoxication in a drug-weary culture. Although taking a drug to improve mental quickness instead of getting bombed certainly seems innocent, nowhere is superstition more rampant than in the marketing claims for drugs that improve memory and general mental acuity. There is truly a desperate need for such drugs in medicine to retard the memory loss caused by Alzheimer's disease and some other forms of dementia. However, despite years of effort, only a few marginally effective drugs have been developed (this is discussed in the "Nicotine" chapter).

The herbal smart drugs are often a concoction of various amino acids and similar compounds. For example, a recent survey of the products hawked on an Internet site included agents containing phenylalanine, Pyroglutamic acid (an amino acid derivative present in fruits and vegetables), Long-sha (a Chinese herb containing a compound related to the neurotransmitter norepinephrine), and vitamin B. All of the compounds were asserted to give a mental boost. Some (tyrosine, vitamin B) are necessary for normal nerve function.

So, why not take "smart nutrients"? First, if you are eating a normal American diet with the typical excess of protein, there is more than enough in your diet to maintain optimal levels in blood and brain. Second, these compounds act over hours to days. They don't simply produce the advertised immediate "energy boost." Finally, even if enough amino acid is provided to boost production of a neurotransmitter, it doesn't automatically mean the neuron is releasing more to have greater effect. Newly made neurotransmitter is simply stored, awaiting the arrival of a nerve impulse to release it. So, simply making more adds to the store that is ready for release. Adding more is effective only if stores are truly depleted. This generally happens only after life-threatening stresses (*not* a bad day at work).

Phenylalanine in this particular ad was reputed to be "the precursor of L-tyrosine, L-dopa and L-dopamine, the body's pleasure chemical and mood regulator." There is some truth to this claim. Tyrosine and phenylalanine are both amino acids that are required for the synthesis of proteins. Tyrosine is the basic building block for the neurotransmitters dopamine and norepinephrine. However, the average American eats enough protein to provide adequate levels of these amino acids. Adding more does not boost production of the catecholamine neurotransmitters. One claim that might have some credence is that providing extra tyrosine could help to prevent the loss of norepinephrine, which occurs when a person takes Ecstasy. There is a rapid loss in this case, which perhaps can be lessened by providing extra precursor. Unfortunately, this does not diminish the dangerous side effects of MDMA at all.

There may be more truth to the claims that taking large doses of other neurotransmitter precursors can influence the production of the neurotransmitter. Choline supplements can indeed enhance the production of the neurotransmitter acetylcholine, which is important for many aspects of brain function, including memory. The death of acetylcholine neurons may help to cause the disabling memory loss of Alzheimer's disease, and supplementing acetylcholine production can produce slight and temporary improvement in the memory of Alzheimer's patients. Unfortunately, in people who take enough choline to actually increase production of acetylcholine, the bacteria in the intestine turn the unabsorbed choline into a compound that gives them a "fishy" smell.

Similarly, tryptophan may increase the production of serotonin in the brain, which can be increased by the tryptophan in high-protein foods, like milk. Since increases in serotonin are speculated to enhance sleep, there may be some truth to the superstition that warm milk enhances sleep.

HAZARDS OF HERBAL DRUGS

Most of the herbal preparations that people use are innocuous, and some are effective. Some have real dangers. Of the group mentioned here, ephedrine poses the greatest risk, because people can easily take enough to cause high blood pressure, strokes, or heart attacks. Often, the marketers of the herbal preparations *recommend* taking excessive doses. Ephedrine is clearly dangerous for someone already experiencing high blood pressure or any kind of cardiovascular problems.

Some of the nutritional supplements can be quite dangerous for people with certain medical conditions, or those taking certain drugs. Taking anything that increases the production of monoamine neurotransmitters (i.e., phenylalanine or tyrosine) is dangerous for someone who is taking a certain type of drug to treat depression (the monoamine oxidase inhibitor class). These drugs prevent the breakdown of monoamine neurotransmitters, and dangerous high blood pressure can result if they are taken in combination with nutritional supplements that increase production of these same neurotransmitters. Furthermore, taking phenylalanine can be dangerous for a person who suffers from phenylketonuria, a disease that prevents the normal metabolism of phenylalanine, which can build up in the blood to dangerous levels.

The long-term effects in otherwise healthy people of taking high doses of these compounds is not known. The current enthusiasm for herbal remedies will provide the data that we need, but, unfortunately, at the likely expense of unwary users of these products.

6

◾

Inhalants

Drug Class: Mixed

Individual Drugs: nitrites (butyl or amyl); anesthetics (nitrous oxide—Whippets, gaseous anesthesia agents used for surgery—halothane, ether); solvents, paints, sprays, and fuels (toluene, gasoline, glues, canned spray paint, etc.)

Common Terms: bolt, bullets, climax, locker room, rush, poppers, snappers, amies

The Buzz: The chemicals in this category have very little in common in chemical structure, pharmacology, or toxic effects, except that they are all taken by inhalation.

The nitrites relax the smooth muscle tissue that regulate the size and shape of blood vessels, the bladder, the anus, and other tissues. The relaxed blood vessels produce a drop in blood pressure, an increased heart rate, and a sense of warmth and mild euphoria. Visual distortions can also occur.

Nitrous oxide is by far the mildest of the anesthetics, and it produces mild euphoria, reduction of pain, and reductions of inhibitions, followed by drowsiness as the concentrations increase. Other anesthetics produce the same effects, but cause major sedation at modest levels.

Solvents produce effects similar to those of alcohol, with stimulation, loss of inhibitions, and mild euphoria, followed by depression. Distortions of perception and hallucinations may occur.

Overdose and Other Bad Effects: The risk of a lethal overdose with inhaled nitrites is small. Because they dilate blood vessels, nitrites cause a reduction in blood pressure. This can produce heart palpitations (rapid, hard heartbeats), loss of consciousness upon moving from lying down to standing up, and headaches. No one who has heart or blood vessel disease should use these compounds without the supervision of a physician. Long-term use of nitrites can produce negative effects that are described later. And when they are eaten, nitrites can cause major medical problems, including death.

The overdose risk for anesthetics ranges from relatively low (nitrous oxide) to very high (modern surgical anesthesia agents). For nitrous oxide, the major risk is not breathing enough oxygen while breathing the gas. For the others, the risk is disruption of heart function and the suppression of respiration, followed by death. Anyone who has inhaled enough anesthetic to become unconscious is in danger and should receive medical attention immediately.

Serious solvent intoxication is like that of alcohol, with muscular incoordination, headache, abdominal pain, nausea, and vomiting. Many of these agents are flammable, so serious burns can occur. The risk of a lethal overdose with solvents is significant. Death usually occurs because the heart rhythm is disrupted (cardiac arrythmia), or due to a lack of oxygen. Accidents and suicide are also significant risks. A significant percentage of people who die from inhalants are first-time users.

Dangerous Combinations with Other Drugs: As with alcohol and sedatives, it is dangerous to combine inhalants with anything else that makes a person sleepy. This includes alcohol and other sedative drugs, such as opiates (e.g., heroin, morphine, or Demerol); barbiturates (e.g., phenobarbital); Quaaludes (methaqualone); Valium-like drugs (benzodiazepines); and cold medicines, including antihistamines.

Combinations of drugs can become deadly when taken together. Even dose combinations that do not cause unconsciousness or breathing problems alone can powerfully impair physical activities such as sports, driving a car, and operating machinery.

CHAPTER CONTENTS

INTRODUCTION

Of all the chemicals and drugs described in this book, it is ironic that those used by the youngest people are the most toxic. Because of their easy access to glues, gasoline, solvents, paints, and sprays, many children begin to use drugs by inhaling these common chemicals. They get a buzz, but along with that buzz comes toxic effects that would horrify any chemical safety expert.

While inhaling substances for highs has been with us since the Greeks, it has only been since the late 1700s, when nitrous oxide was first synthesized, that people used a chemical regularly for this purpose. This "laughing gas" was prominent in England, and was even offered at London theaters for recreational purposes.

As science and industry progressed, a number of volatile compounds, such as gasoline, became readily accessible to the public, and serious inhalant abuse and toxicity became prominent in the 1920s. Beginning in the 1950s, glue sniffing was recognized as a problem, and as more and more chemicals have been marketed, the menu for abuse has grown.

As this is written, about 8 percent of middle school students report using inhalants. Among high school seniors, more than 15 percent report having used volatile solvents at least once in their life.

Because of the diversity of the chemicals in this group, we have divided this chapter into three parts—the nitrites, the anesthetics, and the solvents. The anesthetics and some of the nitrites are made for human consumption, and at least we understand the effects these have on body function. The solvents, including gasoline, sprays, glues, paints, cleaning fluids, and everything else, were never intended for human use. The authors consider these among the most toxic substances used for drug recreation, and we believe that they should never be used by anyone under any circumstances, especially children.

NITRITES

WHAT THEY ARE AND HOW THEY WORK

These chemicals are yellow, volatile, and flammable liquids that have a fruity odor. The nitrites are part of a large class of drugs (including amyl nitrite, butyl nitrite, isobutyl nitrite, and the nitrates like nitroglycerin) that relax the smooth muscles that control the diameter of blood vessels and the iris of the eye, keep the anus closed, and keep us from dribbling urine. When these muscles relax, the blood vessels enlarge and blood pressure falls, more light is let into the eye, and the bowels are let loose.

The medical uses of these compounds have a long and successful history, beginning with the synthesis of nitroglycerin in 1846. That's right, nitroglycerin, the explosive that we all know about, is also a very important drug. The first chemists noticed that just a bit of it on the tongue produced a severe headache (they did not know that this was because it dilated blood vessels), and within a year it was medically used by placing it under the tongue to relieve heart pain caused by blocked blood vessels. Like all of these compounds, nitroglycerin relaxes blood vessels, and today it is very commonly used to relieve the pain that patients with heart disease feel when one of the vessels supplying blood to their heart has a spasm (angina pectoris). Remember the scene in movies when an old person grabs his heart, falls to the floor, and struggles to get his medicine out of his pocket? Then the bad guy takes the medicine away and the victim dies? Almost certainly, it was nitroglycerin that he needed.

The nitrites, like the amyl nitrite "poppers" that some people use for recreation, have the same basic effects as nitroglycerin. They were first synthesized and used medically in 1857, but soon physicians found them to be short-lasting and unreliable, so nitroglycerin under the tongue has remained the medicine of choice. Amyl nitrite is now used clinically only when the very rapid absorption through inhalation is necessary for some cardiac medical procedures.

The side effects of nitrates and nitrites are common and consistent, and they are related to the dilation of blood vessels. When physicians prescribe these drugs, they tell their patients to expect headache, flushing of the skin, dizziness, weakness, and perhaps loss of consciousness if the person changes his body position rapidly.

As with almost all drugs, there is a lot we don't know. In this case, we really don't know exactly why these drugs have the mental effects that make them attractive for some people to use. Users report a physical sensation of warmth, a giddy feeling, and a pounding heart. The psychological sensations are the re-

moval of inhibitions, skin sensitivity, and a sense of exhilaration and acceleration before sexual orgasm. There is a rather common visual disturbance consisting of a bright yellow spot with purple radiations.* These effects may arise
from the dilation of some blood vessels in the brain. Finally, some people use
these drugs not for the mental effects but for their muscle-relaxing properties
to permit anal intercourse.

TOXICITY

Only amyl nitrite is specifically manufactured and packaged for legitimate
medical use in humans. Unless a product is approved by the United States
Food and Drug Administration, it should be considered an industrial chemical not manufactured for human consumption, because even if it is supposed
to be pure, it may contain contaminants that are harmful.

Compared to many drugs, amyl nitrite has less toxicity as long as it is inhaled as intended. Of course, there is always the possibility that the dilation
of the blood vessels will cause someone with blood circulation problems to
have a bad experience. As with all drugs, check with your physician before taking anything.

However, there is a major toxicity problem with nitrites if they are swallowed
rather than inhaled. When they are eaten, nitrites can cause major medical
problems by interfering with the ability of the blood to transport oxygen. Blood
carries oxygen to the tissues by way of the red blood cells, which contain hemoglobin to bind the oxygen and then release it to the cells of the body. If the
hemoglobin cannot bind oxygen, then a person will die rapidly. This is the way
that cyanide (as used in Nazi gas chambers) works. It prevents hemoglobin
from reacting with oxygen, and thus the tissues are suffocated.

Nitrites, when eaten, can have the same effect, although they interact a little differently with hemoglobin than cyanide does. This danger from nitrites
is illustrated by an unfortunate incident that occurred in New Jersey in 1992.
On October 20 of that year, forty children in an elementary school visited the
school nurse because their lips and hands were turning blue, they were vomiting, and they had headaches after lunch. They had a hemoglobin disorder
produced by nitrite poisoning. This was not caused by drug abuse, but by
something much more surprising. The boiler in their school was used to heat
the water, and somehow the boiler fluid, which contained a lot of nitrites, was
mixed with the hot water used for preparing their soup. Fortunately, the kids
received medical care and recovered completely.

Finally, there are some research reports that claim that nitrites can sup-

*This description of nitrite effects is taken from a paper titled "The Psychosexual Aspects
of the Volatile Nitrites" by Thomas P. Lowry, M.D., which appeared in the *Journal of Psychoactive Drugs*, Vol. 14 (1–2), pp. 77–79.

press the immune system. There are very few actual experiments, but some researchers have reviewed the development of a particular kind of cancer that is seen in AIDS patients and correlated the occurrence of that cancer with the use of nitrites. At the time this is written, there are not enough data to reach a valid conclusion.

TOLERANCE AND WITHDRAWAL

Frequent and repeated use of nitrites and nitrates can produce tolerance and symptoms upon withdrawal. Workers in the explosives industry have experienced this. When a worker first goes on the job and is exposed to nitroglycerin in his environment, he might experience headaches, weakness, and dizziness. After a few days these symptoms disappear as tolerance develops. However, when he stops working on the weekend, he might suffer headaches and other symptoms due to withdrawal. A few workers have been found to have cardiac and circulatory problems upon withdrawal, and these were treated by giving them nitroglycerin. Since the advent of the nitroglycerin patch for continuous administration of the drug to heart patients, many people have been continuously exposed to nitroglycerin and have developed tolerance to it. The medical profession has become quite concerned about this because tolerance reduces the effectiveness of the compound and withdrawal can produce cardiac problems.

NITROUS OXIDE AND OTHER GAS ANESTHETICS

WHAT THEY ARE AND HOW THEY WORK

One of the most important drug experiences anyone can have is that of proper anesthesia in the operating room. Most surgery could not be carried out without proper anesthesia because it serves three important functions: pain relief, muscular relaxation, and loss of consciousness. All of the gas anesthetics produce the loss of consciousness, and some of them produce the muscle relaxation and pain relief. The reason for pain relief is obvious. No one would want to be cut and probed without pain suppression, and since most general anesthetics produce only loss of consciousness and not pain relief, then a pain suppressor is added by an anesthesiologist. Muscular relaxation is required so that involuntary muscle contractions will not get in the way of the surgeon's work. Finally, the loss of consciousness provides the patient relief from the anxiety and boredom of the operating room and perhaps some very welcome amnesia for the whole experience. It is probably this characteristic of gas anesthetics that leads to their abuse.

It wasn't always so easy. Until 1847 surgery was carried out without the help of anesthetic agents. Before that there might have been a little help from alcohol or opium, but mostly the patient was held down by an array of strong men while the surgeon worked in spite of his screams. But in 1847 things changed at the Massachusetts General Hospital when ether was first used. Ether had been synthesized recently, and dentists had begun to notice that it had anesthetic properties. A dentist named Morton claimed that he could produce surgical anesthesia with this miracle compound, and that he would demonstrate it at Mass General. With the observation gallery full and the men arrayed to hold down the patient as usual, the dentist appeared with the anesthesia machine he had invented to administer the ether. For the first time a patient underwent major surgery while asleep but with his heart and respiration safely intact. Within a month the word had spread and ether became a powerful part of medicine and surgery.*

Ether was a great general anesthetic because it fulfilled the requirements for anesthesia, but it was quite flammable. Modern nonflammable anesthetic agents, like halothane, are both effective and potent, and anesthesia is achieved by breathing air containing just a small percentage of these gases. This makes them great for the operating room and awful for drug abusers, because it is so easy to overdose with them. As higher levels of anesthesia are achieved, three significant systems are impaired: respiration, blood pressure, and heart contractions.

Breathing is produced by the firing of a group of nerve cells deep in the brain. They are a little resistant to anesthetics, but at high levels their activity is suppressed, and respiration is depressed. Also, the smooth muscle cells that keep blood vessels at a set diameter relax, and this causes a drop in blood pressure. Finally, anesthetics can have a direct effect on the ability of the heart to contract, so it becomes weaker and prone to disruptions of its rhythm. Halothane is particularly tricky because the difference between the concentration that is effective and that which causes problems is small.

Lots of chemicals and gases can be anesthetic agents, ranging from inert gases like xenon to the most modern compounds. Scientists still do not know exactly how anesthetics work. We know that they suppress the firing of nerve cells, and some can relax various muscles. At this point the best evidence is that, in part, they suppress consciousness by increasing the action of the neurotransmitter GABA (see "Brain Basics" chapter for an explanation of GABA), which inhibits excitable activity in neural networks.

When an anesthetic gas is inhaled, the sequence of responses is fairly uniform for many of the agents. There can be a brief period of excitation or stim-

*This description is taken from chapter 13, "The History and Principles of Anesthesiology," of *Goodman and Gilman's the Pharmacological Basis of Therapeutics*, Joel G. Hardman and Lee E. Limbird, eds., 9th ed., (New York: McGraw Hill, 1996).

ulation, like after the first drink of alcohol. That is followed by pain relief, dizziness, weakness, and general depression of functions. At higher levels, reflexes such as eye blink, swallowing, and vomiting can be lost. Finally, heart function and respiration are lost and the person dies. Some agents (such as enflurane) have more excitatory effects at overdose, and at high levels these can cause epileptic seizures. Others produce little in the way of stimulation and only depress the nervous system.

The window of concentration between anesthesia and death is very narrow for these drugs. In medical settings the gases are carefully mixed with oxygen and survival body functions are monitored continuously. The anesthesiologist is completely capable of maintaining breathing for the patient or administering cardiac stimulants if necessary. Even with this level of care, problems do occur. Without this careful approach, a person is at enormous risk of either dying or sustaining permanent brain damage.

Nitrous Oxide

Nitrous oxide was first synthesized in the late 1700s as a colorless and almost odorless gas, and its anesthetic and pain-relieving properties were appreciated almost immediately. For quite a while it remained out of the mainstream of medicine, being used mostly for recreation and entertainment at carnivals. The first medical usage of this gas came in the mid 1800s when dentists found it to be an excellent way to suppress pain.

One cannot easily achieve deep surgical anesthesia with nitrous oxide alone, unless it is applied in an environment where the atmospheric pressure is raised. Now it is used medically only to augment other anesthetics and sedatives, or for minor procedures that do not require the loss of consciousness. When nitrous oxide is inhaled in sufficient quantity, there is a euphoric feeling that comes along with the pain relief. The term *laughing gas* arises from the giddy state that it produces. By comparison to any of the other potentially fatal drugs that people inhale for recreation, nitrous oxide is safer, since it has little effect on critical body functions, including respiration, brain blood flow, and liver, kidney, and gastrointestinal tract processes.

The pharmacological mechanisms of nitrous oxide have not been completely determined. Certainly it acts like a general anesthetic and under high pressure can cause loss of consciousness, so, as we suspect with other anesthetics, it may increase GABA inhibition of nerve cells. Part of its effect may also be through the brain's built-in opiate system—the same receptors that morphine and heroin activate. One of the best bits of data that support this is that the specific opiate antagonist naloxone blocks the pain-relieving properties of this gas in animal experiments. In fact, nitrous oxide has been used to treat opiate and alcohol withdrawal symptoms.

Nitrous Oxide Toxicity and Tolerance

As described above, in clinical settings nitrous oxide is rather free of toxic effects. For recreational users, there are three dangers: not getting enough oxygen; physically hurting oneself by having the gas-delivery device work improperly; or a vitamin B_{12}-related problem that might occur with repeated use.

First, remember that nitrous oxide is an anesthetic gas that can make one unconscious, or at least so disoriented that one loses good judgment. Major problems occur when the user arranges some sort of mask or bag to deliver pure gas and then becomes unconscious and breathes only nitrous oxide. Thus, the person is asphyxiated by lack of oxygen.

Second, there is the physical damage to tissues exposed to any gas that is expanding. Anyone who has ever held her hand in front of an air or gas jet knows that expanding gas is cooling. That's the principle underlying air-conditioning units. Some users try to inhale the gas right out of the tank with no regulation of the flow rate, actually injuring their mouths, tracheas, and lungs from the cooling gas. Also, there is the direct physical risk of overexpanding (blowing up) the lungs as the gas flows at a high volume and pressure.

Finally, there is an odd complication of prolonged nitrous oxide use that is similar to a vitamin B_{12} deficiency. A B_{12}-dependent enzyme is inactivated by nitrous oxide and that leads to destruction of nerve fibers (a neuropathy) and thus neurological problems. These can include weakness, tingling sensations, or loss of feeling. Some dentists who regularly administer this gas have been found to experience just this type of neuropathy.

Tolerance to nitrous oxide can develop, and the euphoric properties diminish with repeated usage. However, in the recreational setting, where it is used only occasionally, tolerance is unlikely.

SOLVENTS

If there were ever a drug category to "Just Say No" to, this is it. This category of chemicals is literally a wastebasket of anything that anyone can get in vapor form and then inhale. It consists of all sorts of industrial chemicals, such as toluene, benzene, methanol, chloroform, freon and other coolants, paints, glues, and gases. **The authors take the position that these compounds are so toxic to both the first-time user and the long-term user that they should never be used under any circumstances.** However, we all know that people do inhale these chemicals, and so in the paragraphs below we will describe a few of the more common agents and talk about their toxicity.

uicide-prone individuals use inhalants to relieve their pain? Both are probably true, as is the case with so many other drugs.

First-time users can and do die. In a British study of one thousand deaths
from inhalant use, about one-fifth of the deaths were to first-time users. The
deaths were from a variety of causes, but each was associated with inhalant use.
This is a remarkable statistic, and it should make anyone wary of ever trying
these chemicals.

So, if a person lives long enough to be classified as a chronic inhalant user,
what are the long-term effects? Many research studies have been published on
this subject, but almost all of them involve case studies of people that were referred with specific medical problems. There are no broad studies covering
large numbers of inhalant users without reported medical problems. So we
don't know from a statistical perspective what the long-term toxic risk is. However, the medical studies of individuals who do report problems are sobering.
One neurological study of abusers referred for medical treatment showed that
thirteen of twenty people (65 percent) studied had central nervous system
damage as revealed by clinical examination and neurological imaging. Another study showed damage in 55 percent of a different group of people.

One of the best-studied chemicals is toluene. It is a common industrial solvent and a component of glues. In one study of chronic abusers, eleven of
twenty-four patients had damage to the part of the brain called the cerebellum.
This area of the brain is well known for controlling fine, delicate muscle
movements, and new studies suggest that it might play a part in learning.
Whether cerebellar impairment clears when the abuse stops has not been determined. Some studies suggest that the cells in this area die. Other brain
areas, including the visual and other nerve pathways, are affected as well, but
we caution that complete and controlled human studies are impossible to do,
since no one is going to agree to take these compounds just for the benefit of
medical research.

Tests of intellectual function show that abusers have problems with memory, attention, and concentration. Like the physical studies, these studies also
considered small numbers of patients who were ill, so we have to be careful
in the interpretation of these results. However, there is no question that some
people get very sick and suffer substantial central nervous system damage
from chronic use of inhalants.

Other body functions also suffer. The combined list of compounds and the
body functions they impair is huge, and it gets larger every day as research
shows new effects of these chemicals. It is enough to say that long-term usage
of inhalants can damage the heart, lungs, kidneys, liver, blood, and many
other areas, in addition to the nervous system. These chemicals are truly not
for human consumption.

What They Are and How They Work

These compounds have only one characteristic in common (otl
toxicity), and that is that they produce more or less the same fee
cohol and anesthetics do.

As with inhalational anesthetics, once the user begins to inhale
levels peak in a few minutes and most of the agents are absorbed b
As blood levels rise, there is dizziness, disorientation, perhaps an init
of stimulation followed by depression, and a sense of being light-heade
users describe changes in their perception of objects or time and/or ha
sions or hallucinations involving any of the senses. Muscular incoord
occurs as levels increase, along with ringing in the ears (tinnitus), dou
sion, abdominal pain, and flushing of the skin. These are followed l
standard symptoms associated with chemical depression of the central ne
system, including vomiting, loss of reflexes, cardiac and circulation probl
suppression of respiration, and, possibly, death.

The most dangerous effect of inhalant use is "sudden sniffing death," whi
occurs during the abuse of coolants and propellants (like Freon), and fu
gases (like butane and propane), which probably induce abnormal hea
rhythms. This may happen because the chemicals depress the excitability o
the heart cells that set the beating pattern, while at the same time increasing
the sensitivity of these and other heart cells to the stimulant epinephrine
(adrenaline).

We do not know exactly how these compounds produce their mental effects. However, based on the physical effects, we can assume that they work
in the same manner as anesthetics.

Toxicity

There is such a large number of diverse compounds that it is impossible to list
all of the toxic effects of every one of them. Also, long-term inhalant users almost always use other drugs, so it is difficult to sort out which toxic effect be-
longs to which drug or which combination of drugs. But there is one common
thread that runs through all of these compounds. Many users are injured, not
from direct toxic effects of these agents but from trauma related to their use.
Disorientation and loss of muscular coordination make accidents more likely,
and because many of these chemicals are flammable, serious burns occur. In
one well-respected study, 26 percent of deaths associated with inhalant use
were from accidents.

Also, people commit suicide under the influence of inhalants. In the same
research study, 28 percent of the deaths associated with inhalant use were
from suicide. Did the inhalants cause depression and suicide, or did the

7

Marijuana

Drug Class: No specific class, but legally considered a Schedule I narcotic

Individual Drugs: low-grade marijuana (1 percent or less delta-9-tetrahydrocannabinol [THC]), high-grade marijuana—sinsemilla (4 to 8 percent THC), hashish (7 to 14 percent THC), hash oil (up to 50 percent THC)

Common Terms: marijuana, reefer, pot, herb, ganja, grass, old man, blanche, weed, sinsemilla, bhang, dagga, smoke (dried plant material); hash, tar (hashish); hash oil, oil, charas (extracted plant resin)

The Buzz: People's experiences with marijuana vary widely and depend upon the potency of the drug taken. In general, smoking marijuana first relaxes a person and elevates his mood. These effects are followed about a half hour later by drowsiness and sedation. Some people experience this as stimulation followed by a relaxed feeling of tranquillity. Users may shift between hilarity and contemplative silence, but these swings often reflect the user's situation.

When hashish or high-grade marijuana is eaten, the effects take much longer to be felt (one to two hours) and may produce a more hallucinogenic response.

Overdose and Other Bad Effects: Lethal overdose is virtually impossible. Occasionally people report feeling anxious or fearful soon after smoking or after a particularly heavy dose. Relaxed and reassuring conversation with the user is often the best treatment for such an episode.

Although no one has ever died from an overdose of marijuana, it does impair judgment and the kinds of complex coordination needed to drive a car. Automobile accidents and stupid mistakes are the largest risks of marijuana intoxication.

People with heart disease or high blood pressure may be at risk because marijuana use increases the heart rate and places a greater work load on the heart.

Marijuana can also endanger unintended users. There have been reports of small children unknowingly eating large amounts of cannabis in cookies and going into coma.

Dangerous Combinations with Other Drugs: There has been very little work on this topic, but possible dangers include interactions with heart or blood pressure medications or with drugs that suppress the function of the immune system. In addition, one recent study shows that the combination of marijuana with cocaine can lead to very dangerous effects on the heart.

CHAPTER CONTENTS

A BRIEF HISTORY

All of the marijuana preparations people use for their psychoactive properties derive from the cannabis plant. The first written accounts of cannabis cultivation appear in Chinese records from as far back as 28 B.C., though the plant was likely cultivated for thousands of years before that. The Chinese writings indicate that the plant was grown for fiber, but they also recognize its intoxicating and medicinal properties. In fact, THC (as well as nicotine and cocaine) was recently identified in an Egyptian mummy from approximately 950 B.C. By around A.D. 1000, use of the cannabis plant as an intoxicant had spread to the eastern Mediterranean region, and European explorers to this area returned with fascinating stories of the effects of hashish.

Cannabis had been introduced to eastern Europe much earlier (around 700 B.C.), but not until Napoleon ventured to Egypt in the early nineteenth century did European culture fully acquaint itself with hashish. By the 1840s, recreational use of cannabis products (as well as a number of other drugs) had grown to be quite chic among the artists and intellectuals of France, many of whom used the drug in their search for new ways to enhance creativity and to view the world.

Although the original European explorers brought cannabis seeds to the New World to cultivate hemp plants for rope and cloth, it was not until the early twentieth century that marijuana began to impact United States society directly.

THE CANNABIS PLANT AND ITS PRODUCTS

Cannabis is a highly versatile plant. Hemp, a strong fiber, comes from the stem and has been used to make rope, cloth, and paper. When dried, the leaves and flowers are used as marijuana for their psychoactive and medicinal effects. The roots of the plant have also been used to make medicines, and ancient Chinese used the seeds as a food. Cannabis seeds are still used for oil and animal feed.

The two most prevalent species of cannabis are *Cannabis sativa* and *Cannabis indica*. In years past people cultivated *C. sativa* to make hemp. Under natural conditions it will grow as high as a lanky fifteen to twenty feet. *C. sativa* still grows wild as a weed across the southern United States. *C. indica* has been cultivated throughout the world mostly for the psychoactive properties of its resins. These plants generally grow to no more than a few feet in height and develop a thicker, bushier appearance than *C. sativa*.

The cannabis plant contains more than four hundred chemicals, and several of them are psychoactive. By far the most psychoactive of these is delta-9-tetrahydrocannabinol (THC), found in the plant's resin. The resin is most concentrated in the flowers. In an unfertilized plant it provides a sticky coating that protects the flowers from excessive heat from the sun and enhances contact by grains of pollen. The vegetative leaves contain a small amount of resin, as do the stalks, but the concentrations in these parts of the plant are so low as to have little intoxicating effect.

Today much cultivation of "drug" strain marijuana plants has occurred, but the amount of THC present in the flowers of individual plants varies considerably. In addition to the genetic makeup of the plant, the growing conditions, timing of harvest, drying environment, and storage environment can all significantly influence the potency of the final product. As the plant matures, the balance of various chemicals in the resin change, as does the amount of resin secreted at the flowering tops of the plant. Early in maturation, cannabidiolic acid (CBDA) predominates and is converted to cannabidiol (CBD), which is converted to THC as the plant reaches its floral peak. The extent to which CBD is converted to THC largely determines the "drug quality" of the individual plant. When the plant matures into the late floral and senescent stages, THC is converted to cannabinol (CBN). A plant that is harvested at the peak floral stage has a high ratio of THC to CBD and CBN, and the psychoactive effect is often described as a "clear," or "clean," high, with relatively little sedative effect. However, some cultivators allow the plants to mature past this peak to produce marijuana with a heavier, more sedative effect. The difference between the feelings associated with peak- versus late-harvested marijuana has been described as the difference between being "high" and being "stoned."

Burning marijuana for smoking produces hundreds of additional compounds. This means that when someone smokes a single joint, hundreds upon hundreds of chemical compounds enter the body. We know that many of these act on various organs and systems in the body, but we don't know what effects most of these compounds may have, either acutely or after prolonged use. This makes it impossible at present to truly understand all of the effects of marijuana. Many scientific studies have, therefore, restricted their attention to THC, allowing us to evaluate at least some of the effects of cannabinoids

on the brain and behavior. But we're left uncertain about the long-term consequences of marijuana use.

DRUG PREPARATIONS: FROM "HEADACHE POT" TO "HOSPITAL POT"

The products made from marijuana plants for psychoactive effects vary
markedly in their THC content and therefore in their psychoactive potency.

Low-grade marijuana is made from all the leaves of both sexes of the plant.
These vegetative leaves contain very little THC compared to the pistillate
flowers of the female plant or to the smaller leaves adjacent to them. The
THC content of such a preparation may be only 1 percent or lower. Smokers
sometimes call this headache pot because smoking it can produce more of a
headache than a high.

Medium-grade marijuana is made from the dried flowering tops of female
cannabis plants raised with and fertilized by male plants. Fertilization limits
the psychoactive potency of the resulting marijuana because the female flowers secrete THC-containing resin only until fertilization. After that time the
flower no longer needs the protective resin, and it begins to produce a seed.

High-grade marijuana is made from the flowering tops of female plants
raised in isolation from male plants. The resulting marijuana is called sinsemilla, which means "without seeds." As the female flowers mature without
fertilization, they continually secrete resin to coat the delicate flowers and
small leaves surrounding them; the flowers grow in thick clusters, heavy with
resin. When these "buds" are harvested and dried, they contain an average of
around 5 percent THC. Some samples of sinsemilla test as high as 11 percent.

Such powerful marijuana has been called hospital pot because occasionally
an unsuspecting smoker, expecting the usual gentle high of medium-grade
marijuana, gets frightened by the sudden and powerful high of sinsemilla,
panics, and winds up in the emergency room. Actually, the best treatment for
such a scare is a calm and reassuring "talk down" by a friend. The feeling of
panic often arises from an unexpected sense of loss of control, and the individual needs only to be reassured that he is safe and that nothing will threaten
him.

It is worth noting that some cultivators in the United States today, using
well-controlled indoor growing conditions, produce marijuana with THC
concentrations as high as 10 percent. The THC content of most marijuana in
the United States ranges from two to 5 percent. Interestingly, during the last
few years it has often been said that United States marijuana is ten times more
potent now than it was in the 1960s and 1970s. This isn't exactly true. Since
the 1970s the THC content of marijuana seized by United States law en-

forcement officials has been measured by the Potency Monitoring Project in Mississippi—a government-funded project. In the early 1970s they generally reported that samples of seized marijuana contained low concentrations of THC—in the range of 0.4 to 1 percent—but those samples often came from low-potency, high-volume Mexican "kilobricks," which probably contained considerably less THC than most of the marijuana that was actually being smoked in those days. Also, it was not until the late 1970s that the higher-potency cannabis products available to smokers, such as buds and sinsemilla, were included in the samples analyzed by the Potency Monitoring Project. Thus, estimates of THC content in the 1970s probably underestimated the average THC content of the marijuana smoked during that period. When independent laboratories analyzed marijuana samples during the 1970s, THC contents were often considerably higher than those reported by the Potency Monitoring Project—in the 2 to 5 percent range, typical of most marijuana samples today. Since 1980 the seized marijuana tested by the Potency Monitoring Project has included more representative samples of what is available on the street, and between 1981 and 1993 the THC content has hovered between 2.3 and 3.4 percent—all within the average range of independently tested samples during the 1970s.

Hashish is produced when the resin of the cannabis plant is separated from the plant material. The purest form of hashish is virtually 100 percent resin. In India this pure material is called charas. Most hashish, however, is not pure resin and contains varying amounts of plant material as well. It often appears as a dark-colored gummy ball that is rather hard, but not brittle. The average THC content of hashish is around 8 percent, but can vary quite a bit, up to 20 percent. Hashish is often smoked in a pipe or rolled into a cigarette along with tobacco or lower-grade marijuana. A more traditional means of smoking hashish is to ignite a small piece and let it burn under a glass or cup. The user then tilts back the glass and inhales the smoke from underneath.

Hash oil is the most potent of the preparations made from the cannabis plant. After the plant is boiled in alcohol, the solids are filtered out, and when the water evaporates, what's left is hash oil. This is generally a thick, waxy substance that is very high in THC content—ranging from 20 to 70 percent. It can be scraped onto the inner rim of a pipe bowl for smoking or used to lace tobacco or marijuana cigarettes.

HOW THC MOVES THROUGH THE BODY

When marijuana is smoked, the rich blood supply of the lungs rapidly absorbs the THC. Since blood from the lungs goes directly from the heart to the brain, the high, as well as the effects on heart rate and blood vessels, occurs

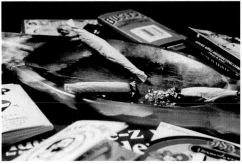
Mexican brown heroin and Southeast Asian heroin.

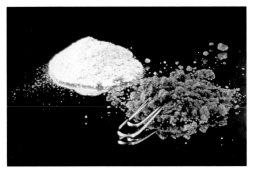
Marijuana rolled into cigarettes for smoking.

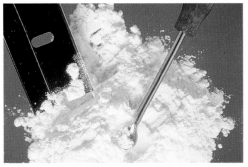
Powdered cocaine.

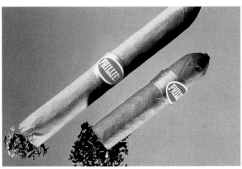
Hollowed-out cigars packed with marijuana, called blunts.

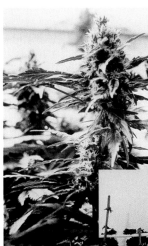
Marijuana abusers prefer the *colas,* or buds of the plant, because of their higher THC content. Leaves are discarded or used as filler.

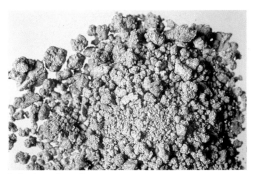
Mexican heroin.

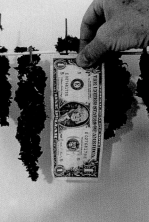
Marijuana buds hung out to dry.

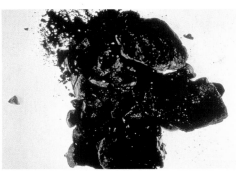
Mexican black tar heroin.

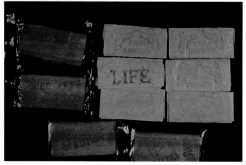

Heroin repackaged for sale on the streets of the United States.

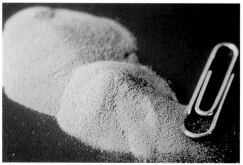

Highly refined Southeast Asian heroin.

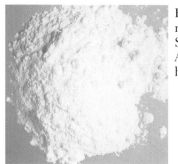

Morphine base.

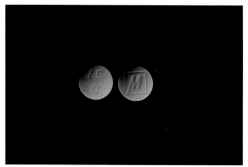

Demerol. Controlled ingredient: meperidine hydrochloride 100 mg.

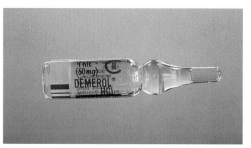

Demerol. Controlled ingredient: meperidine hydrochloride 50 mg/ml.

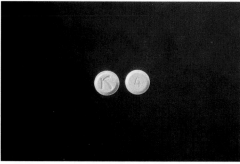

Dilaudid. Controlled ingredient: hydromorphone hydrochloride 4 mg.

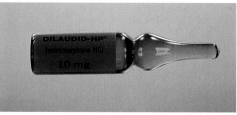

Dilaudid-HP injection. Controlled ingredient: hydromorphone hydrochloride 10 mg/ml.

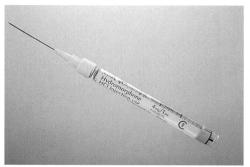

Hydromorphone hydrochloride. Controlled ingredient: hydromorphone hydrochloride 4 mg/ml.

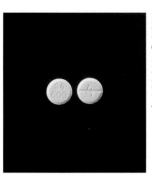

Hydromorphone hydrochloride. Controlled ingredient: hydromorphone hydrochloride 4 mg.

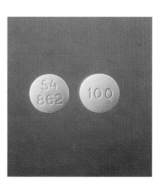

Oramorph SR (an opiate). Controlled ingredient: morphine sulfate 100 mg.

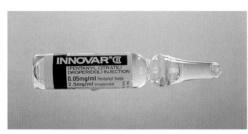

Innovar (an opiate). Controlled ingredient: fentanyl citrate 0.05 mg/ml. Other ingredient: droperidol 2.5 mg/ml.

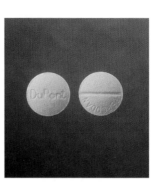

Percodan. Controlled ingredients: oxycodone hydrochloride 4.5 mg; oxycodone terephthalate 0.38 mg. Other ingredient: aspirin 325 mg.

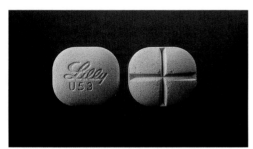

Methadone HCl diskets. Controlled ingredient: methadone hydrochloride 40 mg.

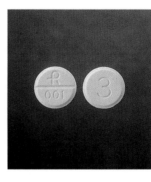

Acetaminophen with Codeine No. 3. Controlled ingredient: codeine phosphate 30 mg. Other ingredient: acetaminophen 300 mg.

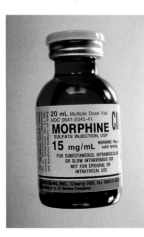

Morphine sulfate. Controlled ingredient: morphine sulfate 15 mg/ml.

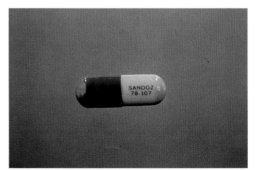

Fiorinal with Codeine (an opiate). Controlled ingredients: codeine phosphate 30 mg; butalbital 50 mg. Other ingredients: aspirin 325 mg; caffeine 40 mg.

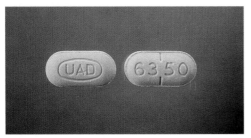

Lorcet (an opiate). Ingredient name: hydrocodone bitartrate 10 mg. Other ingredient: acetaminophen 650 mg.

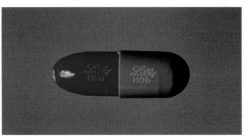

Darvon Compound-65. Controlled ingredient: propoxyphene hydrochloride 65 mg. Other ingredients: aspirin 389 mg; caffeine 32.4 mg.

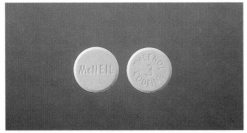

Tylenol with Codeine No. 3. Controlled ingredient: codeine phosphate 30 mg. Other ingredient: acetaminophen 300 mg.

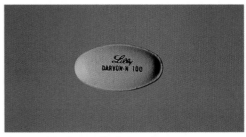

Darvon-N. Controlled ingredient: propoxyphene napsylate 100 mg.

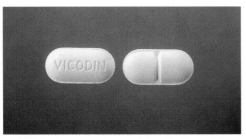

Vicodin. Controlled ingredient: hydrocodone bitartrate 5 mg. Other ingredient: acetaminophen 500 mg.

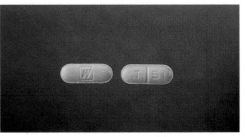

Talwin Nx (an opiate). Controlled ingredient: pentazocine hydrochloride 50 mg. Other ingredient: naloxone hydrochloride 0.5 mg.

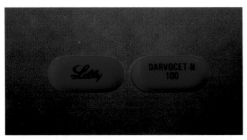

Darvocet-N 100 (an opiate). Controlled ingredient: propoxyphene napsylate 100 mg. Other ingredient: acetaminophen 650 mg.

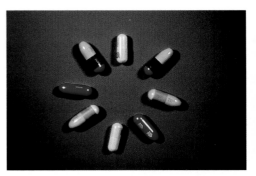

Depressants, or sedatives, widely prescribed to treat anxiety and insomnia.

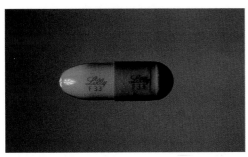

Amytal Sodium (a sedative). Controlled ingredient: amobarbital sodium 200 mg.

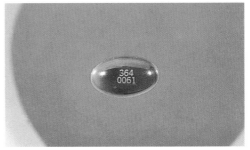

Chloral Hydrate (a sedative). Controlled ingredient: chloral hydrate 500 mg.

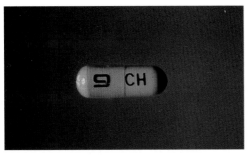

Nembutal Sodium (a sedative). Controlled ingredient: pentobarbital sodium 100 mg.

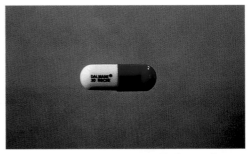

Dalmane (a sedative). Controlled ingredient: flurazepam hydrochloride 30 mg.

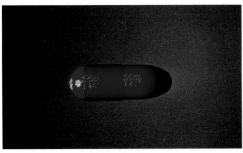

Seconal Sodium (a sedative). Controlled ingredient: secobarbital sodium 100 mg.

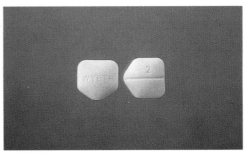

Equanil (a sedative). Controlled ingredient: meprobamate 200 mg.

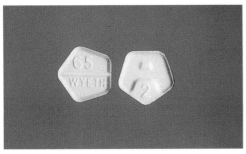

Ativan (a sedative). Controlled ingredient: lorazepam 2 mg.

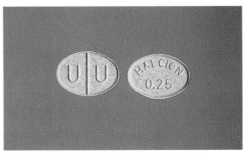

Halcion (a sedative). Controlled ingredient: triazolam 0.25 mg.

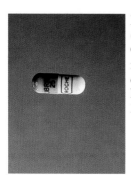

Librium (a sedative). Controlled ingredient: chlordiazepoxide hydrochloride 25 mg.

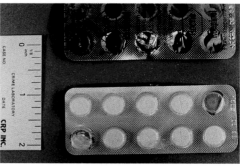

Rohypnol contains the controlled ingredient flunitrazepam hydrochloride. Pictured here is a 2-mg tablet with packaging. "Roofies," as they are known on the street, are sold inexpensively in Mexico. They are smuggled into the United States, where they have recently become a problem among American teens. The problem is rapidly spreading from the American Southwest to other parts of the United States.

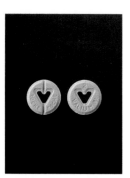

Tranxene (a sedative). Controlled ingredient: clorazepate dipotassium 3.75 mg.

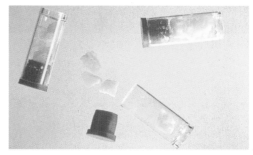

Crack, the smokable form of cocaine, provides an immediate rush.

Valium. Controlled ingredient: diazepam 2 mg.

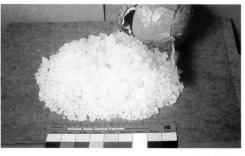

Ice, so named because of its appearance, is a smokable form of methamphetamine.

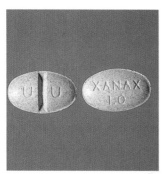

Xanax (a sedative). Controlled ingredient: alprazolam 1 mg.

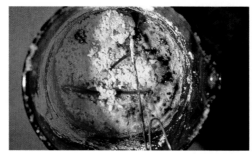

Crude methcathinone, or cat.

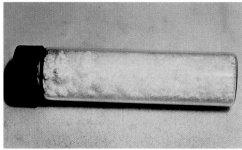

Pure cat.

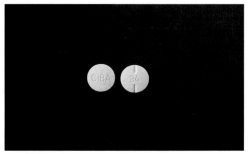

Ritalin. Controlled ingredient:
methylphenidate hydrochloride 20 mg.

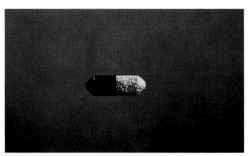

Dexedrine (a stimulant). Controlled
ingredient: dextroamphetamine sulfate 5 mg.

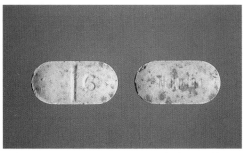

Adipex-P (a stimulant). Controlled ingredient:
phentermine hydrochloride 37.5 mg.

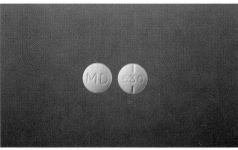

Methylphenidate hydrochloride. Controlled
ingredient: methylphenidate hydrochloride
10 mg.

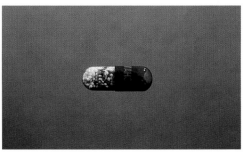

Fastin (a stimulant). Controlled ingredient:
phentermine hydrochloride 30 mg.

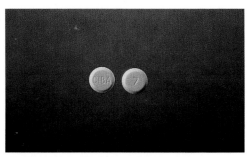

Ritalin. Controlled ingredient:
methylphenidate hydrochloride 5 mg.

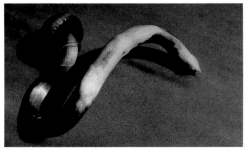

Psilocybin mushroom.

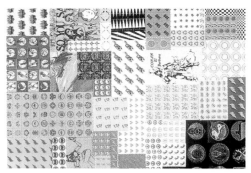

Collage of LSD blotter paper.

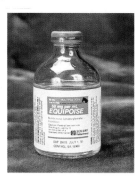

Counterfeiters duplicate packaging for black-market sales.

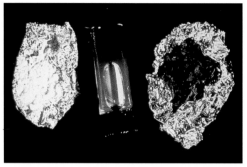

PCP is most commonly sold as a powder (left) or liquid (center), and applied to a leafy material such as oregano (right), which is then smoked.

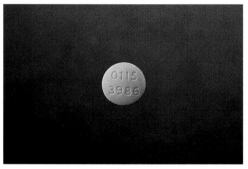

Android-25 (a steroid). Controlled ingredient: methyltestosterone 25 mg.

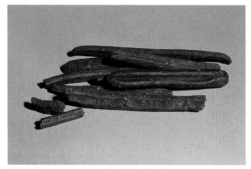

Black, resinous sticks of hashish.

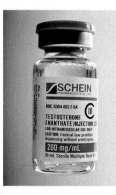

Testosterone. Controlled ingredient: testosterone 200 mg/ml.

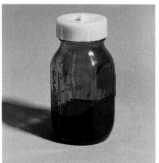

Amber, viscous hash oil.

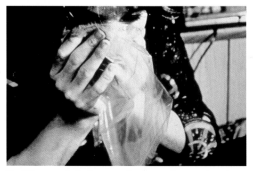

Sniffing an inhalant-soaked rag from a bag is a form of huffing.

within minutes. Much of the THC is actually gone from the brain within a few hours after smoking. However, THC also accumulates in significant concentrations in other organs, such as the liver, kidneys, spleen, and testes. THC readily crosses from the blood of a pregnant woman into the placenta and reaches the developing fetus.

How the smoker smokes makes a difference in how much of the THC from the marijuana actually gets to the body. A cigarette allows for approximately 10 to 20 percent of the THC in the marijuana to be transferred. A pipe is somewhat more efficient, allowing about 40 to 50 percent to transfer, and a water pipe (or bong) is quite efficient. Since the water pipe traps the smoke until it is inhaled, theoretically the only THC lost is what the smoker exhales.

Although much of the high wears off relatively soon after smoking, THC remains in the body much longer. About half of the THC is still in the blood twenty hours after smoking. And once the blood carrying the THC passes through the liver, some of the THC is converted into other compounds that may remain there for several days. Some of these metabolites have psychoactive effects as well, so that although the initial high may disappear within an hour or two, some of the effects of marijuana on mental and physical functions may last for days.

Not only may THC and its metabolites stay in the blood for days; they stay in the fatty deposits of the body much longer. This is because they are very lipid-soluble, meaning that they easily get absorbed into and stored in fat. THC stored in fatty deposits is released from these tissues slowly over a rather long period of time before finally being eliminated. What all this means is that about 30 percent of ingested THC (and its metabolites) may remain in the body a full week after smoking, and may continue to affect mental and physical functions subtly. In fact, the remnants from a single large dose of THC may be detectable up to three weeks later.

All of these rules apply when marijuana is eaten instead of smoked, except that less THC gets to the brain and it takes a lot longer for it to get there. When marijuana (or any drug) is taken into the stomach, the blood that absorbs it goes to the liver before flowing to the rest of the body (including the brain). This means two things. First, the liver breaks down some of the THC before it ever has a chance to affect the brain. Second, the remaining THC reaches the brain more slowly because of its indirect route through the bloodstream. However, because the body absorbs THC more slowly when marijuana is eaten, the peak levels of the drug last longer (though they are lower than they would be if the same amount were smoked).

Whether the user eats or smokes marijuana, and the accompanying differences in the way THC is distributed and metabolized, appear to have a substantial impact on the kind of experience he has. Rather than experiencing a sudden change from being straight to being high, the marijuana eater experi-

ences a slow and gradual shift that lasts longer. Many experienced users report
that what happens after eating marijuana is more reminiscent of a mild mushroom or LSD trip; it's not simply "getting high." Since high levels of THC can
cause hallucinogen-like experiences, people who have eaten marijuana and
reported such feelings may actually have achieved higher levels of THC than
many smokers—despite the fact that some of it is metabolized by the liver before it gets to the brain—because they ate a larger amount than they would
likely have smoked.

EFFECTS ON THE BRAIN

THE BRAIN RECEPTOR FOR THC

Perhaps the most striking finding from research on cannabinoids has been the
recent discovery of a cannabinoid receptor in the brain. This was not the first
time that researchers had located a specific brain receptor for a plant material. The opiate receptor, which was discovered years ago, is involved in the
modulation of pain and possibly of stress in a broader sense as well. But while
it makes sense that our brains have evolved a chemical system for dealing
with pain, it's less clear why it would evolve a receptor for THC and what its
implications are for human beings.

Since the brain provides its own cannabinoid receptors, it must also provide
its own compound to activate those receptors. Anandamide (the name comes
from *ananda*, the sanskrit word for "bliss") is one compound, found naturally
in the brain, that binds with cannabinoid receptors. Another is called 2-AG.
It also activates THC receptors in the brain, and is present there in amounts
170 times greater than anandamide. There are likely several other such naturally occurring compounds, because several different subtypes of cannabinoid receptors have been discovered.

THE HIPPOCAMPUS

Although we must leave it to the anthropologists and ethnobotanists to figure
out *why* we have cannabinoid receptors, we do know *where* they are in the
brain, and that might help us to understand the effects of marijuana. The
hippocampus is critically involved in the formation of new memories (as we
discussed in our "Alcohol" chapter), and has a very high concentration of
cannabinoid receptors. Not surprisingly, the inhibition of memory formation
by marijuana is its most well-established negative effect on mental function.

In animal studies, when rats are given THC they show significant deficits
in memory formation—not the ability to recall previously learned informa-

tion, but the ability to store *new* memories. In fact, an animal treated with THC performs a memory task as poorly as an animal with a damaged hippocampus. Normally the cells in the hippocampus become active and communicate with one another while an animal learns such a task. However, the hippocampal cells in the animals under the influence of THC did not activate in normal ways. These experiments make a compelling case that the memory deficits associated with acute marijuana use are due to the THC suppressing the activity of hippocampal cells and hindering acquisition of new memory. After the animals' bodies eliminated the THC, their memory and hippocampal function returned to normal. The compound 2-AG, which exists naturally in the brain and stimulates THC receptors, also decreases the ability of the hippocampus to carry out some of its memory-related functions.

These studies raise an important question about the effects of chronic marijuana use on the hippocampus. Does marijuana kill brain cells? A number of studies in rats have investigated the effects of THC on various areas of the brain, including the hippocampus, by giving the rats very large doses of THC for very long periods. While some of these studies suggest that some damage can occur, the way the experiments were done raises questions about the relevance of the results. The studies that show these effects on hippocampal cells generally exposed animals to high concentrations of THC nearly every day for several months (a substantial percentage of the life span of a rat). In many animal studies of this kind, the doses given are hundreds of times higher than a human user would take at any given time. When researchers gave lower doses, far less severe effects were observed in the hippocampus, even when the drug was given for more than twice as long. And even the low doses in many of these animal studies were much higher, were administered much more frequently, and were administered for longer periods of time than most marijuana smokers would ever self-administer the drug.

Generally, science of this sort progresses first by finding significant results in rats or mice, and then by attempting to see if the effects show up in non-human primates, such as rhesus monkeys, whose brains (and behavior) are more similar to those of humans. A few years ago some good findings were published: the experiments had used rhesus monkeys to assess the effects of daily exposure to a reasonable amount of marijuana smoke for one year. At the end of the study the animals' brains were examined and no evidence was found of permanent gross changes in neurons or of neuronal death. Chronic exposure to THC could conceivably cause long-lasting changes in the organization of the brain, or in the chemistry of neurons, but that would be hard to detect. If the prolonged THC exposure occurred while the brain was maturing (childhood or adolescence), then the changes might be quite important. At this point no biological data support this. However, as we will see later, some human studies show that prolonged marijuana use can have long-lasting effects even after people quit using the drug, and subtle brain changes may underlie these effects.

So, what do we make of the animal research? It's not perfect and cannot give us final answers, but there are good reasons to take the results seriously. This is particularly true for studies of the hippocampus, because that structure in the rat is remarkably similar to that in the human, both in how it looks and in what it does (i.e., promote memory). Although profound damage to the hippocampus, as observed in those studies, is unlikely to occur in any but the heaviest of marijuana users, less severe effects could occur with more moderate use. The user might risk subtly damaging hippocampal circuits without causing obvious memory deficits. Her circuits might just be less sharp than they otherwise would have been. We don't know for sure.

OTHER BRAIN REGIONS

Two other areas of the brain particularly rich in cannabinoid receptors are the cerebellum and the basal ganglia. These regions help to coordinate and fine-tune our movements, and marijuana is known to disrupt these functions as well. Cannabinoid receptors, however, are not found in the brain stem, which is critical for breathing. That may be why it's virtually impossible to take a fatal overdose of marijuana.

One area of the brain that is involved in the rewarding (and possibly addicting) effects of some drugs is the nucleus accumbens, which contains cells which use the neurotransmitter dopamine (please see the "Addiction" chapter). Until now there was no evidence that THC had any effect on dopamine activity in this region, leading many people to believe that marijuana carried no risk of addiction at all. As we write this book two studies have emerged which show that THC causes the levels of dopamine there to rise. It is important to remember that when it comes to science it is never wise to bank on the results of just a few studies, but recent reports at least raise the possibility that THC has some effect on the brain's reward systems. If so, then marijuana may join the long list of other things that stimulate these circuits, including nicotine, food, heroin, sex, and alcohol. We expect that scientific research will eventually show that anything pleasurable (even a good biscuit) will evoke dopamine, and if the pleasureable experience is repeated enough, then withdrawal from it will produce discomfort. (Who wants to give up tasty food?) But the key here is a matter of degree. Maybe food, sex, and marijuana release some dopamine in the reward circuit, but cocaine is so much more effective that it is therefore much more addicting. As we continue to emphasize, good information is critical to making healthy decisions, and just because someone concludes that marijuana may stimulate the reward circuit, one should not

infer that this drug is the pharmacological equivalent of other drugs like cocaine or heroin.

EFFECTS ON OTHER BODY PARTS

THE IMMUNE SYSTEM

THC receptors are located in many different places outside the brain and affect body functions in a range of ways. One of these is the immune system —
the complex of structures, cells, and chemicals that fight infection and disease.
In fact, two different main types of cannabinoid receptors have been identified:
one that is highly concentrated in the brain, and one that is highly concentrated in certain immune-system cells.

Some animal studies indicate that THC can reduce immunity to infec-
tions, but the doses used in these studies were far greater than any human user
would take. Unfortunately, at present, there are not enough reliable studies of
the effects of THC on human immune function to make a convincing case
either way. Still, a lot of basic research is being conducted that *suggests* that
THC may compromise the function of immune cells. We will simply have to
wait to see if these early studies prove to be relevant to the human marijuana
user.

THE HEART

Smoking marijuana increases the heart rate. Laboratory studies have shown
that this increase measures in the general range of twenty to thirty beats per
minute. Relatively frequent smokers do develop some degree of tolerance to
this effect, but even tolerant individuals experience substantial increases in
heart rate after smoking. Clearly such an increase in heart rate could pose a
risk for some individuals, particularly those with heart disease or high blood
pressure, or those who take medications that alter heart rhythms. Still, there
is no clear evidence that marijuana smoking leads directly to heart disease or
produces heart attacks.

THE LUNGS

Two separate and important questions bear on this topic: Does chronic marijuana smoking impair the functioning of the lungs? Does chronic marijuana
smoking promote lung cancer?

The answer to the first question is yes. Some studies of chronic, heavy marijuana smokers show that their lungs do not produce as much airflow as the
lungs of the nonsmoker do. In addition, solid studies have found both an ab-

normal clinical appearance and an abnormal organization of cells in the airways of heavy marijuana smokers relative to nonsmokers and to those who smoked tobacco alone.

Although there have been rumors that marijuana smoke is ten or even one hundred times more toxic to the lungs than tobacco smoke is, the truth is that marijuana smoke and tobacco smoke are rather similar. Many of the toxic compounds, such as tar, carbon monoxide, and cyanide, are found in comparable levels in both types of smoke. One known carcinogen, benzopyrene, is found in both but occurs in greater concentration in marijuana smoke, while tobacco-specific nitrosamines appear only in tobacco. So far, no definitive evidence links marijuana smoking with lung cancer, but eventually such a link will probably be established. One study measured DNA damage (thought to be a precursor to the development of cancer) in lung cells from marijuana smokers, tobacco smokers, and nonsmokers. The study found a trend toward DNA damage in cells from marijuana smokers regardless of whether they also smoked tobacco. This suggests that marijuana smoking alone might predispose a person to develop lung cancer. Finally, a recent study of lung cancer patients suggests that people who smoke *both* tobacco and marijuana regularly may run a greater risk of developing lung cancer, and at an earlier age, than smokers of tobacco alone.

But how much marijuana smoke will prove to represent a risk? Very few marijuana smokers inhale even a significant fraction of the amount of smoke a typical cigarette smoker does in a given day. On the other hand, marijuana is smoked differently than tobacco. The amount of marijuana smoke inhaled per puff is two-thirds larger than a typical puff of a tobacco cigarette. Marijuana smoke is also inhaled more deeply into the lungs, and is held in the lungs four times as long. So, the toxins in the marijuana smoke get greater access to the lungs and may do that much more damage than cigarette smoke. One study showed that a marker for carbon monoxide in the blood measured five times higher after smoking a marijuana cigarette than it did after smoking a tobacco cigarette of comparable size. The amount of tar inhaled from the marijuana cigarettes was three times higher, and of that amount, one-third more was retained in the respiratory systems of the subjects who smoked marijuana than in those who smoked tobacco.

Finally, one recent study, which has not yet been confirmed by other laboratories, indicates that chronic marijuana smokers who smoke three to four joints per day suffer from chronic bronchitis as often as cigarette smokers who smoke a pack or more per day. People in these two groups also showed comparable changes in the structure of their lung cells. These changes do not indicate the presence of lung cancer, but many investigators believe that such changes may foreshadow later development of lung cancer.

THE REPRODUCTIVE SYSTEM

Although marijuana does not make people sterile, as some rumors have asserted, long-term use of marijuana does have some effects on reproductive function. Through its effects on the brain, marijuana suppresses the production of hormones that help to regulate the reproductive system. In men this translates to decreased sperm counts and, occasionally, erectile dysfunction (impotence) from high doses over a long period of time. A woman who uses marijuana regularly over a long period of time may experience irregular menstrual cycles. Though these effects almost never cause complete infertility, they could decrease the probability of conception.

Another hormonal effect of marijuana in men may result in the development of breast tissue (the scientific term for this is *gynecomastia*), an effect that is generally not enjoyed by men. This is caused by marijuana's ability to increase secretion of the hormone prolactin.

SUBJECTIVE EFFECTS: THE "INTERNAL" EXPERIENCE

As a drug, marijuana defies characterization. It does not fit neatly into any of the general categories into which most other psychoactive drugs can be placed. However, it shares characteristics with many of them. So, rather than try to squeeze the effects into a simple category, we will first describe the range of effects and then try to unify the information in a practical way.

Many, perhaps most, people don't even get high the first few times they use marijuana. This unusual lack of effect may be due to the need to learn the techniques of smoking, such as inhaling the proper amount and holding the smoke in the lungs. It also appears that the user has to *learn* how to appreciate or perceive the high that the drug provides. This is in marked contrast to most drugs, whose effects lose power with repeated use (tolerance).

People's subjective experiences of THC vary widely. Most people report that the high is either intellectually interesting, emotionally pleasing, or both. The "interesting" aspect of the high may relate to what many people call an improvement in sense perception. Some people say that they hear subtleties in speech or music that they wouldn't have recognized without the drug. To some, visual images may seem more intense or more meaningful. Likewise, feelings often seem more intense to the user, or differ from what she'd feel without the drug. Generally, the user interprets these changes in cognition and feeling as positive, but the interpretation also depends on the situation in which they occur. A sense of emotional well-being and intellectual stimulation could switch to something less pleasant in other surroundings.

It's difficult to assess the accuracy of reports of enhanced perception, cognition, or emotional insight because the high does not generally translate well into straight language. Many people who report having tried to write down the subtleties of their thoughts and feelings while on marijuana find afterward that the words they wrote just don't convey the experience. Even if, while they were high, they thought they had captured the moment, the resulting account seems to miss the substance of the experience.

Still, what does this translation problem mean? Are the feelings and thoughts that one has while high not as profound as they seem in the moment? Are they just what one would have thought or felt otherwise, but given a false importance by the drug? Perhaps the drug produces a relaxed and open state in which normal feelings and thoughts can be experienced more fully; but the effect can't be due to relaxation alone because drugs like Valium clearly do not impact perception, thinking, and emotion the way marijuana does. The difference could relate to the effects of THC on memory and the perception of time.

A number of early research reports indicated that marijuana altered the user's perception of time, seeming to slow it down. Users sometimes refer to being on "pot time," when rather brief events seem to stretch on and on; that might be due to wandering concentration or disjointed memory. Perhaps because THC makes it harder to remember one's ideas and feelings, only the most salient or important parts stick in the memory, changing the user's interpretation of the experience.

TOLERANCE, DEPENDENCE, AND WITHDRAWAL

Although users do develop a tolerance to marijuana, this development is not as simple or as clear-cut as it is in the case of some other drugs. Frequent smokers generally report less of a feeling of being high than infrequent users after smoking a marijuana cigarette or taking oral THC. Interestingly, frequent users also report feeling high after smoking an inactive placebo cigarette (though less so than after a real one). These findings indicate that tolerance to the subjective effects of marijuana does develop, and that there is a significant learning effect associated with chronic marijuana use. Perhaps frequent smokers associate the feeling of being high with the various environmental stimuli that surround the act of smoking, so that smoking a joint (even an inactive one) and expecting to get high leads them to feel high despite the lack of drug.

Dependence can be measured in a variety of ways, but in general it seems that even heavy marijuana users do not become dependent. One way to assess dependence is to determine if the individual craves the drug so much that it comes to control much of her behavior. The dependent person will have difficulty in controlling her use of the drug and will sacrifice much to get it. The number of people who have this level of difficulty with marijuana is very small, and there does not appear to be a significant degree of craving associated with marijuana. Some individuals have reportedly experienced psychological dependence, but these cases are hard to assess since each is unique and there have been no truly well-controlled studies.

Withdrawal occurs when, after chronic use, a drug is abruptly withdrawn and the user suffers a kind of rebound of unpleasant, often dangerous effects. The classic cases are the agitation and illness associated with opiate withdrawal and the anxiety, and sometimes tremors and seizures, associated with alcohol withdrawal. Even after the most intense exposure, the effects associated with marijuana withdrawal are mild. For example, in one study people consumed 10- or 30-milligram doses of THC by mouth every three to four hours around the clock for up to twenty-one days. These are *very* large doses (even taken orally), given continuously over a long time, and do not model the intake of any but the most extreme users of marijuana. When they stopped, the subjects most frequently showed irritability and restlessness. Less prominent symptoms were insomnia, sweating, and mild nausea. When THC was readministered to these subjects, the symptoms went away, indicating that they had been the result of the THC withdrawal.

EFFECTS ON MEMORY AND OTHER MENTAL FUNCTIONS

ACUTE EFFECTS

Although researchers cannot stick electrodes into the brains of human subjects to see exactly how marijuana affects memory, some have conducted revealing studies on the memory effects of acute marijuana intoxication. In general these studies show what the animal studies predicted they would. While people are high, they are significantly less able to store new information than when they aren't. In fact, the single most common and reproducible cognitive effect of marijuana is this interference with memory processing. It is important to emphasize that, as with alcohol exposure, the deficit is not in the ability to recall old, well-learned memories, but rather in the ability to form new ones.

For example, twenty years ago researchers found that after smoking one joint, people in their twenties were significantly impaired in their ability to recall the details of a story that they both read and listened to while high. However, if they learned the story the day before they smoked the joint, then the subjects could recall the story with no trouble. So, it's probably the case that marijuana compromises the ability to learn new information but not the ability to recall previously learned information.

"Residual" and Chronic Effects

Since THC remains in the body (and thus the brain) for so long after exposure to marijuana, it is important to know how long memory (and other cognitive functions) may be affected. Although researchers have undertaken a considerable number of studies, most of them are flawed because they fail to control for influences, such as smoking experience or intelligence, that make the results difficult to interpret. Still, when all the findings are boiled down, it does appear that marijuana has residual effects on cognitive functions (including memory) for up to forty-eight hours after smoking. It is therefore probably not wise to take a challenging test or to fly an airplane within a day or two after smoking marijuana. However, there is no good evidence of residual effects on mental function lasting beyond two days.

Although a lot of research in this literature is flawed, one very recent study that was well done studied a group of people of considerable interest—college students. The investigators recruited students in two distinct groups: "heavy" users (those who had used marijuana nearly every day during the month before the study and had THC in their blood when they came to the laboratory), and "light" users (those who had used marijuana on average only once in the thirty days before coming to the laboratory and had no THC in their blood when they arrived). The students spent the night under supervision and were given a battery of mental tests the next morning. The intent was to assess the cognitive function of the heavy users, but a number of interesting differences (and similarities) appeared between the backgrounds of the light-and heavy-using groups. The heavy users tended to come from more affluent families with higher incomes. There were no differences between light and heavy users in psychiatric history: neither group had more psychological problems than the other. However, when their present emotional state was assessed, the heavy users were happier (remember, though, that they still had THC in their systems).

The mental tests revealed two important findings. First, the heavy users showed much less mental flexibility in problem solving than did the light users. They often made the same mistake over and over again on one test, indicating that they tended to become locked in to a particular problem-solving strategy and had a hard time generating new ones even when the current one no longer worked for them. The heavy users also showed impaired memory function, but this problem did not appear on all of the memory tests that they took. They were as good as light users at remembering a short story that was read to them. However, male heavy users (but not female heavy users) did not perform as well as light users at recalling figures that they were shown and then asked to draw from memory. The heavy users also had significantly more trouble learning lists of words over time.

So, what we know from this study is that about one day after their last dose, people who smoke daily are significantly impaired on some measures of memory for words and pictures, and make more errors than would be expected on a problem-solving test that requires mental flexibility. But since none of the light users had THC in their systems when they came to the lab, we do not know the effects of marijuana one day after use in people who use the drug less than daily. The other thing we don't know is how long the residual impairment of heavy users lasts, or if there is any permanent impairment that is due to brain damage rather than residual THC in their brains.

This study did try to address the second question. The investigators looked a bit more closely at the light users and found that although they had all used marijuana very little during the month before the study, some had used it more than others across their lifetimes (and some quite heavily earlier in their lives). When the light users were divided up into subgroups based on their life histories of marijuana use, there was no relationship between the scores they got on the mental tests and how much marijuana they had used in the past. With no THC in their systems at the time of testing, it did not matter how much these subjects had smoked in the past—there were no apparent permanent effects. But once the light users were subdivided, the numbers of subjects in each subgroup became rather small. So, from a purely statistical point of view, the lack of effects should be interpreted cautiously until more studies are done with larger numbers of subjects.

DOES MARIJUANA PROMOTE AGGRESSION?

In a word—no. In the late 1920s and 1930s, as United States society was beginning to recognize marijuana use, articles appeared in some newspapers associating marijuana with crime. Some government agencies of the time promoted the idea that marijuana use led to aggressive behavior. Even *Scientific American* wrote in 1936 that when marijuana was combined with other intoxicants it made the smoker vicious and prone to kill. (It is interesting, given the political climate of the time, that the editors of *Scientific American* chose to attribute the viciousness to the effects of marijuana and not to any of the other "intoxicants," which included alcohol.) This image of marijuana effects is very inconsistent with the 1960s image of a dreamy-eyed, smiling young woman at Woodstock offering a joint to the camera. Though there lingers some debate about the effects of marijuana on aggressive behavior, a clever laboratory study conducted recently shows clearly that, if anything, marijuana *decreases* aggressive behavior in people when they are provoked. The study is worth explaining.

Researchers brought young men into the laboratory and showed them two buttons on a table. They were told that by pressing button A they would accumulate points that would result in a reward. They were also told that pressing button B would remove points from another subject in a different room who would be engaged in the same task (there was actually no other subject). As the men worked at pressing their buttons, every so often they would see that they were losing points. This was attributed to the actions of the other (fictitious) subject. The experimenters could arrange to have more or less points removed in order to create the impression that the other subject was being mildly or highly aggressive to the actual subject. As one might expect, as the fictional subjects became more aggressive, the real subjects began to press button B to retaliate. After a while the subjects smoked either a marijuana cigarette or a placebo cigarette that tasted like marijuana but had no THC. After smoking the marijuana cigarettes the subjects showed a clear *decrease* in aggressive response to the highly provoking actions of the "other subjects." Although this was obviously not a study of aggression on the street, it does have the scientific advantage of well-controlled treatments and well-defined measurements. Moreover, it is consistent with the vast majority of anecdotal reports about marijuana effects, which claim that it makes people more peaceful.

EFFECTS ON MOTOR PERFORMANCE AND DRIVING

Some people believe that marijuana does not impair the ability to drive. The truth is that it does. The decrease in attention and concentration that marijuana produces can be very dangerous when one is operating any kind of heavy machinery. A marijuana smoker's reflexes may be in good enough shape to control a car, but they may not be of much use if she stops paying close attention to the road. Similarly, the marijuana-induced changes in perception and sense of time may be entertaining on the couch in the living room, but could be deadly on the highway. Laboratory studies using driving simulators have shown that marijuana significantly impairs both the ability to concentrate and the ability to make corrections. This appears to be true on the real road as well. One study showed that young people who reported driving frequently while on marijuana were twice as likely to be involved in accidents than their nonsmoking peers. The best bet is never to drive while using any drug (legal, illegal, or prescription) known to impair motor or cognitive skills.

ARE THERE MEDICAL USES?

This is a hot-button issue. When medical professionals discuss the possible medical uses of marijuana, their emotions seem to escalate, and when passions run high, otherwise fair and reasonable thinkers can sometimes interpret data and draw conclusions in ways that they normally would not. In trying to make sense of the debate, we want to present simply what the scientific and clinical literature tells us about the potential usefulness of marijuana as a medicine. And in general, the literature tells us that there are indeed valid medical uses for cannabis products.

Prior to 1900, cannabis products were used frequently as appetite stimulants, muscle relaxants, and analgesics (pain relievers). In the early twentieth century, though cannabis was still used, its prevalence began to decline as competitive drugs became available. Finally, in 1937, the Marijuana Tax Act effectively stopped all legal medical use. Marijuana is currently categorized in Schedule I under the Controlled Substances Act, passed in 1970. This schedule is meant to list drugs that have a high potential for abuse, lack an accepted medical use, and are unsafe for use even under medical supervision. In 1972 the National Organization for the Reform of Marijuana Laws (NORML) began a campaign to have marijuana moved to Schedule II so that it could be legally prescribed. NORML asked the Bureau of Narcotics and Dangerous Drugs (now called the Drug Enforcement Administration—DEA) to begin the process of rescheduling the cannabis products. It took more than a decade, but the required public hearings were initiated in 1986. After two years of hearings, the administrative law judge for the DEA, Francis L. Young, wrote that marijuana was "one of the safest therapeutically active substances known to man" and that marijuana fulfilled the legal requirement of currently acceptable medical use. However, his order that marijuana be moved to Schedule II was overruled by the DEA.

APPETITE

As the debate progressed, the demand for marijuana for medical uses grew, and the Food and Drug Administration (FDA) was persuaded to issue a handful of approvals for patients under a special permission called an Individual Treatment Investigational New Drug Application (sometimes called a Compassionate Use IND). By the late 1980s the number of requests for Compassionate Use INDs increased markedly as AIDS patients and their physicians asked for permission to use marijuana to enhance appetite to combat the physical wasting associated with AIDS. However, in 1991 the program was halted because it was at odds with the Bush administration's anti–drug abuse policies. Many AIDS patients were left in the position of having to break the law to use marijuana to fight their physical wasting. As of 1997, a group of physicians and researchers in San Francisco, who have been trying to initiate controlled studies of the clinical effectiveness of marijuana for this purpose, estimates that there are two thousand AIDS patients in San Francisco alone who are currently using marijuana in this way.

Two of the chief concerns about smoked marijuana as a medical treatment are the risk to lung function and the presence of carcinogens. Although cancer patients might use marijuana only once every few weeks, AIDS or glaucoma (see below) patients could use it much more frequently. The proponents of medical usage argue that water pipes would address the concern about the smoke's effect on the lungs to some degree, and that researchers, if allowed, might develop a nonsmoking system for delivering marijuana vapors. For example, it might be possible to extract the therapeutic compounds from marijuana into a fluid suspension delivered with an inhaler. Another concern relates to possible toxic effects to the immune system, particularly in AIDS patients who are already immune-compromised. Although this is a subject of current debate in the medical literature, one large-scale study of HIV-infected men found no evidence that marijuana accelerated the process of immune-system failure.

NAUSEA

One of the more unpleasant side effects of cancer chemotherapy (treatment with drugs to kill the cancer cells) is that the medicines make many people feel quite nauseated. THC clearly helps to control this side effect. In fact, THC has been available since 1985 in capsule form for use by cancer patients under the brand name Marinol (dronabinol), categorized by the DEA under Schedule II. Marinol has been shown to help control nausea and also to help patients gain weight. However, some physicians and patients argue that, compared to marijuana (which they use illegally for the same purpose), Marinol's dosage and duration of effect (because it is taken orally rather than smoked) are harder to control and that it is simply not as effective. This might be so because cannabidiol, a component of natural marijuana that is not present in Marinol, has antianxiety effects that patients find helpful in addition to THC's purely antinausea effects. Proponents argue that until a synthetic THC preparation can be made that truly reproduces the effects of the various cannabinoid compounds in marijuana, marijuana cigarettes should be made available for medical use. A 1990 survey showed that 44 percent of oncologists (cancer specialists) had suggested the use of marijuana to some of their patients to help relieve the side effects of their chemotherapy.

GLAUCOMA

Research in the 1970s found that marijuana significantly reduced the pressure of the fluid within the eye that is too high and potentially damaging in glaucoma patients. At present, however, neither marijuana nor Marinol is used as a treatment.

Marijuana is by no means the only drug that is effective in treating the conditions mentioned above, but there certainly is a strong argument for the value of marijuana as medicine. Multiple sclerosis and other disorders that produce spasticity with impaired muscle control (marijuana works as a muscle relaxant), seizures, chronic pain, and migraine headaches have also been reported to respond positively to marijuana. The proponents of marijuana as medicine point out that it is hard to beat in terms of safety. As we described above, it is next to impossible to overdose on marijuana, and its lack of addictive properties makes it safer on that score than many medicines currently used as muscle relaxants or for pain management.

RECENT LEGISLATIVE ACTIONS

In November 1996 Arizona and California passed propositions related to the medical use of marijuana. In California, *the Compassionate Use Act of 1996* (Proposition 215) passed by a margin of 56 percent to 44 percent. Essentially, the proposition states that patients or defined caregivers who possess or grow marijuana for medical treatment as recommended by a physician are exempt from laws that otherwise prohibit possession or cultivation of marijuana. It also states that physicians who recommend the use of marijuana shall not be punished in any way for doing so. It is important that the language of this proposition is such that marijuana need only be "recommended" by a physician, and that it does not specify the conditions for which it may be recommended. The proposition goes on to state that persons using marijuana for medical purposes can still be held liable if they engage in conduct that endangers others or if they divert marijuana for nonmedical purposes. Still, it is clear from a reading of the proposition that California voters endorsed a very loose interpretation of which uses might be considered "medical."

In Arizona, the Drug Medicalization, Prevention, and Control Act of 1996 (Proposition 200) passed by a vote of 65 percent to 35 percent. This proposition offers a similar bottom line as far as it concerns the medical use of marijuana, but it goes considerably further in that it enables physicians to recommend use of other drugs currently grouped with marijuana under

Schedule 1 of the DEA classification. Schedule 1 drugs include LSD, heroin, and other notorious drugs of abuse. Many people believe that marijuana should not be listed on Schedule 1 in the first place, arguing that it is not addictive and is far less powerful than most of the drugs on the list. Aside from that debate, however, the Arizona proposition has raised serious concerns about other Schedule 1 drugs potentially being used as medicine.

Within two months of the passage of these two propositions, the United States Congress conducted hearings on the issue, and the Clinton administration crafted a response. The Drug Enforcement Administration (a federal agency) has always issued licenses to physicians that allow them to prescribe has controlled substances that are approved for medical use, so that without this DEA license, a physician would be limited in terms of what drugs she could prescribe. To discourage physicians in California and Arizona from recommending marijuana for medical use, the federal government has stated that it may investigate physicians who recommend marijuana and potentially withdraw their DEA licenses. Several physicians, health organizations, and patients have sued the government in response.

Some of the people and agencies who have taken stands against the Arizona and California propositions believe that these are thinly veiled maneuvers toward legalizing drugs. The concern is that once a drug (or a group of drugs) is approved for medical use, the next step could be legalization for nonmedical uses. Whether or not this is a legitimate concern, the potential usefulness of marijuana as medicine, and the initiatives in Arizona and California, have added considerable fuel to another, even more emotional debate: the legalization of marijuana.

THE QUESTION OF LEGALIZATION

The subject of the legal status of marijuana (and all drugs of abuse, for that matter) evokes strong emotional responses. It is important to try to put aside the emotion of the debate and look closely at the issues from a broad perspective, which includes pharmacological, social, and economic viewpoints. The legal status of any drug depends heavily on the culture in which that drug is evaluated and the prevailing social conventions relative to that drug. For example, in the United States today we choose to have marijuana categorized as a Schedule I narcotic, and to keep it illegal, while we allow the sale and advertisement of known addictive drugs such as nicotine and alcohol. Other societies have chosen to prohibit alcohol consumption vigorously while placing little or no sanction on the use of cannabis products. We should recognize the two principle factors that change attitudes and laws about drugs: culture and time.

MARIJUANA IN THE TWENTIETH-CENTURY UNITED STATES

What had been a fascination with marijuana in the nineteenth century among artists and intellectuals was quickly overshadowed in this country by fears about an association between marijuana and crime, particularly violent and sexual crime. Although we now know that there is no such relationship, by the mid-1920s the popular media had seized on this idea and concern began to grow. Although then, as now, there were no scientific data to support the conclusion that the use of marijuana led to violent behavior, by the mid-1930s all the states of the union had laws regulating the use of marijuana. As we mentioned above, even magazines devoted to interpreting the science of the day got on the bandwagon. Both *Popular Science Monthly* and *Scientific American* published articles in 1936 portraying marijuana as a "menace" to American society, particularly to the young.

A major player in elevating marijuana to the status of "national menace" was Harry Anslinger, who served as commissioner of Narcotics in the 1930s. Mr. Anslinger began something of crusade against marijuana, skillfully using congressional testimony, the medical establishment, and the popular media to warn of the dangers of marijuana to American society. He was successful, and in 1937 congressional hearings were held to address the association between marijuana and crime. By this time it was clear that Congress was ready to limit the use and possession of marijuana, and it passed the Marijuana Tax Act of 1937, which did not outlaw marijuana but created a tax structure around the cultivation, distribution, sale, and purchase of cannabis products, which made it virtually impossible to have anything to do with the drug without breaking some part of the tax law.

Interestingly, almost immediately after the passage of the Marijuana Tax Act, the pendulum began to swing the other way. In the early 1940s studies were published that indicated that marijuana was relatively harmless and that any relationship to criminal behavior was likely due to marijuana's association with the use of alcohol, which proved to be the prime cause of aggression. Other studies during that time began to show that although acute marijuana use impaired cognitive function, it did not change the personality of the user, and that it affected thinking and feelings more than behavior. By the late 1960s, when the Marijuana Tax Act was ruled unconstitutional by the United States Supreme Court, Mr. Anslinger's assertions about the relationship between marijuana and violent crime were discredited. Still, marijuana was illegal, and this label alone implied "dangerous" for most people. What has developed since that time has been an interesting tension between a legal status that implies danger and a scientific literature that consistently suggests that marijuana (used in the ways it is generally used) is a relatively safe drug.

Little scientific work was done with marijuana through the 1950s and

1960s, though its use increased. The media during the 1960s increasingly focused on "hard" drugs such as LSD (which was legal until 1966, and placed on Schedule 1 in 1967), while marijuana became a symbol of youthful rejection of "the establishment." The acceleration in marijuana use began in the late 1960s and by the spring of 1970, the National Institute of Mental Health estimated that as many as 20 million individuals had used marijuana at least once.* In December of 1970, the Gallup organization estimated that 42 percent of college students had smoked marijuana. Perhaps the social association between marijuana and hallucinogens during the 1960s can account for its continued inclusion with LSD and heroin under the category of Schedule I narcotics, despite the profound differences in the potency of its effects on (and risks to) individuals. The use of the drug decreased in the 1980s as social and political conservatism grew, but now it is strongly on the rise so far in the 1990s as the perceived risks of using it have again dropped.

THE CONSEQUENCES OF ILLEGALITY

There are two main consequences of the illegality of marijuana: crime and a loss of credibility for the authorities who present marijuana as dangerous. Since people continue to use marijuana and cannot buy it at the corner store with their coffee, cigarettes, and beer, criminal distribution networks have evolved to meet the demand. Growing out of the competition within these networks comes the violent crime so common to our daily news reports in recent years. At the same time, users, by definition, become criminals. We spend a considerable amount of money each year to apprehend, prosecute, and imprison people on marijuana charges. These costly laws have apparently not hindered the marked increase in marijuana use, particularly among young people, during the early 1990s. Clearly, as a society we are not ready to endorse the use of marijuana by selling it in the corner drugstore, but both conservative and liberal sectors are increasingly calling for a dramatic rethinking of marijuana laws and policies.

Aside from the criminal issue, many people feel they have been lied to by the government agencies responsible for educating and interpreting science to the lay public. In the 1960s, as more and more young people tried mari-

---

*Drug use data were not well collected until the 1970s, but this estimate was based on multiple surveys and presented by Stanley Yolles as a "Statement for the National Institute of Mental Health" to the Subcommittee on Public Health and Welfare of the Interstate and Foreign Commerce Committee, U.S. House of Representatives, 91st Congress, 2nd Session, February 4, 1970 (U.S. Government Printing Office, Washington, D.C., 1970, p. 181). This reference and a complete discussion of the issue is presented in Chapter 57 of Licit and Illicit Drugs, by Edward M. Brecher and the editors of Consumer Reports, (Little, Brown and Company, Boston, 1972, p. 422).

juana and discovered that it did not turn them into insane, violent killers, they began to resent and distrust the authorities who had presented those images. Authority began to lose its credibility relative to drugs in those days. Thirty years later, that credibility has not been regained, in part because the scientific truth about marijuana (and other drugs) is often lost among political and moral agendas.

VOICES FOR DECRIMINALIZATION

In 1970, a commission that was formed to take a closer look at marijuana laws recommended that the private possession of small amounts of marijuana for personal use no longer be considered offenses, but that selling marijuana or driving under its influence still be punishable. The same year that that report was released, the American Medical Association and the American Bar Association suggested the reduction or elimination of criminal penalties for possession of very small amounts of marijuana. Soon thereafter, individual states began taking steps to decriminalize marijuana for personal use, and in 1977, President and Mrs. Jimmy Carter called for the decriminalization of possession of small amounts of marijuana. The general view of many who supported decriminalization in the 1970s was that the laws against marijuana were more harmful than the drug itself.

THE SWINGING PENDULUM

The "Reagan Eighties," however, brought a new get-tough attitude to the issue of illegal drug usage. The trends toward decriminalization were abruptly reversed and replaced by the "War on Drugs." States began to reinstitute tougher policies and penalties. During the 1980s the number of people aged eighteen to twenty-five who reported using marijuana steadily decreased while alcohol usage increased and the use of powder, and then crack, cocaine began to skyrocket. Crack is now a major scourge of the urban underclass, and for both pharmacological and social reasons is a major contributor to violent urban crime.

Still, since the early 1990s marijuana use has significantly increased, and this trend appears to be continuing, particularly among young people. In just the two years between 1992 and 1994, the use of marijuana by adolescents twelve to seventeen years of age nearly doubled. Perhaps this is just the pendulum swinging back from the more conservative and reactionary 1980s. Or maybe a new generation of users is now exploring drugs. Cocaine was the drug of the 1980s, a decade that more than a few financial writers refer to as the "Go-go Eighties." Cocaine is clearly a "go-go" drug, whereas marijuana has a considerably more mellowing and contemplative effect, perhaps reflecting a change in the spirit of the times.

WHAT WILL HAPPEN NEXT?

As a society we have much bigger drug problems to deal with than marijuana. A rational and convincing chorus of voices across the political spectrum, including medical and scientific professionals, political pundits, and members of the business community, are urging a restructuring of our legal response to recreational drugs. Some call for total legalization of all drugs, some for less radical changes, but it's clear that something needs to change. The legal debate over marijuana is still complicated. On one hand there are now clear medical uses for the drug, and it obviously does less social and medical harm than our legal drug of choice, alcohol. It is also the leading cash crop in a number of states already, and the revenues from its controlled cultivation, sale, and taxation could be significant, turning the loss of resources for prohibition and prosecution into gains in the legal economy and national and state coffers. Legalization would eliminate the need for a criminal production and distribution network, along with its violent and antisocial consequences.

On the other hand, marijuana is not harmless, as some of its proponents would claim. Just because it is not as harm*ful* as other drugs that are now legal does not mean it should go unregulated. It has relatively long-lasting effects after even a single dose, and the jury is out on whether or not it produces brain damage or increases the risk of lung cancer after heavy and prolonged use. Finally, despite its benign profile relative to other drugs, marijuana is currently illegal and that label alone is a difficult obstacle to overcome in the public (and political) mind.

So, the debate remains open and passionate, but our guess is that all drug laws are going to change significantly in the not-too-distant future and that marijuana laws will be a part of that change. The reform of marijuana laws may also lead the way because, while there aren't many good reasons to legalize a number of other recreational drugs, there are some good reasons to change marijuana laws.

8

Nicotine

Drug Class: No specific class—prescription and nonprescription medication for smoking cessation. Legal for use by adults in any form.

Individual Drugs: tobacco, nicotine chewing gum (Nicorette), nicotine skin patch (NicoDerm), chewing tobacco, snuff, cigarettes, cigars, pipe tobacco

The Buzz: Nicotine is a specific kind of stimulant that increases attention, concentration, and (possibly) memory. Many people also report that nicotine has a calming or antianxiety effect as well.

Overdose and Other Bad Effects: Dangerous overdose from nicotine is quite rare but it is possible. A serious overdose would cause tremors (shaking) and convulsions that could paralyze muscles needed for breathing and kill a person. Less serious nicotine poisoning results in dizziness, weakness, and nausea, which disappear as the drug is eliminated. Many people experience such side effects when they first smoke or when they use nicotine gum for the first time in a smoking-cessation program (the gum delivers quite a bit more nicotine than a cigarette).

As with many drugs, nicotine reaches the fetus in a pregnant woman and can cause permanent damage. If the mother smokes, then the bad effects specific to smoking also impact the fetus.

Dangerous Combinations with Other Drugs: Nicotine powerfully stimulates the heart and circulation. It can cause problems in combination with other drugs that increase heart rate or blood pressure, or that reduce the oxygen-carrying capacity of the blood.

Nicotine and cocaine taken together put far more stress on the heart than either drug alone does. This combination increases the risk of sudden death from heart attack.

CHAPTER CONTENTS

A BRIEF HISTORY

Like many drugs that are used recreationally today, nicotine has a history of being used as medicine. In the 1500s tobacco was used to treat a number of ailments, from headaches to colds. So revered was tobacco for its medicinal properties during that time that it became known as a holy plant. In 1828 French chemists isolated the active ingredient in tobacco and called it nicotine. Although tobacco continued to enjoy rave reviews from some quarters for its supposed medical properties, others were beginning to voice the concern that it might be bad for people's health. By the 1890s nicotine was no longer a compound prescribed as medicine in the United States.

All this was before smoking tobacco became at all popular in the United States. In the mid-1800s the vast majority of tobacco factories produced chewing tobacco rather than tobacco for smoking. It was not until the early 1900s that smoking began to replace chewing, at first in the form of cigars, which provided a transitional opportunity to both chew (the cigar is often left in the mouth, allowing nicotine to be absorbed orally) and smoke at the same time.

Cigarettes did, however, catch on, and per capita sales of cigarettes to adults in the United States reached a peak in the early 1960s when about 40 percent of U.S. adults were smokers. Since then smoking has decreased, and in 1990, only about 25 per cent smoked. This decline is likely due to compelling research showing that smoking causes cancer and other health problems; the use of these research findings in truthful and believable public educational campaigns about smoking; and the ban on TV advertising for cigarettes. Even so, since 1990 the percentage of American adults who smoke has stabilized at around 25 percent and has not declined further since then.

SMOKING BY YOUNG PEOPLE

While older people have stopped smoking, smoking by people under eighteen remains a problem. The number of middle school and high school students who say they have smoked during the past thirty days has been increasing steadily since 1991. In 1991 about 14 percent of eighth graders, 20 percent of tenth graders, and 28 percent of twelfth graders had smoked within the past month. By 1995 those numbers were 19 percent, 27 percent, and 34 percent, respectively. Obviously, a significant proportion of young people are choosing to use cigarettes despite the wealth of information on their negative effects.

Why? We don't know, but it could be a combination of effective non-TV advertising and the sense among many young people that they are not vulnerable to the health effects of cigarettes. They may have a parent or other relative who has suffered those ill effects, but believe that those are "old people." This is a tough point to argue with because the negative health effects *are* relatively far off for the young smoker. But the young person *will* get older, and the time will come when health decisions made in high school may powerfully impact on quality of life. Nicotine is clearly an addictive drug, and it appears that people who start smoking as adolescents put themselves at very high risk for addiction. In fact, almost all addicted smokers started as adolescents. By the time the young smoker begins to think about the future or feel some of the ill effects of smoking, the addiction is probably in place. Quitting is then a problem—not impossible, but a problem.

HOW NICOTINE MOVES THROUGH THE BODY

GETTING IN

The speed and efficiency with which nicotine enters the blood and is transferred to the brain depends very much on how it is administered. When a person smokes tobacco, nicotine is absorbed very rapidly into the blood through
the lungs and passes within seconds to the brain. The amount of nicotine in
a typical cigarette is enough to kill a child or make an adult very sick, but because not all of it gets into the blood through the lungs—most of it is lost in
exhaled or uninhaled smoke—a cigarette does not threaten an overdose.

If a person takes nicotine by mouth in the form of snuff (smokeless tobacco), the absorption of nicotine may be more complete than it is with smoking, but the dose is delivered over a much longer period of time. For example,
the typical dose of nicotine from a cigarette is about 1 milligram. However, a
plug of snuff maintained in the mouth continuously for thirty minutes delivers a dose in the 3- to 5-milligram range. The mucous membranes of the
mouth are a good site for absorption because a lot of blood flows nearby, but
the process is still much slower there than it is in the lungs. So, while snuff delivers a larger total dose over time than a cigarette does, they both result in
about the same peak concentration of nicotine in the blood.

Nicotine gum delivers less nicotine than snuff. Even if it is chewed for
thirty minutes continuously, nicotine gum generally delivers only about 1.5
milligrams of nicotine.

Cigars present an interesting case in nicotine absorption, because generally
the smoker doesn't inhale. Although some of the smoke still makes it to the
lungs, most of it comes into contact with membranes in the mouth and upper
airways, across which nicotine can be absorbed. How much nicotine gets absorbed through the direct contact of the cigar tobacco with the mouth depends
largely on the style of smoking. Those folks who stick a cigar in their mouth
and leave it there until the end looks like the end of a dipstick from an old lawn
mower engine will absorb much more nicotine through the mouth than those
who hold the cigar in their hand and puff intermittently.

GETTING AROUND

Once nicotine is absorbed, how is it distributed? Again, this depends on how
it is taken. Smoking a cigarette results in a peak concentration in the lungs,
blood, and brain within about ten minutes. But these concentrations decline
rapidly as nicotine is redistributed to other body tissues. Twenty minutes after
smoking, the nicotine concentration in the blood and brain is down to half of
what it had been just ten minutes earlier. With snuff the distribution is slower,

but the peak nicotine concentrations are quite similar to those obtained after smoking a cigarette.

GETTING OUT

Studies on animals that have very closely followed the concentrations of nicotine in the brain have shown very high levels five minutes after administration, declining to near nothing thirty minutes later. Nicotine's rapid absorption from the lungs, coupled with this pattern of distribution to the brain, allow the smoker a lot of control over the peaks and valleys of nicotine exposure. In this sense, cigarettes offer a very effective drug delivery system.

These characteristics also set up the smoker for addiction in two ways. First, nicotine's rapid route to the brain provides a quick and potent hit. Second, the rapid redistribution out of the brain means that the brain areas that control the behaviors associated with smoking are ready for more nicotine soon after the smoker finishes the last cigarette.

After nicotine is absorbed and distributed throughout the body, the liver breaks most of it down into two inactive metabolites, cotinine and nicotine-N-oxide. The kidneys eliminate these metabolites through the urine. Cotinine is the marker used in urine screens for nicotine because it stays in the body for several days.

EFFECTS ON THE BRAIN

Before the 1980s it was not at all clear how nicotine affected the brain. We now know that nicotine stimulates a specific subtype of receptor for the neurotransmitter acetylcholine—the *nicotinic acetylcholinergic receptor*. These receptors are distributed rather widely on nerve cells throughout the brain, so nicotine has effects on a wide variety of brain structures. In general, it excites nerve cells and increases cell-to-cell signaling. Several studies have shown that nicotine increases the activity in brain regions that are associated with memory and other mental functions, as well as in some structures involved with physical movement.

When acetylcholine receptors in the brain are blocked, animals (and people) have a difficult time remembering new information. Conversely, some reports show that stimulating these receptors improves memory somewhat. Since nicotine promotes the release of acetylcholine and also activates its own subtype of acetylcholine receptors, some investigators have predicted that nicotine might enhance memory function. While this has not been proven, studies are under way to determine if nicotine can help patients with memory deficits, like those with early Alzheimer's disease.

IS NICOTINE ADDICTIVE?

Yes. There is currently discussion about this question as the FDA considers regulating nicotine as a drug. Cigarette companies find themselves under fire for allegedly manipulating nicotine content. Any honest and thorough appraisal of the scientific and medical literature on nicotine must conclude that this is a drug that causes physical dependence and addiction. At least three related lines of evidence lead to this conclusion.

REINFORCEMENT

In the language of psychology, a reinforcer is something that motivates an individual to work toward getting more. Nicotine is known to promote the release of the neurotransmitter dopamine in brain regions that mediate reinforcement (see the "Addiction" and "Stimulants" chapters). It is not surprising, then, that animals will work for nicotine. When rats have the opportunity to press a bar in order to self-administer small doses of nicotine, they will do so.

Humans, too, will work for nicotine once they have been smoking for a while. In fact, all smokers do, given that they spend their money on cigarettes. The willingness to work for them was typified in an old advertisement for cigarettes that centered on the phrase "I'd walk a mile for a Camel."

TOLERANCE

Studies have demonstrated the rapid development of tolerance to the effects of nicotine. When people begin to smoke they experience a range of rather unpleasant effects, such as dizziness or nausea, but these disappear over days or weeks as the smoker continues to smoke. Tolerance to other effects of nicotine develops even more rapidly. For example, when a group of smokers was given two equal doses of nicotine sixty minutes apart, they experienced more pronounced elevations of their heart rates and reported greater subjective effects from the first dose compared to the second.

WITHDRAWAL

On reporting for his first morning of smoking-cessation treatment after a required day of abstinence, one of my patients summed up his feelings by saying, "I want to hurt something." As I scanned the room for sharp objects I realized that he was in nicotine withdrawal. Although not all smokers are so extreme (or honest) in their feelings soon after quitting, most report powerful cravings and irritability during the first two to three weeks after their last cigarette. These are clearly symptoms of withdrawal.

As with tolerance, withdrawal from nicotine has both short- and long-term aspects. For example, most smokers report that their first cigarette of the day is the one that makes them feel best. This effect can be seen as the termination of a miniwithdrawal after the overnight abstinence.

SUBJECTIVE EFFECTS

Although nicotine, particularly as administered by smoking, is clearly addictive, it also clearly differs from many other addictive substances. It lacks the obvious mind-altering effects of alcohol, stimulants, or opiates. People don't use nicotine because it provides a rush or a high. Rather, most users report that it calms them and reduces anxiety. But even these effects are more complicated than they may seem.

Since the vast majority of nicotine users obtain it by smoking, we should consider the effects of smoking as a particular kind of drug delivery. Many people derive considerable comfort and calming from small personal habits or rituals—such as tapping a foot or humming to themselves—and many such habits become *associated* with nicotine delivery during smoking. Lighting up, holding the cigarette, moving it to and from the mouth and puffing—any or all of these small rituals could calm the smoker in and of themselves and become associated with the pharmacological effects of nicotine. Adding these habits to nicotine delivery makes it hard to determine what role the nicotine alone plays in the reported calming effect. Another consideration is that the people who report the antianxiety and calming effects of smoking are most often people who have been smoking for a while. Thus, it is hard to know whether the calming is a primary effect of nicotine or simply the reduction of an addicted person's craving.

Another commonly reported effect of smoking is the suppression of appetite. Again, it is not clear if this effect is principally due to the nicotine or the smoking, but animal studies show that nicotine can reduce eating when it is given in the absence of smoke. In humans, smoking one cigarette has been shown to diminish hunger contractions in the stomach. It is also possible that the appetite is suppressed in part because smoking reduces the function of the taste buds in the mouth. Other possibilities include the effects of smoking on energy metabolism and blood-sugar levels. The fact is that we do not know exactly why smoking suppresses appetite, but it seems clear that for some people it does. Of course, there is another side to this coin: when a smoker quits smoking, his appetite often increases and he gains weight. This could be due to the effects of the physical withdrawal of nicotine from the system or to the need to replace the oral habits associated with the act of smoking.

EFFECTS ON MENTAL FUNCTION

In recent years a number of studies have suggested that nicotine may enhance mental function. This early work was promising enough that some studies were initiated involving people in the early stages of Alzheimer's disease to determine if nicotine might improve their failing memory capacity. In such studies researchers generally administer nicotine either by injecting it or by using a patch that allows it to be absorbed slowly through the skin. Although it's still uncertain whether nicotine may be of use to Alzheimer's patients, some convincing studies show that nicotine does improve some mental functions for at least a brief time after its use. In a study that used the nicotine patch, the Alzheimer's patients showed increased capacity for learning verbal material while exposed to nicotine. With nicotine injections, some patients experienced an enhancement of short-term acquisition of memory as well as improved attention and concentration.

This does not mean, however, that a person should smoke cigarettes or chew nicotine gum while studying or during an exam or other activity that demands concentration or memory. The carbon monoxide in the cigarette, combined with the lack of oxygen exchange in the lungs due to the smoke, would likely lead to other side effects, such as dizziness, which could easily overpower any potential attention- or memory-enhancing effects of the nicotine. In addition, chewing nicotine gum often delivers enough nicotine to make even experienced smokers feel nauseated the first time or two.

Another potential medical use for nicotine is in the treatment of adult attention deficit hyperactivity disorder (ADHD). Although work on this problem is just beginning, one study indicates that nicotine patch treatments reduce ADHD symptoms in both smokers and nonsmokers.

Although these studies appear promising and may lead to more effective treatments for these disorders, it is critical to remember three things. First, the studies we mentioned are very recent and have not yet led to any routine medical uses for nicotine. Second, several of the studies have involved *injections* of nicotine, which, of course, should never be undertaken without medical supervision. Third, those results should *never* be interpreted as a reason to smoke. The health costs of smoking far outweigh any potential health benefits of nicotine.

SMOKING AND EMOTIONAL FUNCTION

A recent study has shown that adolescents who are smokers are twice as likely as nonsmoking adolescents to suffer an episode of major depression, and that teens with long-term depression were more likely to be smokers than teens without depression. Although these findings do not tell us *why* a teen smoker is more likely to become depressed or vice versa, they may provide valuable warning signals. A young person who has problems with depression may be at higher risk than normal for smoking, and it may be wise for such people to take special care to avoid situations in which smoking is prevalent. Likewise, a teen who smokes may be more susceptible to depression and should watch for early signs of it so that antidepressive treatment can be started, if necessary.

EFFECTS ON THE HEART

It is well known that smoking causes lung cancer and other chronic lung diseases. What is less well known is that smoking also contributes to diseases of the heart and vascular system, which actually kill more people in the United States annually than any cancer. Nicotine affects the heart in several ways. The heart is a big muscle, and like all muscles it needs a rich supply of oxygen to do its work pumping blood throughout the rest of the body. When nicotine is in the system, it results in the release of adrenaline, which increases heart rate and blood pressure. The heart then needs more oxygen in order to increase its workload, but its oxygen supply doesn't increase, so it must do extra work with no extra help.

What's worse, the carbon monoxide in smoke also decreases the ability of the blood to carry oxygen, making the situation even more stressful for the heart. Repeatedly stressing the heart in these ways leads to damage and compromises its function. The newest data also suggest that cigarette smoke is directly toxic to the inner lining of the blood vessels. Something in the smoke makes them hard and inflexible, adding to the cardiovascular problems. It is estimated that as many as 30 percent of the deaths attributed to heart and vascular disease relate to smoking.

All of these negative effects on heart and circulatory functions may have another, less dangerous, but unwanted effect. Smokers develop thinner skins. A 1997 study of identical twins in which one twin smoked and one did not showed that the smokers had skin that was thinner than that of their twin siblings. Investigators think that this may be why some smokers tend to have more wrinkles and look older than they are. One possible explanation for this effect on the skin is that smoking can decrease the blood supply to the topmost layer of the skin and thus damage it.

SECONDHAND AND SIDESTREAM SMOKE

There are two sources of smoke from cigarette smokers: the smoke they exhale (secondhand) and the smoke rising off of the lit cigarette, cigar, or pipe itself (sidestream). It is worth knowing that sidestream smoke has a higher concentration of carcinogens than either secondhand smoke or the smoke that a smoker takes into his lungs through a cigarette filter. Whatever the source, smoke can cause disease. The Environmental Protection Agency, after considerable study of this issue, determined that secondhand smoke is indeed a carcinogen in and of itself and is responsible for a significant number of lung cancer deaths each year in the United States. Of course, the amount of exposure to secondary smoke is a critical factor in the risk of developing lung disease (as is the smoker's own amount of exposure), and a few parties in smoky rooms will probably not kill anyone. However, people who spend a lot of time in smoky places, like bars, or who live with smokers are clearly placing themselves at some risk for lung disease.

The effects of secondhand smoke on the development of heart disease is even more alarming. A ten-year study published in 1997 shows that regular exposure to secondhand smoke can double a person's risk of heart disease. This study of more than thirty thousand women suggests that as many as fifty thousand people may die each year in the United States as a result of heart attacks related to secondhand-smoke exposure.

PRENATAL AND POSTNATAL EFFECTS

As with most drugs, nicotine passes to the fetus in the blood of the pregnant woman who smokes (or otherwise uses nicotine). Babies born to smoking moms have recently been shown to have levels of cotinine in their urine that are nearly as high as those of active smokers. As time passes after birth and their nicotine levels fall, these babies show symptoms of nicotine deprivation. The pregnant smoker also passes along cyanide and carbon monoxide to her baby, both of which are very bad for the developing fetus. Remember that carbon monoxide reduces the ability of blood to carry oxygen and thereby depletes body tissues of oxygen. Also, nicotine constricts blood vessels bringing blood to the fetus, further limiting oxygen supply. In the fetus, this oxygen depletion is thought to account for the fact that babies born to smoking mothers are smaller, lighter, and have smaller head circumferences than babies born to nonsmoking mothers. In addition, as with alcohol, smoking during pregnancy likely has lasting (perhaps permanent) effects on the brain and mental function of the child after birth. Some studies have linked maternal smoking with difficulties in verbal and mathematical abilities and hyperactivity during childhood.

Once a baby is born, an immense amount of brain development is still going on. Exposure of babies and small children to secondary smoke should also be avoided. For example, some studies have suggested that there is an increased risk of sudden infant death syndrome (SIDS) in babies of smoking mothers and that this could be due to smoke in the environment. It is also possible that this could be due to damage that the baby suffered before birth due to the mother's smoking or to the combination of prenatal and postnatal exposure.

Recent research also indicates that the children of fathers who smoke are more likely to develop childhood cancers than children of nonsmoking dads. Based on the Oxford Survey of Childhood Cancers, the study of some three thousand parents showed that fathers who smoked twenty or more cigarettes per day had a 42 percent increased risk of having a child with cancer, and that those who smoked ten to twenty cigarettes per day increased the risk by 31 percent. The risk was increased by 3 percent for fathers who smoked less than ten cigarettes per day. These results suggest that smoking may damage sperm in ways that could lead to cancer-causing alterations of the DNA.

The message is very clear—smoking and babies just don't mix.

HEALTH RISKS OF SMOKELESS TOBACCO

We should also stress that the chewing of tobacco and snuff represent significant health risks in their own right. In addition to the nicotine they deliver, their prolonged use can increase the likelihood of cancers of the mouth and esophagus. Many users develop thickening lesions in the mouth that may develop into cancer of those tissues. Smokeless tobacco also causes gum disease, which can result in inflamed and receding gums and can expose the teeth to disease. In short, smokeless tobacco is not a safe substitute for smoking.

QUITTING

Not so many years ago, the prevailing wisdom was that the ability to quit smoking was a matter of simple willpower. This attitude implied that smoking was not *really* an addiction, that no special techniques were required for quitting, and that one who could not quit simply lacked the internal fortitude to do so. We now know that none of this is true. Nicotine is an addictive drug, and quitting is a complicated change of behavior that is not easy.

Many former smokers report having quit on their own, but there are also plenty of treatments available to help. Unfortunately, there is no one treatment that works for everyone. Probably because the behavioral *habits* of smoking are tied up with the physiological addiction to nicotine, many people require a number of different treatment strategies to address the whole problem. On the behavioral side, these can include educational counseling, group or individual smoking-cessation training, hypnosis, or stress-management training. On the medical side, they can include the use of nicotine chewing gum or nicotine skin patches. Also, a medication called Zyban, which was previously used as an antidepressant under the name Wellbutrin, has recently been approved for use in smoking cessation.

With all these options, how does one choose? The best first step is to get a referral from a physician, psychologist, or pharmacist to an established smoking-cessation program. Sometimes these are run in hospitals or clinics, but they may also be operated as part of a community mental health clinic or by a private practitioner. In any case, the people in charge of the program should be trained professionals prepared to discuss the various options in detail.

The bad news is that although most of these programs can help people to quit for a brief time, many people return to smoking within six months. It appears that programs that use multiple approaches (such as behavior training and hypnosis) have a somewhat better record of keeping people off cigarettes longer than single-method programs do. Still many people in multiple-approach programs return to smoking within a year. Why is this the case? We're not sure, but it probably has to do with how much behavioral habit the act of smoking involves, and how many places, people, and things out in the real world the smoker has associated with the act of smoking over the years. The very uncomfortable cravings for nicotine diminish rapidly within days of quitting, and nicotine gum or skin patches can help during this time. The first few days are clearly the worst, but most people report that by about two weeks the cravings are mostly gone. What remain are all the cues that used to be associated with smoking—the morning cup of coffee, the evening beer, the talk with a friend on a break at work, the after-dinner smoke (the list can go on and on).

These are powerful stimuli that can exert considerable control over behavior. Many people will report that they felt well on their way to really kicking the habit when an old friend with whom they used to smoke came back for a visit, or that they went back to a bar where they used to smoke and drink and have fun, and before they knew it, the cigarette was back in their hand. A smoking-cessation program must anticipate these situations and provide strategies for dealing with them. It's a valuable help to schedule follow-up sessions to talk such things over, learn strategies, and get support. This can be particularly helpful because it has been shown that stressful conditions can lead to relapse as well.

One final point on quitting: if at first you don't succeed, try again. Every person is different and every addiction is different. If trying on one's own did not work, a treatment program might. If one treatment program did not work, a different one might. Enough types of help are available that there is a good chance one will work for any motivated person who wants to quit smoking.

9

■

Opiates

Drug Class: Opiate analgesics

Individual Drugs: opium, heroin, morphine, codeine, hydromorphone (Dilaudid), oxycodone (Percodan), meperidine (Demerol), diphenoxylate (Lomotil), hydrocodone (Vicodin), fentanyl (Sublimaze), propoxyphene (Darvon)

Common Terms: Chinese molasses, dreams, gong, O, skee, toys, zero (opium); Big H, dreck, horse, mojo, smack, white lady, brown (heroin), speedballs (opiates and cocaine)

The Buzz: People who inject opiates experience a rush of pleasure, then sink into a dreamy, pleasant state in which they have little sensitivity to pain. Their breathing slows, and their skin may flush. Pinpoint pupils are another hallmark of opiate effects. Opiates taken by ways other than injection have the same effect, except that a pleasant drowsiness replaces the rush. Nausea and vomiting can accompany these effects, as well as constipation. An injected heroin/cocaine combination (speedball) causes intense euphoria, the dreaminess of heroin, and the stimulation of cocaine.

Overdose and Other Bad Effects: Opiate overdose can be lethal. This is not a cumulative effect of years of misuse, but can happen the first time you take the drug. Breathing simply slows to the point that it ceases. Fortunately, hospital emergency rooms can offer a rapid and completely effective treatment for opiate overdose: the opiate antagonist naloxone (Narcan) can reverse the dangerous effects of opiates. Opiate overdoses are most common with injectable forms of drug, but can occur with any dosage form if enough is taken. Medical attention is critical.

Dangerous Combinations with Other Drugs: Opiates are especially dangerous when used in combination with other drugs that suppress breathing. These include alcohol, barbiturates (e.g., phenobarbital), Quaaludes (methaqualone), and Valium-like drugs (benzodiazepines).

CHAPTER CONTENTS

WHERE OPIATES CAME FROM

No less a cultural icon than Dorothy of *The Wizard of Oz* has experienced the effects of opiates (remember the field of poppies?). As was apparent in *The Wizard of Oz*, you pretty much have to lack a brain to resist the effects of opiates. For those with a more classical bent, morphine derives its name from Morpheus, the Greek god of dreams, who was often depicted with a handful of opium poppies. Use of opiates began in prehistoric times, probably with teas prepared from opium poppies. The oldest historical references to the medicinal use of opiates arise from the Sumerian and Assyrian/Babylonian cultures (about four thousand years ago). The smoking of opium has been documented between 1000 and 300 B.C. from opium-smoking pipes recovered from archeological sites in Asia, Egypt, and Europe. Arab traders introduced opiates to China between A.D. 600 and A.D. 900. Paralleling developments in Europe, medical use gradually evolved into recreational use and the numbers of opium addicts grew. The importation of opium into China became a major source of trade for England, and helped start a war between China and England when China banned this importation in the early nineteenth century.

Use (and abuse) in Europe was popularized during the Middle Ages. One agent of its popularity was Paracelsus, who coined the term *laudanum* for an opiate preparation, meaning "to be praised." Later, many of our favorite poets (Samuel Taylor Coleridge, Elizabeth Barrett Browning, among others) used and abused opium. Coleridge reported an opium experience in his famous "Kubla Khan."

Opium has been used widely in the United States throughout its history. It was popular long before the wave of Chinese immigration introduced opium smoking to this country. Since opium was a major ingredient in many of the patent medicines available before the FDA was started, the average housewife was a major consumer. As in the story of cocaine, the rising availability of increasingly potent preparations led to greater recognition of the drug's toxicity and addictive qualities.

In 1805, morphine, the major active ingredient in the opium poppy, was purified; in 1853 the invention of the hypodermic syringe followed. The first major wave of addiction to injectable narcotics resulted from the wide use of injected morphine during the American Civil War. The final improvement came courtesy of the Bayer Company in 1898, when the company's scientists discovered a way to add an extra chemical group into morphine to make it more soluble in fat, so that it would enter the brain faster. This improvement produced heroin.

WHAT OPIATES ARE

Opiate drugs are any drugs, natural or synthetic, that produce the characteristic opiate actions: the combination of a dreamy, euphoric state, lessened sensation of pain, slowed breathing, constipation, and pinpoint pupils.

Opium refers to a preparation of the opium poppy *(Papaver somniferum)*. It is obtained in a very low-tech, labor-intensive manner throughout the world. Opium farmers cut the developing seed pod of the opium poppy and collect the gummy fluid that oozes out of the cut over the next few days. The sap is refined in several ways. It may be dried into a ball and used directly (gum opium), or dried and pounded into a powder (opium powder). Raw opium appears as a brown tarry substance. Opium can also be made into an alcohol-water extract that is called tincture of opium. This is the famous laudanum of your great-great-grandmother's era, or the paregoric of that age.

The easiest way to develop a clinically useful drug is to use naturally occurring compounds, and pharmacologists have done just that with the opium poppy. There are at least five important opiate analgesics that are either direct products of the seed pod or minor modifications of it.

Morphine is a major constituent of the seed pod. This is a potent opiate, and is used in injectable form after surgery or in pill form. Codeine, on the other hand, is a much less potent opiate, and is used mainly in pill form for milder pain. Many people have encountered it as a Tylenol-codeine preparation that is used commonly for dental pain or in prescription cough medicine (Robitussin A-C, terpin hydrate with codeine, cheracol, etc.). Despite the lower potency of codeine, a four-ounce bottle does contain enough for a pleasurable experience. These cough syrups used to be available over-the-counter until recreational use became too popular. Now most states require a prescription for codeine-containing cough syrups.

Other compounds are prepared by chemically modifying substances in the opium. These are hydromorphone, oxycodone, and hydrocodone. Hydromorphone (Dilaudid), a very strong opiate, is an effective analgesic that is widely abused. Oxycodone is synthesized from a nonanalgesic in opium (thebaine) and ranks intermediate between morphine and codeine in its effectiveness against pain. It is marketed in combination with aspirin under the prescription name Percodan. Hydrocodone (Vicodin) is a moderately strong opiate which has recently been "discovered" and is now widely abused.

And, of course, there is heroin, the most infamous product of the opium poppy. It is usually provided in bags of loose powder. In the United States, the basic unit of illegal consumption is a clear plastic bag containing about 100 milligrams of white powder. The actual color can range from white to brown. The user either snorts the powder directly or dissolves it in saline and injects it. The actual composition of the powder depends upon the supplier and can range from 10 to 60 percent heroin (in combination) with various contaminants, including talc, quinine, and baking powder, making up the balance.

Ironically enough, heroin is one product that has defied the normal course of economics, having improved in quality as the price has fallen. The purity of heroin supplied in the open market has increased in recent years to the point that the powder can be smoked or snorted and enough can be absorbed to provide a high. The national average purity of heroin seized by the police has increased from 3.6 percent in 1980 to 37 percent in 1992, with some markets reporting purity of 60 to 70 percent.

As mentioned above, heroin is actually just morphine that has been slightly changed chemically. In fact, once heroin enters the brain, it is converted back to morphine. However, the improved fat solubility gets heroin into the brain faster. Many physicians are lobbying for its use in terminal cancer patients due to this difference in clinical effect. The government may well base its decision, however, not just on medical benefit but on the long and unpopular legal history of this compound.

Have scientists improved upon mother nature? The answer is probably no, but they certainly have diversified. The original hope was to find a drug that would eliminate pain but not cause tolerance or addiction. That mission has been unsuccessful, as all the effective opiate analgesic drugs are also addictive. However, the attempt has led to some alternative man-made opiates with very desirable characteristics for particular clinical uses.

Meperidine (Demerol) is an opiate that is used like morphine for intense postsurgical pain. Its advantage is that it works orally or by injection (unlike morphine, which really is most effective after injection). Meperidine has a definite downside: it can cause seizures at high doses. Methadone is a uniquely long-lasting opiate that can be taken in pill form. It offers a treatment for opiate addiction. Methadone provides a sort of surrogate that replaces illegally obtained, intravenously injected heroin with an active drug that keeps the addict from going through withdrawal. But its gradual and mild onset of action also keeps the addict from getting high. Methadone also can offer relief from chronic pain, although tolerance and physical dependence clearly develop. Doctors must weigh this against the potential benefits. Fentanyl (Sublimaze) is a *very* fat-soluble, *very* fast-acting analgesic that anesthesiologists use when they put patients to sleep. It is also used in patches that release the drug slowly through the skin to provide more long-lasting pain relief. In its injectable form, fentanyl is also used by many drug addicts, and commonly causes overdose. Fentanyl's high comes on fast, and is intense, brief, and just a step away from fatal suppression of breathing. Finally, there is propoxyphene (Darvon). This drug is such a poor opiate that many clinical studies find it to be no more effective than a placebo. However, some people swear by it, although it's really little stronger than aspirin.

The differences among these drugs are in how quickly they reach their site of action (the opiate receptors), and then in how much it takes to activate the receptors (potency). All the opiate drugs bind to the same molecule in the brain. However, they do so with varying degrees of success. Below is a list of drugs that bind very well, bind okay, and bind poorly. The clinical use of these drugs is determined in large part by this characteristic. Obviously, a drug like codeine won't do much good with the pain associated with major abdominal surgery, and hydromorphone would be overdoing it for a simple headache. Therefore, the form in which each of these is prepared and administered is tailored to its typical use.

OPIATE DRUGS

High Efficacy	*Medium Efficacy*	*Low Efficacy*
morphine	hydrocodone	codeine
hydromorphone	oxycodone	propoxyphene
meperidine		
fentanyl		

HOW PEOPLE TAKE OPIATES

Most opiate drugs are easily absorbed into the body from many different routes, mainly because they dissolve in fatty substances and so can cross into cells. Snorting heroin works because it can be absorbed across the mucosal lining of the nose. Most other opiates cannot be absorbed well after snorting. However, some opiates can form a vapor if heated, so they can be absorbed into the body if they are smoked. This was the basis of the historical "opium pipe" with which opium was administered in the early history of the United States and in Asia and Europe. Almost all opiates can be absorbed from the stomach, although injection is a much more efficient route for some, like morphine, that are more poorly absorbed from the stomach than others.

Until recently, the most common route for recreational use of opiates was injection. Since intravenous injection is more difficult and more dangerous than other routes, many users do not start this way. Instead, they start by skin-popping—injecting drugs subcutaneously (just beneath the skin). Heroin powder is dissolved and injected. Morphine, fentanyl, and meperidine almost always appear as legally prepared injection forms that have been diverted from medical use, although there is some fentanyl production from underground laboratories. Recently, snorting heroin has replaced injection, especially by new drug users. In part, users are avoiding the stigma—and risk of AIDS—that come with injecting a drug. In part, they may believe—mistakenly—that they cannot become addicted if they don't inject drugs. Codeine and propoxyphene are the preparations most often used orally. Among the stronger opiates, hydromorphone (Dilaudid), oxycodone (Percodan), meperidine (Demerol), and, of course, methadone (Dolophine) are available as pills. Sometimes drug users resort to grinding up pills of codeine, hydrocodone, or methadone and injecting the suspension in desperation if they cannot get opiates any other way. This is an extremely risky business, as the other pill components were not designed to dissolve in saline, or to be injected directly into the bloodstream. Injecting particles into a blood vessel can irritate the blood vessel, thus setting off a chain of reactions that leads to vascular in-flammation and permanent damage. In addition, the pill particle can lodge in a small vessel and block off the blood supply to an area of the body.

GETTING OFF, COMING DOWN: ABSORPTION AND ELIMINATION

The rate at which opiates enter the body depend mainly on how they are ad-ministered. The fastest and most popular way to get high is to inject the drug directly into the bloodstream. The second fastest is to smoke it. When opiates are smoked or injected, peak levels in the brain occur within minutes, al-though the time varies a little from drug to drug. Fentanyl is the most fat-soluble, and achieves maximum brain concentrations in seconds (hence its popularity). Heroin is a little slower; it takes a couple of minutes. Morphine is slower still (five minutes), but not by much. The faster the buzz, the greater the danger of death by overdose, since drug levels in the brain can rise so quickly. Heroin that has been snorted is absorbed more slowly than after in-jection because the drug must travel through the mucous membranes of the nose to the blood vessels beneath.

How about after taking a pill? Here, the high is a much slower proposition, as the drug must be absorbed from the small intestine into the bloodstream, then pass through the liver, which can metabolize much of a dose, before it ever gets into the circulation. This all takes about thirty minutes, so there's no rush after oral administration. In fact, the absence of this rush provides some of the basis for the utility of methadone as a heroin treatment.

There is much less diversity in how long this buzz lasts than in how quickly it starts. Most of the drugs mentioned above last for four to six hours. The exact duration of action may vary from two hours (morphine) up to six or so (propoxyphene), but all opiates are pretty similar. There are only two main ex-ceptions. Methadone lasts for twelve to twenty-four hours, so it can be given as a single daily dose. Fentanyl goes to the other extreme: the effects are over within an hour.

OPIATE EFFECTS ON THE BRAIN

"Morphine hits the backs of the legs first, then the back of the neck, a spread-ing wave of relaxation slackening the muscle away from the bones so that you seem to float without outlines, like lying in warm salt water. As this relaxing wave spread through my tissues, I experienced a strong feeling of fear. I had the feeling that some horrible image was just beyond the field of vision, moving, as I turned my head so that I never quite saw it. I felt nauseous. A series of pictures passed, like watching a movie: a huge neon-lighted cocktail bar that got larger and larger until streets, traffic and street repairs were included in it; a waitress carrying a skull on a tray; stars in the clear sky. The physical impact of the fear of death; the shutting off of breath; the stopping of blood. I dozed off and woke up with a start of fear. Next morning I vomited and felt sick until noon." The character in William Burroughs's novel *Junkie* describes his first experience with morphine fairly accurately. The only thing missing from this description is the rush that comes with intravenous injection that most users compare to orgasm.

All opiates cause a pleasant, drowsy state in which all cares are forgotten (nodding off), and there is a decreased sensation of pain (analgesia). The feelings are the most intense after injection, which brings the rush. After the orgasmic feeling, usually sexual feelings diminish, and people experience decreased sexual desire and performance. This happens because opiates affect the release of many hormones and neurotransmitters, including those involved in the regulation of sexual behavior. People under the influence of opiates will often say that they just don't worry about their troubles anymore: they are in a special, safe place where cares are forgotten. The allure is understandable, and at the beginning it is impossible to understand the misery of addiction and withdrawal.

OPIATE EFFECTS ON THE REST OF THE BODY

So, what is going on below while the opiate user is in a dreamy, pleasant state? Breathing slows, pupils are constricted, and many users experience nausea and perhaps even vomit. Although the effects on breathing can be quite dangerous, the other physiologic effects are fairly benign. For example, opiates do not produce big changes in blood pressure in healthy individuals. Most of the effects are caused by the way opiates act on the brain, specifically on opiate receptors in the parts of the brain involved with the control of breathing and other involuntary functions. For example, opiate users vomit because morphine stimulates a center in the brain (the chemoreceptor trigger zone) whose job it is to cause vomiting in response to ingestion of a toxic substance. So, in the movie *Pulp Fiction*, the injection of adrenaline into the heart to reverse opiate overdose was *not accurate*. The effects on breathing that were causing the woman to OD were mediated in the brain, and injecting a drug directly into the heart to get it started again were good theater, but bad pharmacology. Injecting an opiate receptor blocking drug (naloxone, or Narcan) into the bloodstream instead would have effectively treated the OD.

One very important effect of opiates *is* caused by its actions in the body, and this fact has made life easier for generations of foreign travelers. Opiates increase the tension in certain muscles in the gastrointestinal tract so much that the normal propulsive movements that move food along cannot operate effectively, hence their well-known ability to cause constipation. This can be a good thing if you are in Mexico and have traveler's diarrhea. Diphenoxylate (Lomotil) utilizes a neat chemical trick to stop diarrhea without affecting the brain. This is a very safe, very effective medicine that numerous pharmaceutical companies have tried to improve upon with little success, and indeed it is widely used to treat mild diarrhea. Through a similar action, opiates constrict the muscles of the urinary bladder, and can cause difficulties in urination.

HOW OPIATES WORK IN THE BRAIN

The unique efforts of the opium poppy to make opium alkaloids may reflect ingenious plant evolution to match the biology of their predator/pollinators. The poppy plant figured out how to make a compound that acted on a class of neurotransmitter receptors in the brains of mammals. Opiates act by binding to specific receptor molecules for the endorphin/enkephalin class of neurotransmitters in the brain. These endogenous opioids are among the chemical neurotransmitters that control movement, moods, and physiology. They help to control many bodily activities, including digestion, regulation of body temperature, and breathing. They also seem to be involved in the function of the reward circuits (see "Addiction" chapter), which is why stimulating them makes you high. When you think of it, the ability of a plant to produce a substance that induces such a unique and, perhaps, pleasurable state is amazing. The poppy is not alone, as the marijuana plant, as well as the mushroom *Amanita muscaria*, both make psychoactive compounds.

Many different neurons in different parts of the brain release endorphins or enkephalins, but normally each neuron is simply doing its job, firing away only if stimulated by other neurons. So, activation of all the endogenous opioid neurons virtually never happens. Taking heroin is like every endogenous opioid neuron in the brain firing all at once.

Which of the many endogenous opioid neurons in the brain are responsible for this high? The first is a small group of neurons in the hypothalamus of the brain. The neurons that use the main endorphin neurotransmitter beta-endorphin all start here, and they spread out throughout the brain. There is a theory that these neurons are activated during extremely intense stress, with the purpose of calming us down. The theorists speculate that in the body's most extreme time of stress, when it is on the verge of death, a sense of calm relaxation is about all that is called for. The beta-endorphin neurons fire like crazy and induce an opioid-like pleasant state. This is a great hypothesis, and we are part of the way toward proving that beta-endorphin can do this. We do know that injecting beta-endorphin in the brain creates many aspects of this state, including slowed breathing, analgesia, and a drowsiness.

The enkephalins are a different story. Many different kinds of neurons use enkephalins to communicate with other cells. They appear in parts of the brain involved in processing painful sensations, controlling breathing, and other actions influenced by the opiates. They are also found in the gastrointestinal tract, where they regulate digestive function. Most important, they are found in several places involved in the reward system, and may be important there. However, they probably do not function as a cohesive unit the way the endorphin neurons seem to occur.

Endorphins and enkephalins seem to be different members of a closely related "family" of neurotransmitters that have similarities in structure. There is a third member of the family, the dynorphins, which share some actions, like analgesia, but actually cause unpleasant rather than pleasant feelings. These three neurotransmitters share receptors. This is perhaps a resourceful evolutionary trick played by the brain to get the most "bang for the buck" out of neurotransmitters and their receptors. By combining different opioid peptides with their receptors, a large number of possible combinations can produce a great diversity of effects. There are three different kinds of receptor molecules that the enkephalin/endorphin neurotransmitters share.

The main opiate receptor (named with the Greek letter mu) provides the major effects of opiates: analgesia, euphoria, respiratory depression—almost everything opiates do. The main backup receptor (delta) probably cooperates with mu in some places to help produce these same effects. There is a third receptor (kappa), and this is the weird one. The drugs that are specific for this receptor produce analgesia, but they do not produce a high. This should be it, you might think: the perfect nonaddicting analgesic drug. There is only one problem: stimulation of this receptor alone causes the opposite of euphoria, or dysphoria. Unfortunately, the addicting properties of opiates cannot be distinguished from their pain-killing properties. All of the other clinically useful drugs we use now are specific for the mu receptor, and they are all addictive.

NATURAL HIGH: OUR OWN ENDORPHINS

Was John Denver right? Are the joys of nature (music, sex, meditation, whatever) as great as drugs? There may be a crumb of truth in this, in the end. As we discussed above, the brain produces its own opiates—the enkephalins and endorphins. If we inject these into animals, they cause the same effects as morphine or heroin. The big question is, are they released in circumstances in which we feel great? Even bigger, can we learn to release them ourselves? The latter question is a premise of a somewhat recent science fiction book, *Earth*, by David Brin, which depicts a future world where drug abuse no longer exists: the new social outcasts are the brain addicts who have learned to release their own opioids. Can we learn to do this?

Do naturally released endorphins contribute to behavioral state? Of course. We have lots of information from studies on animals and from some done with humans that this is so. For example, one enterprising scientist measured endorphin levels in animals undergoing experimental acupuncture and measured increased release during the procedure, lending credence to this ancient Chinese healing technique. Can we learn to release more endorphins intentionally? How can we tell if we are doing it right? First, we could give a drug like naloxone (Narcan), and see if the endorphin high stopped. This approach has actually been tested on people listening to their favorite music who found that they didn't enjoy the music as much if they were treated with an opiate antagonist (we're not sure if the same principles apply to Beethoven and Metallica). The alternative is to collect cerebrospinal fluid from people who are engaged in some pursuit that is supposed to release endorphins and measure the endorphins. This is obviously an implausible strategy to use on people. Since not much of either form of research has been done, the honest answer to the question is—we don't know.

How about runner's high? Do endorphins kick in at the end of a marathon? The only way to know, as described above, would be to sample the CSF at the end of a marathon, or to give a runner the opiate antagonist naloxone during the race. Not too many runners would likely volunteer for these experiments.

So, is all this speculation about endorphins a bunch of mythology? Absolutely not! Endogenous opioids play an important role in suppressing pain and in promoting reward. Recent studies showed that animals with no beta-endorphin will not take care of their babies, implicating endorphin as a critical element in nurturing behavior as well. These neurotransmitters are crucial to an important and related group of behaviors essential to human survival.

ADDICTION, TOLERANCE, AND DEPENDENCE

While the buzz from opiates might sound alluring, it comes at a cost. Opiate drugs stimulate all opioid systems simultaneously. The problems with crude approaches like this is that there are many unwanted effects that accompany the desirable ones. One of these is certainly the cycles of withdrawal that opiate users experience. People who take opiates for a while (weeks) can develop significant dependence and addiction, and undergo withdrawal when they stop. Most opiate addicts use heroin or other opiates several times a day. With this pattern of use, tolerance develops to many of the actions of opiates, but it develops to different effects at different rates. Unfortunately for pain patients, tolerance develops easily to the ability of opiates to suppress the sensation of pain. (However, it has been argued that patients experiencing intense, chronic pain like that associated with terminal cancer actually show little tolerance to the analgesic effects of opiates in this circumstance.) It also develops fairly well to the suppression of breathing (which is why opiate users can tolerate higher and higher doses). However, the constipation remains, and the pinpoint pupils are slow to change. The latter is fortunate, as it offers a useful sign of OD in a comatose patient, and can help to identify even a chronic user. While tolerance develops to opiate-induced euphoria, the drug keeps providing enough pleasure to continue to be reinforcing.

Part of the tolerance results from chemical changes in how cells respond to opiates. The normal chain of events initiated by heroin adapts to the continuous presence of the heroin. The adaptation becomes so thorough that cells function normally even though heroin is present. Another part of tolerance is purely a conditioned response. Pharmacologists have learned from animal studies that if you give animals a dose of heroin every day in the same room, they tolerate higher and higher doses. However, if you move them to a strange environment, the dose that they usually tolerated kills them: we think that conditioned responses permit their bodies to anticipate and counter the effects of the drug.

This conditioning effect probably does apply to humans. Frequently, very experienced opiate users who OD do so in an unfamiliar environment: they couldn't get drug from their usual source and had to go somewhere else.

Opiate withdrawal is miserable but not life-threatening (unlike alcohol withdrawal). Again, in *Junkie*, William Burroughs provides a good description: "The last of the codeine was running out. My nose and eyes began to run, sweat soaked through my clothes. Hot and cold flashes hit me as though a furnace door was swinging open and shut. I lay down on the bunk, too weak to move. My legs ached and twitched so that any position was intolerable, and I moved from one side to the other, sloshing about in my sweaty clothes. . . . Almost worse than the sickness is the depression that goes with it. One afternoon I closed my eyes and saw New York in ruins. Huge centipedes and scorpions crawled in and out of empty bars and cafeterias and drugstores on Forty-second Street. Weeds were growing up through cracks and holes in the pavement. There was no one in sight. After five days I began to feel a little better."

The earliest signs of withdrawal, as described above, are watery eyes, runny nose, yawning, and sweating. When people have been using opiates heavily, they experience mild withdrawal as soon as their most recent dose wears off. As withdrawal continues, the user feels restless and irritable and loses his appetite. Overall, it feels like the flu, and as withdrawal peaks, the user suffers diarrhea, shivering, sweating, general malaise, abdominal cramps, muscle pains, and, generally, an increased sensitivity to pain; yawning and difficulty sleeping gradually become more intense over the next few days. The worst of the physical symptoms abate after a few days.

If flu symptoms were all that happened when addicts stopped using, treating heroin addiction would be easy. Unfortunately, there is another symptom that is more intangible but probably much longer-lasting. There is a dysphoria (the just-feeling-lousy feeling), which may be the reverse of opiate-induced euphoria. Withdrawing opiate addicts just feel *bad*, and they feel bad in a way that they know opiates will solve. The craving for a fix can last for months, long after the physical symptoms have abated.

Why do these withdrawal symptoms happen? We discussed earlier how withdrawal from any drug often resembles the opposite of acute drug effects. It would make sense, then, that opiates that cause constipation would cause diarrhea upon withdrawal. The body of the addict assumes a certain level of intestinal tract movement in the presence of a constipating agent. Remove the constipating agent, and the underlying processes that were counteracting it to keep things normal suddenly find themselves unhindered. The character in the movie *Trainspotting* experienced this effect, which necessitated his mad dash for the bathroom in one scene. This represents the sort of yin-yang response the body has to any disruption. (If you shiver and feel cold when you are withdrawing from opiates, what do opiates usually do to body temperature?)

There is a big argument among addiction researchers about how much the desire to avoid withdrawal maintains addiction. Obviously, when people first get addicted, they haven't been taking the drug long enough to go through withdrawal if they stop. However, after several months or years, the withdrawal is stronger and may contribute more to an addict's continued drug taking. If you know drug will solve the problem, it seems an easy solution, doesn't it?

PATTERNS OF USE: ARE YOU A JUNKIE?

Many people use opiates occasionally for the high. They take a pill, drink cough syrup, or inject heroin or fentanyl, for example. Some people develop a habitual pattern of daily use that accelerates over a period of time, then stabilizes at a certain level. These people take opiates every few hours. After the first week or two, they are resistant to (tolerant of) many of the effects of the drug, and every time the drug wears off, withdrawal signs begin and the cycle of use starts again.

What pattern of use means that you are an addict? Can a person be addicted after the first dose? The answer for opiates isn't very different from the answers for all the other drugs we discuss. It is not determined by whether a user injects drugs, or uses them only on weekends, or has never shared a needle, or has ever blacked out. The answer is that he's addicted when he has lost control of use: when he must continue to pursue whatever pattern of use he has set. For some, this loss of control might come from smoking heroin; for some, injecting or snorting; and for some, even drinking cough syrup.

Is a person an addict if he goes through withdrawal? Or, conversely, if he doesn't go through withdrawal, is he not a junkie? This is a common rule of thumb many people use. As we have said, an opiate user will go through withdrawal if he has been taking the drug regularly enough that his body has adapted to it. This is a clear indication of tolerance. Usually, such adaptation means he *is* in a regular use pattern, but a user can be addicted before he has taken the drug long enough to show strong withdrawal signs. Conversely, a pattern of use might be compulsive but low (drinking cough syrup), and the withdrawal might be so mild it isn't noticeable.

What pattern of use clearly indicates addiction? The National Institute of Drug Abuse has accumulated statistics about "addiction careers," or the typical drug-use pattern of someone who is addicted to opiates. Usually, use begins with occasional experimentation, often with skin-popping first, or weekend use, and then gradually accelerates over a period of months to continuous administration at intervals of four to six hours. The surprising part about opiate addiction careers is that they end. Many opiate users follow this pattern for about ten to fifteen years and then quit, often without prolonged treatment. The reasons are not entirely clear, but probably include a host of social and physical reasons.

OPIATE OVERDOSE AND TOXICITY

SHORT-TERM EFFECTS

The other downside to taking opiates is that there are many physical side effects of stimulating all opiate receptors in the body simultaneously. Death by overdose is a major possibility. The most dangerous thing about the opiate drugs by far — and the usual cause of death — is the suppression of breathing, which can be fatal within minutes after an injection. It's not the result of cumulative toxicity, but can happen with a single dose. Usually at this point the patient has become so sedated and sleepy that he is in a coma, and he has pinpoint pupils. The most common reason for overdose with opiates is that the user has received a dose that is much higher than expected. The composition of street heroin varies widely, and is never known to the user. In some inner cities it can be as high as 60 percent pure or as low as 10 percent. Tolerance is not adequate to compensate for such a difference in dose. Seizures can develop with extremely high doses, especially in infants and children who have OD'd by ingesting drug intended for an adult. Seizures are much rarer in ordinary adult users, but obviously can be very dangerous.

If breathing continues after an opiate dose, there is relatively little else to worry about. The other side effects of opiates are uncomfortable but not dangerous: nausea and vomiting, constipation, difficulty urinating. Sometimes opiates cause a flushing of the skin and tremendous itching. This happens because morphine probably releases histamine, one of the molecules involved in allergic reactions, in the skin.

If opiate addicts were in perfect health, these would be little to worry about. Unfortunately, this is often not the case. Addicts are frequently undernourished, generally in ill health, and often addicted to alcohol or other drugs. For example, in most people the effects of opiates on blood pressure are minor. However, these effects can be worse in people who already have problems with their cardiovascular systems. Similarly, the constriction of the bile ducts can cause them to spasm, which is extremely painful in users with bile duct problems.

The existence of contaminants in illegally prepared injectable forms of heroin represents another major hazard. Depending upon the source (which is almost never known), heroin can be contaminated with quinine or other contaminants, including talc and mannose. Some apparent heroin overdoses are actually problems caused by these contaminants.

LONG-TERM EFFECTS

What are the long-term effects, and which of them are dangerous? The answer might surprise you. One of our teachers, a wise and ancient British pharmacologist named Frederick Bernheim, was fond of getting up in front of the medical school class and saying that if you didn't mind being impotent and constipated, opiate addiction really wasn't too bad. Of course, he couldn't say that today, but there is some truth to this assertion.

The long-term consequences for your major body systems of taking opiates every day are, as our teacher implied, somewhat benign. Yes, addicted men can become impotent, and sexual and reproductive function can be impaired in men and women addicts. Women often stop having menstrual cycles, and in men sperm production falls. The people who use opiates over the long term are also chronically constipated, as he described. Users typically lose weight because they spend so much time chasing down the drug, they don't eat well. Otherwise, the opiates themselves are not damaging to organ systems, in marked contrast to regularly ingested alcohol. The recent death of Jerry Garcia of the rock group the Grateful Dead is a case in point: he was a long-time opiate addict, but he died from complications of his diabetes, not from the heroin.

None of this sounds too bad. However, there are other major considerations. First of all, with any pattern of compulsive drug use, the user tends to ignore anything but obtaining the drug. Therefore, he tends to neglect his health, usually eats poorly, and suffers all the other complications of not taking care of oneself. Furthermore, addicts often engage in risky behaviors associated with obtaining and using the drug. For example, many women addicts engage in unprotected sex to obtain money for their next fix, and thereby increase their risk of contracting sexually transmitted diseases. Many people who inject drugs share the needles, which greatly increases their risk of contracting HIV and hepatitis. In New York City, a substantial percentage of all heroin addicts who inject heroin are infected with HIV. In fact, the recent popularity of snorting heroin is motivated in large part by the desire to avoid needles. These people don't avoid addiction, but they do avoid a potentially lethal side effect from needle-transmitted disease. In the context of HIV and other sexually transmitted diseases, the potential effects of opiates on the immune system present a real concern. Opiates do seem to suppress immune function, and most immune cells are loaded with opiate receptors: numerous recent studies have shown changes in immune-cell function if they are exposed to opiates.

There are some other toxicities associated with long-term opiate use. As mentioned earlier, injecting particles or using unsterilized needles can cause inflammation of veins. This can cause serious damage to blood vessels. And there is a somewhat unexpected result of very long-term use on the brain. Although opiates themselves are not particularly toxic to neurons (unlike alcohol), the repeated suppression of breathing that is caused by continuous opiate use can produce changes in the brain associated with hypoxia (low blood oxygen). Long-term addicts simply don't breath enough to maintain normal levels of blood oxygen. While this problem is not unique to opiates, it is a potential side effect that could have long-term consequences.

TREATMENT FOR OVERDOSE AND ADDICTION

As we mentioned earlier, injecting adrenaline directly into the heart is not the way to reverse an opiate overdose. There is a far simpler and completely effective treatment. The opiate antagonist naloxone (Narcan) will almost immediately reverse the life-threatening suppression of breathing.

Treating opiate addiction is another matter. As with other addictions, there is no easy solution. People have tried many of the strategies used for alcoholics. A number of groups, such as Narcotics Anonymous, emphasize abstention, attendance at meetings, etc. The other major approach used in the

United States is to provide long-acting methadone, administered on an out-patient basis to patients in treatment programs. The idea of this strategy is to allow the addict to avoid withdrawal and the constant need to procure drug. The other advantages of methadone are that the drug is given orally, without the risks of IV administration, and that the dose is controlled and can gradually be worked down. Although some complain that this method just substitutes one addiction for another without addressing the social and psychological reasons for the addiction, patients' lifestyles do improve.

10

Sedatives

Drug Class: Sedative, hypnotic, anxiolytic

General Sedatives: barbiturates (phenobarbital, pentobarbital [Nembutal], secobarbital [Seconal], amobarbital [Amytal]); chloral hydrate (Notec, Somnos, Felsules); glutethimide (Doriden); others (Equanil, Miltown, Noludar, Placidyl, Valmid, methaqualone [Quaaludes]).

Benzodiazepines: flunitrazepam (Rohypnol), diazepam (Valium), chlordiazepoxide (Librium), and a variety of other similar benzodiazepines with the following brand names: Ativan, Dalmane, Xanax, Serax, Tranxene, Verstran, Versed, Halcion, Paxipam, Restoril (there are hundreds more)

GHB: Gamma-hydroxybutyrate (GHB, Liquid X, Easy Lay)

The Buzz: All of the sedatives produce about the same psychological effects. First there is a sense of relaxation and a reduction of anxiety—a general "mellow" feeling. At higher doses, this is followed by lightheadedness, vertigo, drowsiness, slurred speech, and muscle incoordination. Learning is impaired, and memory for events that occurred while under the influence of these chemicals, especially the benzodiazepines, may be impaired. The duration of action can vary from a couple of hours to more than a day, so it is important to be alert to the possibility of prolonged impairment. Unexpected side effects (just the opposite of what the drug is expected do) occasionally occur, such as anxiety, nightmares, hostility, and rage. All of these drugs impair the ability to drive, and, in general, their effects are increased by alcohol. A person who has had a sedative and a drink of alcohol should never drive.

Overdose and Other Bad Effects: With benzodiazepines the risk of fatal overdose is small if they are taken alone. High doses simply cause prolonged sleep and perhaps memory impairment for the period they are active. However, if they are combined with any other sedating drug, benzodiazepines can cause fatal suppression of respiration. If a person has taken a benzodiazepine and is difficult to arouse, it is best to assume that some other drug may be present and to seek medical attention immediately.

Almost any of the sedatives except the benzodiazepines will cause death by suppression of breathing and heart failure if taken in sufficient quantity. The progression of symptoms is as follows: drowsiness and muscular incoordination with slurring of speech; deep sleep from which the person cannot be aroused; loss of reflexes such as eye blink, gag, and withdrawal from a painful stimulus; suppressed breathing; and death. If a person has taken a sedative and cannot be aroused, seek medical attention immediately.

Dangerous Combinations with Other Drugs: As with alcohol, opiates, and inhalants, it is dangerous to combine any sedative, including benzodiazepines, with anything else that makes a person sleepy. This includes alcohol and other drugs that have sedating properties, such as opiates (e.g., heroin, morphine, or Demerol), general anesthetics (nitrous oxide, halothane), or solvents. Some cold medicines include antihistamines, and sedatives consumed in combination with them can produce depression of heart rate and breathing.

Even drug combinations that do not cause unconsciousness or breathing problems can powerfully impair physical activities such as sports, driving a car, and operating machinery.

There are reports that GHB and flunitrazepam (Rohypnol, or "roofies") have been added to drinks to cause sedation leading to seduction. If a person begins to feel weak, dizzy, lightheaded, or mentally confused after a drink that should not produce such feelings, consider getting that person medical help.

CHAPTER CONTENTS

INTRODUCTION

For all of recorded history, people have sought ways to reduce their anxiety and make themselves peaceful and calm: through meditation, religious practice, psychotherapy, and all kinds of chemicals. Historically, the chemical of choice has been alcohol, and for many it still is. But as biology and medicine have progressed in this century, there has been a growing understanding of how we can manipulate our feelings with very specific drugs. This has occurred as societies have become much more complex and anxiety-provoking, so just as the new drugs have arrived, the demand has risen.

The modern pharmacology of sedation began in the mid 1800s with the synthesis of chloral hydrate, a sedative that is still used today. It was followed by barbital, the first of the barbituates, in 1903. The barbiturates turned out to be a wonderful group of compounds, because small modifications to the chemical structure of the basic compound produced a variety of sedatives with different properties. For example, phenobarbital had antiseizure properties at doses that did not make patients too sleepy. Some barbiturates were extremely short-acting, while others produced anesthesia sufficient for surgery. More than twenty-five hundred barbiturates were synthesized, and at least fifty reached the commercial market. Not only was this an important milestone for patients and physicians but it also demonstrated to scientists that slight changes in a basic molecule could create drugs with very different effects.

Other general sedatives were developed after the barbiturates, but even those used today still share the same problem—at a certain level they depress all brain function, including that which supports breathing. Large doses of barbiturates can and do kill people.

As important as the early sedatives were, this deadly side effect was a major risk, and thus they could not be safely prescribed to anxious and depressed individuals who might use them to commit suicide. This changed in 1957 with the synthesis of the first benzodiazepine-like compound (chlordiazepoxide, or Librium). It quickly became clear that this was a remarkable group of drugs.

They could specifically reduce anxiety without making a person too drowsy, and best of all, they did not excessively suppress respiration. They were much safer. Even though at that time no one knew how these drugs worked, they clearly worked very well, and a huge number of different variations of these compounds were synthesized (more than three thousand).

GENERAL SEDATIVES

WHAT THEY ARE AND HOW THEY WORK

Almost all the general sedatives that are used for recreational purposes are compounds that have been manufactured for medical use and are diverted from legitimate sources. These drugs are obtained by illegal prescriptions, by theft, or by importing them from countries where they can be bought without a prescription. Thus, they almost always appear as pills, packaged liquids, or preparations ready for injection. There is nothing distinctive about their appearance.

There are a number of different general sedatives that are often used for experimentation and recreation, and they are listed in the summary on the first page of this chapter under the heading "General Sedatives." There are no characteristics that separate them enough to justify discussing any of them separately. However, it is important to know exactly what drug one is taking because the potency of drugs in this group can vary considerably.

Our best understanding of the general sedatives comes from studies of the barbiturates. The barbiturates and other drugs act by increasing the function of GABA at its binding site on the nerve cells (see the "Brain Basics" chapter for a discussion of GABA). So, if a signal comes along that releases a bit of GABA onto a cell or network of cells, then in the presence of the barbiturates, that same packet of GABA can be much more effective. They do this by increasing the time that the channels in the cell membrane are open. If they are open longer, then more inhibiting ions flow, and the cell is inhibited from firing action potentials for a longer time. If there is enough GABA and enough barbiturate, then the cells cannot fire at all, and the network shuts down.

With a sedative, shutting down is exactly what we want to have happen, but only in certain areas. What we don't want is for those areas responsible for life to shut down, and there is the secret to good pharmacology—finding a drug that will do exactly what you want and not what it must not do. The barbiturates and other general sedatives are terrific if one knows just how to use them, and they can be deadly if one doesn't.

For instance, the barbiturate phenobarbital is a great barbiturate if one wants mild sedation and perhaps an antiseizure medicine. A clinically appropriate dose of phenobarbital will make one feel a little drowsy and maybe a bit less anxious. More of it will make one sleep, but it takes quite a bit to stop critical life functions such as respiration, and it is not good for surgery. Now assume that a person has experience with phenobarbital and knows how many pills he can take, but cannot get it, so he takes pentobarbital instead. Pentobarbital tends to have a much greater effect on GABA inhibition and is great for surgery, but it does not spare the nerve networks that control respiration. The same dose of pentobarbital that would be appropriate for phenobarbital can fatally suppress breathing. Our experimenter is in real danger of having a lethal overdose.

The message from this is that all of these sedatives are alike in their mechanism of action, but they can be very different in their potency, and maybe even in their specific potency on critical life-support networks. Anytime one takes a sedative, one should know exactly what she is taking and the appropriate dose for that drug.

TOXICITY

The barbiturates, being manufactured for human consumption, do not contain known toxic agents, and in general their toxicity is not great if they are used at clinically appropriate doses. We have already talked about what can happen at high doses—death by respiratory depression. At normal doses, the major concern is that they can have effects that outlast their sleep-inducing properties. For example, driving, flying an airplane, or other activities requiring muscle coordination can be impaired for up to a day after a single dose. Also, as with any drug that sedates, there is the possibility that excitation rather than sedation will develop. No one knows why this happens, but it seems that some people react as though some part of their nervous system is actually stimulated.

If barbiturates are used for a long period of time, the liver systems that metabolize them become enhanced. This may cause some tolerance to develop, but it also causes other drugs to be metabolized more effectively, including steroids, ethanol, and vitamins K and D. So, if one is taking barbiturates with other prescribed drugs, there may be a problem with getting an adequate concentration of those other drugs, and one's physician might increase their dosage.

Chloral hydrate is a liquid that can irritate mucous membranes in the mouth and stomach and may cause vomiting. It can also cause disorienting feelings, like lightheadedness, vertigo, muscle incoordination, and even nightmares. There are also reports that chronic users can experience sudden death, perhaps due to overdose, or to liver damage. (When the liver becomes damaged, its ability to metabolize and detoxify a compound is impaired, and what may be a normal drug dose becomes toxic.)

In general, all of these drugs are safe if taken under the guidance of a physician and not mixed with other sedating compounds. People who experiment with any of them should be aware that the safety window between the effective dose and the lethal dose may be rather small.

TOLERANCE AND WITHDRAWAL

Tolerance will develop to all sedatives if they are used in sufficient doses for a period of weeks or more. There is a real risk with sudden withdrawal, because the central nervous system adapts to the drugs by turning down the inhibitory systems that these drugs enhance. It's like the brakes have been on in a car, the driver has been compensating by pressing the accelerator more, and then suddenly the brakes are off and the driver cannot let up on the gas. The car goes faster and faster and then out of control. That's what happens to the brain. The GABA system stops being enhanced and is in a weakened condition, so the brain, out of control, becomes overexcited and can have electrical discharges that produce epileptic seizures.

Then there is the problem of psychological dependence, or, simply, learning to live in a sedated state. Some people who are chronically anxious or agitated may get some relief from these drugs, but upon withdrawal, they are miserable because they have not cured their problems, but only suppressed them.

BENZODIAZEPINES

WHAT THEY ARE AND HOW THEY WORK

The benzodiazepines are remarkable because they are one of the closest drugs we have to a "magic bullet" for anxiety. Used in the proper way, benzodiazepines can provide significant relief from anxiety without disrupting normal functions. Most important, they are quite safe from the risk of overdose if they are used alone and *not* in combination with any other sedating drug, including alcohol. While there are a few deaths from benzodiazepines, in the vast majority of these cases the person had used them with something else.

The mechanism of action of these drugs is just about the same as that of the general sedatives—the enhancement of GABA inhibitory systems. So, the question arises, why don't they suppress respiration and cause death? It's because they work through a special benzodiazepine binding site on the GABA receptor molecule (the place where GABA interacts with the nerve cell), and the nerve cells that control respiration and other important functions do not have many benzodiazepine sites on their GABA receptors. It's a miracle. Almost the perfect drug, because the receptors are on cells that participate in thinking and worrying, but not on those that keep us alive. It is no wonder that these are among the most prescribed drugs on earth.

PROBLEMS WITH BENZODIAZEPINES

So, is it a perfect class of drugs? No. First, benzodiazepines make one sleepy and uncoordinated, at least during the first few days of use. So operating machinery such as cars and airplanes and saws is a really bad idea. Also, they cause problems with learning, and some of them can cause amnesia. Finally, significant tolerance develops and increasing doses are required, along with a long withdrawal period when one decides to stop taking them.

Because they enhance inhibition in the central nervous system, benzodiazepines can impair the process of neuroplasticity that we talk about in the "Brain Basics" chapter. That is, they can prevent the brain from recording and adapting to new information and changing its wiring pattern. Read the paragraph about how long-term potentiation of synapses may underlie learning. Benzodiazepines suppress this process. The general sedatives do this too, but few people take them chronically, while a lot of people take benzodiazepines for prolonged periods. So general learning is a problem, and someone who needs to learn new information should never use these drugs and expect to do so to their full potential.

The really dark side of not learning is amnesia—not remembering something important. Benzodiazepines can cause amnesia, and this is part of the major controversy about their abuse in social situations. There are increasing reports that benzodiazepines are being put into the drinks of women who are then seduced but have amnesia for the whole event. This may have become more prominent because of the availability of flunitrazepam (the brand name is Rohypnol, commonly called roofies), which is an especially potent benzodiazepine. A very small amount (2 milligrams) will easily disappear in a drink but be quite effective. This is the worst kind of drug abuse because it is inflicted on someone who does not choose it.

There has been a lot of publicity about flunitrazepam lately because it is being widely distributed in the underground market and the government has banned importation of it. In fact, it is being treated almost hysterically as an evil drug. It is nothing more than a very potent benzodiazepine. As far as we can determine, it does exactly what the far more common Valium does and nothing more. It's just that it takes about 2 milligrams of flunitrazepam to do what 10 milligrams of Valium will do. The only characteristic that makes it more dangerous than any other benzodiazepine is that it more easily disappears into a drink. However, if it is put in someone's drink after she has had a lot of alcohol already, then it could lead to a serious overdose.

As for other problems with benzodiazepines, they are about the same as those for the general sedatives—lightheadedness, vertigo, poor muscle coordination, nightmares, etc.

GHB

When a drug makes *Time* magazine, it's a hot topic. GHB made it on September 30, 1996, as *Time* reported the death of a seventeen-year-old Texas girl. An outstanding athlete and a highly responsible student, she went to a dance club, had a couple of soft drinks, then went home complaining of a headache and nausea. Twenty-four hours later she was dead from an overdose of GHB. There was no other toxic agent in her body, and no evidence that she knew she took the drug. The speculation is that GHB was slipped into her drinks.

GHB is just arriving in social circles and is rapidly gaining in popularity. The Internet is full of descriptions (many very inaccurate) about the effects of the drug, and there are even instructions for making it in home laboratories. GHB can be lethal, it is easy to manufacture, and it is difficult to detect in a drink—a perilous and dicey combination.

What It Is and How it Works

GHB—gamma-hydroxybutyrate—is most often available as an odorless and colorless liquid, perhaps with a salty taste. It is used as a general anesthetic in Europe, and it has been sold in health-food stores for body building, but that is now illegal in most areas, having been banned by the United States Food and Drug Administration for over-the-counter sales in 1990. Now most of the market is found in nightclubs and at raves.

Until recently this drug was thought to work by binding to the GABA receptor on nerve cells and activating that receptor. It may do that, but new studies suggest that GHB may itself be a neurotransmitter in the brain. It meets many of the requirements that neurobiologists have established for a transmitter. It is synthesized in the brain, it has specific receptor sites and specific receptor locations, and its effects can be blocked by specific receptor antagonists. Thus, it may have a very specific role in the brain, although we don't know what that is. Even so, there is nothing very remarkable about this and it should not make much difference to anyone but neuroscientists, except for one unusual fact—it easily crosses from the blood to the brain.

Under normal circumstances, the brain is remarkably insulated from the rest of the body by the blood brain barrier. To get into the brain, substances must dissolve easily in fat to move through tissues. Most neurotransmitters will not cross the blood brain barrier, and so no matter how much of them one takes in, they never reach the brain. This is a very important property of the body because neurotransmitters are present in much of what we eat, and if we had meals that included a huge amount of a particular neurotransmitter, we would die of either overexcitation or too much inhibition.

So, what does it mean that GHB can cross from the blood to the brain? Although we are not sure yet, it could mean that whatever role GHB plays in normal brain function, that role is going to be modified by added GHB moving into the brain. Instead of having a normal circuit that is wired and functioning in an orderly manner, the circuit could become disordered as the GHB receptors get randomly activated as the drug courses through the brain. This is a bit different from other sedatives that simply increase the activity of a receptor, more or less preserving the orderliness of the network.

Whatever the neuropharmacology of GHB turns out to be, it is clearly a potent drug. In general, it can be thought of as a major sedative on the basis of its effects. It produces relaxation, mild euphoria, then headache, perhaps nausea, drowsiness, loss of consciousness, seizures, and coma or even death. We don't know about other, more subtle effects on learning and memory, but given the sedative nature of the drug, such mental functions are probably impaired.

Some research has suggested that GHB interacts with opiate systems and cocaine-sensitive processes and that it has PCP-like effects. The best research available as this is written indicates that GHB is different from all of these drugs in both site of action and effect. The good news is that it does not seem to be very reinforcing, and thus it might not be addictive. (See the "Addiction" chapter for a discussion of addiction and reinforcement.) Monkeys given the opportunity to administer the drug to themselves through intravenous injection in one research study did not consistently choose to do so, suggesting that the drug was not too attractive. But the human experience with this drug is still limited and proper studies with humans are not yet available.

TOXICITY

As illustrated by the *Time* article, GHB can be quite toxic. We do not know anything about long-term effects of its use, but the short-term effects are clear. Overdose can occur easily, and we suspect that alcohol and other sedatives increase the effects of GHB. The overdose signs are similar to those for other sedatives, with drowsiness, nausea, vomiting, headache, loss of consciousness, loss of reflexes, and suppression of breathing, leading up to death. Epileptic seizures may also occur. Please be aware that normal toxic screens in the emergency room are not yet set up to detect GHB. Therefore, if anyone shows signs of these problems, it is critical to get medical help and tell the medical personnel that GHB may be present.

Tolerance and Withdrawal

There is also little data about tolerance with continued use of GHB, or about any withdrawal effects. However, given that GHB is a sedative, prolonged use almost certainly will cause tolerance, and abrupt withdrawal would result in hyperexcitability of the central nervous system.

Note

Because GHB is growing in popularity, easy to manufacture, readily found in nightclubs, and hard to detect in a drink, it is important to be alert to the possibility that someone may add it to a drink. If a person begins to feel weak, dizzy, lightheaded, or mentally confused after a drink that should not produce such feelings, consider getting that person medical help. At this point, there is no FDA-approved antagonist for GHB. Good medical support early on can prevent most of the problems that ingesting GHB will cause.

11

Steroids

Drug Class: Anabolic steroids

Individual Drugs: testosterone, methyltestosterone, boldenone (Equipoise), methandrostenolone (Dianobol), stanozol (Winstrol), nandrolone (Durabolin, Dex-Durabolin), trenbolone (Finajet), ethylestrenol (Maxibolin), fluoxymesterone (Halotestin), oxandrolone (Anavar), oxymetholone (Anadrol)

Common Terms: steroids, roids, juice

The Buzz: Steroids do not cause a buzz immediately when they are taken because they don't take action for hours. After a typical stacking regimen of some weeks' duration, some users report feelings of euphoria, great energy, and increased combativeness/competitiveness. Such users complain of depression when they stop using anabolic steroids.

Overdose and Other Bad Effects: Anabolic steroids do not cause death by acute overdose in the same way that opiates or other drugs that act on the brain do. However, they cause many changes in body function that can cause serious injury or death. Serious heart damage, and even death from heart attacks or stroke, have occurred in people using anabolic steroids.

WHAT ARE ANABOLIC STEROIDS?

Testosterone and drugs that act like testosterone in the body are called anabolic steroids. The term *steroid* refers to their chemical structure, and the
term *anabolic* refers to their ability to promote muscle growth. Testosterone
production during adolescence and after is responsible for both sexual maturation and the growth in height and muscle mass that men experience at this
time. Medically, anabolic steroids are used mainly in men who have inadequate testosterone production; illegally they are used by many athletes, both
professional and amateur, for their ability to increase muscle mass. Most of the
steroids used illegally by athletes have been diverted from appropriate medical
or veterinary use, or have been prepared by bootleg labs and packaged in a way
that resembles the real product. They appear as pills (white, yellow, or pink)
or as injectable solutions.

There are other natural steroid hormones, but they are not anabolic steroids.
Estrogens and progesterone are the steroids that are present in females, and
cortisol is the steroid that is normally released by the adrenal gland under
conditions of stress. Cortisol is a catabolic hormone that tends to break down
muscle. Normally, the only anabolic steroid present in the body is testosterone. Obviously, men have much more than women, but women produce
a tiny amount of testosterone as well. The steroids that people take to treat
asthma are not anabolic steroids; instead they are variations on cortisol. So
asthma sufferers who take steroids for their asthma should not worry that they
are using a dangerous drug.

In a normal man, testosterone is present from the time of fetal life. During
fetal development, it is responsible for the development of the male genitalia
and the maturation of the parts of the brain responsible for reproduction and
other aspects of brain function that are different in men and women. During
puberty, testosterone production increases dramatically, causing the rapid
growth in size, the thickening and coarsening of body hair, the lowering of the
voice, genital development, acne, and the muscle growth that happens at that
stage of life. It influences the production of fat-carrying proteins in the blood
and lowers levels of the "good" lipid-carrying protein that can protect against

heart disease. Testosterone also contributes to the increase in libido that occurs at this age. Once puberty is over, testosterone levels tend to be fairly constant through adult life.

The effects of taking anabolic steroids during puberty are more dramatic in women. During normal puberty, the rise in estrogen and progesterone is responsible for female characteristics emerging—the development of breasts, for instance. Since women usually only make a tiny amount of testosterone, the very high levels that appear after taking anabolic steroids lead instead to the emergence of masculine characteristics: extra muscle deposits, a deeper voice, thicker and coarser body hair, and an enlarged clitoris. And where the steroids have caused anatomical changes, as with the deeper voice and enlarged clitoris, these effects are irreversible.

Medically, testosterone is used to treat men whose bodies don't produce enough; they tend to be anemic, and this can be a serious condition that is easily reversed with hormone treatment. It is also occasionally used for its anabolic properties to facilitate tissue regrowth in burn patients, but that is the only exception.

Testosterone had been used for decades in this way by doctors, and rarely presented a problem. However, the cold war changed all that. The Communist countries of Eastern Europe started using anabolic steroids to improve performance in both their men and their women athletes in the fifties and sixties, and the improvement in performance was not lost on the rest of the world. Some of the athletes (for example, women swimmers from East Germany) have since claimed that they were given these substances without their knowledge, although they recognized that they were receiving a very active drug because of the dramatic changes they noticed in their bodies. Other countries caught on, and by the mid-1960s the use was common. By the early 1970s almost three quarters of the athletes involved in middle-or short-distance running or in field events admitted to using steroids, and most of the weight lifters also used steroids. The use of anabolic steroids was banned in 1976, but use continued unabated among professional weight lifters.

Now the use of anabolic steroids has left the mainstream and entered the underground world. If anything, this has increased availability of these substances. Some estimates of use by weight lifters run as high as 80 percent. The increased success of testing has somewhat limited use, but mainly resulted in a "shell game" in which athletes either use products that are not yet recognized by testers, or learn how to stop use long enough before a tournament to avoid detection. A recent survey found that up 11 percent of adolescent boys had used anabolic steroids. Of them, 80 percent were involved in competitive sports. Growing concerns about the rapid spread of anabolic steroid use led Congress to place them under the Controlled Substances Act in 1991.

HOW ARE ANABOLIC STEROIDS USED AND ARE THEY EFFECTIVE?

Normally, testosterone is released constantly by the testes, and when doctors try to treat male patients who have inadequate testosterone, they try to provide steady, low levels. This is not how steroid users typically use them. Usually, they take them in a stacking regimen: a cycle that lasts four to eighteen weeks, starting with low doses of several steroids, gradually increasing the dose every few weeks, then taking some weeks off. The amounts they take are huge in comparison to normal regimens used by doctors. A normal replacement regimen would be about 75 to 100 milligrams of testosterone a week, while a comparable regimen of self-administered testosterone can be up to 1 gram a week, or ten times the normal dose.

The huge doses that users take may explain the difference between public perception and scientific results. For many years, the scientific establishment denied that anabolic steroids could cause any real improvement in athletic performance. However, these controlled scientific studies were done on men who were not particularly fit and who already had optimal levels of testosterone. They put them all on an exercise regimen and gave some men testosterone and others a placebo. All the men usually improved in performance because of the exercise regimen. And since the male body makes about the optimal amount of testosterone, adding a little usually has little impact.

The situation for bodybuilders and others who use anabolic steroids is quite different—they are maximally fit to start, just looking for that slight edge, and taking huge amounts probably does improve performance just a little. Although normally testosterone works only on its own receptor to build muscle, when such huge amounts are taken, scientists have speculated that it "spills over" onto the catabolic steroid receptor and prevents the effects of cortisol. So, instead of just muscle building, huge amounts of anabolic steroids might prevent muscle breakdown, too. Finally, it is possible that just the psychological boost of taking a performance-enhancing drug can have a real impact on performance in sports. In a highly competitive environment of optimally trained athletes, the appearance of advantage may be all that is necessary.

Anabolic steroids definitely improve muscle deposition in women, even in normal amounts; in the amounts taken by athletes, the improvement in muscle deposition can be dramatic. As muscle deposition promoted by testosterone tends to be greater in the upper body, this provides the greatest effects (and therefore the greatest likelihood of abuse) for sports like swimming, which rely on upper-body strength.

WHAT ARE THE HAZARDS OF ANABOLIC STEROID USE?

There is no question that anabolic steroid use can cause bad health consequences. However, extravagant claims on both sides of this argument have flown back and forth in the media. What is the scientific evidence? In women the evidence is clear-cut. There are permanent "virilizing" effects on the voice, hair (including male pattern baldness), and genitalia that do not reverse when anabolic steroid use stops. Also, women experience changes in the profile of blood proteins that promote heart disease, and lose the normal protective effects of their gender on the heart and blood vessels. Similarly, in adolescent males, use of anabolic steroids can cause a premature end to puberty, including a stop to the rapid growth stimulated in part by testosterone during this phase of life. Some of the effects in adolescent boys, like those in women, are irreversible. Normally, the rise in testosterone during puberty stimulates skeletal growth and finally stops it by causing the growing ends of the bone to "close over" and stop lengthening. When this closing over has happened, no further increase in height is possible. Use of anabolic steroids can speed up this process, leading ultimately to a shorter height than expected.

In adult men, huge doses suppress libido and halt sperm production. A growing number of isolated cases indicate that damage to the heart occurs in some users. It is also clear that levels of fat-carrying proteins in the blood of both men and women users change to a pattern that promotes heart disease, although this pattern reverses when steroid use is stopped. There are isolated cases of liver disease and liver cancer that have been attributed to the use of particular steroids. On rare occasions, anabolic steroids cause the appearance of blood-filled cysts in the liver that can rupture and cause dangerous internal bleeding. Finally, testosterone can actually cause some feminizing effects in men. Breast development is the most common. This happens because a very little bit of the testosterone in the body is converted to the female hormone estradiol. This condition commonly develops in weight lifters who use anabolic steroids.

What about the much-touted "roid rage"? Do anabolic steroids really make people incredibly aggressive? There is no more controversial effect of these drugs. There is no question that anabolic steroids can have effects on behavior. As we note below, stopping use can cause depression, and they have even been used successfully to treat depression in experimental studies. Furthermore, there have been a number of cases of anabolic steroid–induced manic episodes.

However, evidence for specific effects of testosterone on aggression is hard to find in controlled studies in humans. There have been small, much-publicized studies showing that testosterone levels were high in a subset of criminals who were known to have committed particularly violent crimes. There are many studies in rats and some in monkeys that show that large levels of steroids can affect aggressive behavior in specific tests. The behavior they describe is not the sort of irrational destructiveness that is so popular in the lay press. Instead, animals often simply compete better, or fight more quickly when provoked. To extrapolate from these studies to explain the behavior of individual men requires a long leap. For the moment, we are left with reports of users who describe their own absolutely uncharacteristic aggressive behavior while under the influence of anabolic steroids. Learning from the wrong conclusions scientists drew from their first inadequate experiments with muscle deposition, we should take these reports seriously.

ARE ANABOLIC STEROIDS ADDICTIVE?

Anabolic steroids certainly are taken in the absence of medical need, and despite the users' knowledge of negative health consequences. This was the basis for their being placed under the Controlled Substances Act. But are they addictive? Users do feel differently when they take steroids, and the feelings are mostly positive. They also experience a withdrawal syndrome when they stop. Some users report fatigue, depression, loss of appetite, insomnia, and headaches as the effects of the drugs wane. But animals certainly don't self-administer them, and they don't provide the typical euphoric rush when an injection is taken. There are no recognizable effects of taking an injection. In comparison to cocaine and heroin, it is difficult to call anabolic steroids addicting, as there is no scientific evidence that they cause the kinds of changes in the brain caused by other addictive drugs. However, it is clear that people develop a compulsive reliance on them, and willingly experience negative health consequences when they are using them—both of which are criteria for drug dependence. However, their inclusion under the Controlled Substances Act probably had more to do with concerns about the distribution to an increasingly broad array of people, including schoolchildren, than with the addictiveness of the drugs. Yet given the real health problems caused by these drugs, this ban does make sense. In the end, the normal male body produces optimal amounts of testosterone for health and vitality, and providing suprapharmacologic amounts provides a scant benefit in terms of slightly better muscle deposition at a great health cost. The focus on success at any price even in amateur athletics has certainly encouraged use of anabolic steroids worldwide, and better education about the consequences should offset some of the messages that encourage this use.

, a tonic containing a (still) secret formula that included cocaine. An-
r pharmacist, Asa Candler, realized the financial potential of this con-
ion and purchased the rights to the formula. The rest is history, as his
a-Cola company became a fixture in the American landscape and now
world.

igmund Freud, known to most as the father of psychoanalysis, was also one
e major forces in the popularization of cocaine in Europe. Freud studied
ine using the well-accepted practice of the time—self-experimentation:
ook the drug and recorded his experiences. His initial reports were over-
lmingly positive: he enjoyed the sense of euphoria and energy, and found
e in the way of toxic effects. His enthusiasm caused him to encourage his
nd Ernst von Fleischl-Marxow to try cocaine in an attempt to free himself
n morphine addiction. This turned out to be a misguided idea, as his
nd quickly substituted cocaine dependence for morphine dependence.
pattern of use escalated to intravenous injections of larger and larger doses
til he developed psychotic symptoms, one of the first recorded cases of
nulant psychosis. Freud was also responsible for noting the ability of co-
ne to produce local anesthesia (numbing), and his mention of this quality
a friend, opthamologist Carl Koller, led to the widespread use of cocaine in
tain types of eye, ear, and nose operations that persists to the present day.
So, why isn't there still cocaine in Coca-Cola? It would be reassuring to
nk that the hazards of cocaine use became so widely understood that its use
s simply banned. The truth is slightly more complicated than that, and the
e is familiar in today's environment of public activism about product safety
d government regulations. During the early 1900s, unregulated sales of
nics" containing potent ingredients such as opium and cocaine boomed.
me of these formulations contained so much cocaine (hundreds of mil-
grams per milliliter instead of the 0.5 milligrams per milliliter in the origi-
l Parke-Davis formula) that toxicities became widespread. The medical
tablishment finally took note. Unfortunately, a scare campaign with racist
ertones also contributed to the public furor. Reports that cocaine made
frican-Americans powerful and uncontrollable contributed to the wave of
ublicity. In 1906, the Pure Food and Drug Act required that manufacturers
st the ingredients on all tonics, and in 1914, the Harrison Narcotic Act of
914 imposed severe restrictions upon the distribution of opium and cocaine
roducts. Today, Coca-Cola contains only caffeine, and clinical cocaine use
restricted to a few surgical procedures.

THE STORY OF EPHEDRINE AND AMPHETAMINE

The story of ephedrine and amphetamine is not dissimilar. The Chinese drug
nahuang was long known to help treat the breathing symptoms of asthma.

12

Stimulants

Drug Class: Stimulants

Individual Drugs: cocaine, amphetamine, methamphetamine, ephedrine, methylphenidate (Ritalin), methcathinone

Common Terms: coke, blow, candy, crack, jack, jimmy, rock, nose candy, whitecoat (cocaine); crank, bennies, uppers (amphetamine); meth, crystal, crystal meth, ice (methamphetamine); Ritalin (methylphenidate); cat, khat, crank, goob (methcathinone)

The Buzz: Stimulants are aptly named: these drugs cause a sense of energy, alertness, talkativeness, and well-being that users find pleasurable. At the same time, the user experiences signs of sympathetic nervous system stimulation, including increased heart rate and blood pressure and dilation of the bronchioles (breathing tubes) in the lungs. These drugs also cause a stimulation of purposeful movement that is the reason for their description as psychomotor stimulants. When injected or smoked, these drugs cause an intense feeling of euphoria. With prolonged and high-dose use, the locomotor activity often becomes focused in repetitive movements like drawing repeating patterns.

Overdose and Other Bad Effects: There are two kinds of dangers with the stimulants. First and most important, at high doses (these are doses a person could take accidentally), death can result with any of these stimulants. High-dose cocaine use can lead to seizures, sudden cardiac death, stroke, or failure of breathing. Lethal doses of amphetamine sometimes cause seizures, but more often can cause lethal cardiac effects, and/or hyperthermia (fever). Death from Ecstasy (MDMA) or ephedrine intoxication, like amphetamine, probably results from effects on the heart and/or body temperature. Like opiates, any of these drugs can cause death with a single dose, and this is particularly easy with cocaine. With repeated use of high doses of stimulants over days to weeks, a psychotic state of hostility and paranoia can emerge that cannot be distinguished from paranoid schizophrenia. Finally, profound addiction can develop to any stimulant.

Dangerous Combinations with Other Drugs: Stimulants can be dangerous when taken with over-the-counter cold remedies that contain decongestants because the effects of the two can combine to raise blood pressure to a dangerous level. Also, stimulants can be dangerous in combination with the antidepressants known as monoamine oxidase inhibitors, because they will enhance the effects of the stimulants. Cocaine is dangerous with anything that would affect the heart rhythm, such as medication taken for certain heart diseases, because these drugs would act in an additive way with the effects of cocaine on the heart. Cocaine also is dangerous in combination with anything that makes people more sensitive to seizures, such as the prescription medication buspirone or extremely high levels of xanthines, like caffeine or theophylline.

CHAPTER CONTENTS

THE HISTORY OF STIMULANT USE

THE STORY OF COCAINE

The yuppies of the eighties certainly did not invent cocaine ephedrine have been used for centuries—cocaine by the America and ephedrine by Asian cultures. Amphetamine, o was the product of the pharmaceutical industry, the result tempts to improve upon ephedrine as a drug for treating asth

Cocaine is a substance that appears in the leaves of several including a shrubby plant (*Erythroxylon coca*) that lives in the America. Cocaine use as early as the sixth century is docum logical relics from South America, but it probably started m natives of South America used cocaine as an important part o Cocaine leaves were chewed for their alerting effects and th crease endurance, particularly at the high altitudes in whicl peoples lived. This practice continues to the present day. Whe conquered the Incas in the sixteenth century, they attempted until they realized that the Indians working in the silver mii harder if given their daily allotment of cocaine.

With the importation of cocaine to Europe and its purificati man scientist Albert Niemann, a new era began. The Corsica gelo Mariani was partly responsible for popularizing the use o Vin Mariani, a coca wine that became the rage of Europe. So the American pharmaceutical industry took note, and Parke manufacturing a cocaine-containing tonic. The success of this a host of imitators, including Georgia pharmacist John Pemb

Dr. K. K. Chen of the Eli Lilly company in the 1920s identified the compound ephedrine as the active agent in mahuang, and ephedrine quickly became an important treatment for asthma. Ephedrine is experiencing a comeback today as an "herbal" treatment for asthma and other diseases that harkens back to the public enthusiasm about cocaine in the late nineteenth century. (We'll see below the drawback to this approach.) At the time, there was not an easy way to make synthetic ephedrine, so it had to be extracted from the native plant, which was in short supply. A few years later, a chemist named Gordon Alles synthesized amphetamine in an attempt to develop a synthetic form of ephedrine. Little did he realize that he had succeeded too well. As a result, amphetamine became easily available in a volatile form that could be inhaled directly. Nasal amphetamine inhalers (Benzedrine) gained quickly in popularity, in part because amphetamine proved to do much more than simply dilate the bronchioles—it produced a stimulation and euphoria that ephedrine lacked almost completely. Abuse of amphetamine for these properties spread rapidly during the 1930s, fueled in part by the very short memories of the medical establishment, which had apparently forgotten the wave of cocaine addiction in the late 1800s. Amphetamine in pill form was given to British and Japanese soldiers in World War II to maintain alertness in long tours of duty. By the end of World War II, amphetamine was an unspoken fixture on the pharmaceutical landscape, and its popularity endures today among truck drivers and college students. The original formulation of the inhalers probably spurred amphetamine abuse because of the euphoria produced by rapid delivery to the brain. Although inhalers are no longer used, it is no surprise that over the next twenty years, intravenous use of amphetamine would grow in popularity among users striving not just to stay awake to study but to obtain the rush produced by rapid delivery of the drug. Finally, in the 1960s, use had become widespread enough that the dangerous effects of stimulants were rediscovered and given voice in the slogan "Speed kills."

Our lack of national memory is remarkable: as a culture we keep rediscovering the beneficial and toxic effects of locomotor stimulants. As soon as the popularity of amphetamine waned, the cocaine abuse of the 1970s began. The widespread availability of a volatile form (crack) that could be inhaled led to a remarkable rise in addiction and toxicity, in a manner reminiscent of the Benzedrine craze of the 1930s. Then, as the dangers of crack emerged and its popularity dwindled, a new drug appeared on the horizon. "Ice," the volatile form of methamphetamine (an amphetamine derivative), has been spreading rapidly during the mid-1990s, sparking a new wave of addiction and toxicity. Amphetamine-related emergency room admissions increased 460 percent from 1985 to 1994 in California alone.

WHAT ARE STIMULANTS TODAY?

The major stimulants used in the United States today (aside from caffeine, discussed separately in its own chapter) are cocaine, amphetamine, and methamphetamine. Ephedrine is rising in popularity as an herbal stimulant, and abuse of methylphenidate (Ritalin), normally prescribed to treat attention deficit disorder, is rising.

On the street, the two most common forms of cocaine are the white powder, which is either snorted or dissolved for injection, and crack, a solid chunk of cocaine that is heated directly in a pipe to form a vapor that is inhaled into the lungs. Both powdered cocaine and crack are prepared originally from leaves of the coca plant, which are mixed with solvents and processed through several steps to remove the cocaine from the leaves and purify it as crystals. Crack is prepared from the powder by boiling it with sodium bicarbonate. Chunks of cocaine base precipitate from this solution. This simple process has a tremendous impact on the speed with which cocaine is absorbed, as we will see below.

The powdered form of cocaine is usually diluted with other white powders, such as cornstarch, talcum powder, lactose, or mannitol, and/or with other local anesthetics, caffeine, or, sometimes, amphetamine. The purpose of the inert powders is economic: to dilute an expensive drug with cheap substances. These ingredients provide some semblance of the sensations associated with cocaine but with cheaper drugs — caffeine or amphetamine for alertness, and local anesthetics for the numbing sensation that users associate with real cocaine. Obviously, the actual ingredients of any substance sold as cocaine are rarely known except by the dealer. Cocaine is used medically as a local anesthetic, and it rarely appears on the street in its medicinal formulation, a solution in glass vials.

Powdered cocaine is usually snorted, where it is absorbed through the mucous membranes and into the blood vessels of the nose. Sometimes it is applied to other places, including the mouth, rectum, penis, or vagina. The purpose here is the same, although the site of application is generally less popular!

Amphetamine and methamphetamine appear in diverse forms: pills, powders of varying colors, or chunks that look like cocaine. Like cocaine, amphetamine appears most commonly from bootleg synthetic labs. It is marketed in many different forms, including loose forms like powders or "rocks," as well as capsules or tablets of various types. Pills marketed as amphetamine are also diverted from approved medical use for attention deficit disorder by patients who sell their pills to others. This pattern of use is becoming epidemic among students. Similarly, methamphetamine is also used occasionally to treat attention deficit disorder, and these pills appear on the market. However, the majority of methamphetamine is made in bootleg labs, and the freebase form, which appears as chunks called ice, which are heated and smoked like crack, is becoming one of the most common forms in circulation. Ephedrine is usually marketed as pills or as an herbal tea preparation.

Methylphenidate (Ritalin) is the well-known drug prescribed to treat attention deficit disorder. It is also a locomotor stimulant that is abused by a growing number of students. Most users obtain it in pill or tablet form from someone who has a valid prescription for its use, or from underground sources who have diverted it from clinical use.

There is an alphabet soup of amphetamine derivatives, including trimethoxyamphetamine (TMA), 2,5 dimethoxyamphetamine, 4-methamphetamine (or Serenity, Tranquillity, Peace), methoxyamphetamine (STP), methylenedioxyamphetamine (MDA), and paramethoxyamphetamine (PMA), which are all chemically related to amphetamine. These are mainly synthesized in bootleg laboratories and appear in diverse forms. Most of these drugs have effects like those which MDMA or hallucinogens produce rather than amphetamine and will be discussed later.

Khat (also spelled *qat* or *quat*) is a stimulant derived from a leafy plant that grows in Africa. For centuries it has been used recreationally by native peoples in Africa and the Middle East in social settings to promote conversation and improve social interactions. In recent years, with the urbanization of many native populations in Africa, khat use in certain groups has extended to Europe, Great Britain, and, recently, the United States. The active ingredient in khat is cathinone, a mild amphetamine-like stimulant. A synthetic variant of cathinone—methcathinone—is rapidly becoming popular. It is a much more potent stimulant with amphetamine-like actions. Both cathinone and methcathinone are prepared in bootleg labs and appear on the street either as an off-white or colored powder or in capsule form. In a reprise of the history of cocaine, the mild stimulant properties of chewing khat leaves have been replaced by the most intense high, which is caused by the pure chemical substance.

Finally, there are a number of synthetic stimulants that enjoyed temporary popularity as appetite suppressants or asthma medications until their abuse potential became recognized. Bootleg versions of many of these are available in some places (4Methylaminorex [4-MAX, U4EU] and pemoline are two such drugs).

GETTING OFF AND COMING DOWN: HOW STIMULANTS GET INTO AND OUT OF THE BODY

COCAINE

The difference in the ways that powdered cocaine and crack are prepared have a huge impact on how they are delivered to the body. Because cocaine constricts the very blood vessels that are absorbing it, snorting is a relatively slow way to deliver cocaine to the bloodstream. Blood cocaine levels rise relatively gradually, and don't reach a peak until about thirty minutes after snorting. Crack, in contrast, forms a vapor when heated that is delivered very quickly to the circulation, as fast as injecting the drug intravenously. Maximum levels are attained within a minute or two, and blood levels of cocaine at this time are much higher than ever observed after snorting comparable doses. Users often come to prefer the fast and intense rush that results from smoking crack. However, this rapid delivery of more drug also means greater risk of addiction or overdose.

Regardless of how cocaine is delivered, about half of a dose is removed from the body in about an hour. This means that a user is usually ready for another dose in about forty minutes or less. The rapid rise in blood levels, followed by a rapid fall—a rush followed by a crash—often leaves the user wanting to reexperience the original high. This rush-and-crash phenomenon can lead the cocaine user to keep taking additional doses until blood levels accumulate to toxic levels. This "run" often continues until the user either runs out of drug or has a seizure or some other sign of toxicity.

If cocaine is swallowed, it can be absorbed, but the process is slower, and much of the drug is metabolized. For this reason, the average blood levels of cocaine in people chewing leaves is very low compared to amounts present in the blood after smoking crack or snorting powder. Similarly, single doses of the original patent formulas, like Vin Mariani, with fairly low levels of cocaine (6 milligrams per ounce), probably resulted in relatively low blood levels of the drug with a single dose.

AMPHETAMINE; METHAMPHETAMINE

Amphetamine and methamphetamine, like cocaine, enter the bloodstream very quickly when they are smoked or injected. This leads to a rapid high and to greater likelihood of toxicity. Amphetamine and methamphetamine are also effective if they are swallowed as pills because they escape destruction in the liver and enter the circulation effectively. Unlike cocaine, amphetamines are long-lasting: the effect lasts for two to four hours. This leads to less of the rush-and-crash pattern of injecting the drug, although there are intravenous users who will use amphetamines in this way.

EPHEDRINE

Ephedrine appears in two forms: as pills, and in a bewildering array of herbal mahuang formulations, including pills and leaves that are brewed as teas. The active ingredient in all forms is ephedrine. Ephedrine is almost always ingested, as either a pill or tea, and it is well absorbed from the stomach and small intestine. Ephedrine reaches its peak effect in about an hour, and lasts for three to six hours.

METHYLPHENIDATE

Methylphenidate is usually taken as a pill. It is well absorbed from the intestine. The mild high produced lasts two to four hours. Addicts have been known to crush the pills and inject them. This practice is extremely dangerous because the other components in the pill can lodge in tiny blood vessels in the lung and eye and cause serious damage. Students have tried to crush the pill and snort it in the hopes that a high would result. However, absorption from this form is slow enough and the dose of most pills low enough that the buzz, if any, is not very much greater than taking a pill.

CATHINONE

Cathinone is usually snorted, although it can be injected intravenously. It is well-absorbed if swallowed, but this choice of route is rare.

WHAT STIMULANTS DO TO THE BRAIN

Amphetamines and cocaine are best known for their ability to increase attention, cause alertness, and eliminate fatigue. Amphetamines are widely used in the United States simply to increase attention and delay sleep and as medical treatments for attention deficit disorder and narcolepsy (a disease in which the patient falls asleep repeatedly during the day). Even Freud commented that the most probable use of cocaine would be for these properties: "The main use of coca will undoubtedly remain that which Indians have made of it for centuries: it is of value in all cases where the primary aim is to increase the physical capacity of the body for a given short period of time and to hold strength in reserve to meet further demands . . . coca is a far more potent and far less harmful stimulant than alcohol, and its widespread utilization is hindered at present only by its high cost."* People who are experiencing the effects of stimulants are often talkative and full of energy, movement, and confidence to the point of being restless and grandiose in thinking that they can accomplish anything.

If stimulants simply increased energy and alertness, they indeed would be the miracle medicine that Freud proposed. However, these drugs cause an un-

---

*Freud's comments are from *Uber Cocaine,* quoted by S. H. Snyder in *Drugs and the Brain* (New York: W. H. Freeman and Company, 1995).

mistakable euphoria and sense of well-being that is the basis of addiction. People who inject or smoke cocaine describe a rush of intense physical pleasure that can only be compared to orgasm. When these drugs are taken in a form that is absorbed more slowly (snorting or taking a pill), this feeling is much less intense and may simply be recognized as a feeling of well-being.

Stimulants also cause a stimulation of movement, which is the reason for their name. People who have taken stimulants are not just alert but are in constant motion—talking, moving, exploring, and generally fidgeting. At higher stimulant doses, this motion becomes a more focused, repetitive, "stereotyped" action. People who have taken high doses of amphetamine will doodle in repetitive patterns or engage in repetitive tasks. This same effect is observed in laboratory animals. At low doses, amphetamine causes animals to move incessantly about the cage, as if they are constantly searching the environment. After a high dose, animals will sniff back and forth in one spot in the cage, or engage in a repetitive grooming or chewing.

Cocaine is sometimes used in combination with heroin or other opiates. In this case, the effect on the brain and behavior is somewhat like the addition of the two. The dreaminess of opiates is added to and cuts the edginess and arousal caused by cocaine. This particular combination can be particularly dangerous: often people who are injecting cocaine slow down their intake of drug when the jitteriness gets too great, but in the presence of heroin, these feelings are not so obvious, increasing the risk of an overdose (on either cocaine or heroin). This is the combination of drugs that John Belushi was taking when he died.

Cocaine and amphetamines decrease appetite through actions in the brain. These drugs were the first diet pills, and were popular for this use in the 1950s and 1960s. Their dependence-producing effects became a real problem in their use as diet aids, and locomotor stimulants are not used for this purpose today, as nonaddicting alternatives have been developed.

WHAT STIMULANTS DO TO THE REST OF THE BODY

If this is all that stimulants did, then the aphorism "Speed kills" would never have appeared in the drug subculture. Unfortunately, this is not the case. Most of the locomotor stimulants, and especially cocaine and the amphetamine derivatives, have additional effects on other body functions. Cocaine and amphetamines mimic the effects of the sympathetic nervous system: they initiate all the bodily responses of the flight-or-fight syndrome. These drugs increase blood pressure and heart rate, constrict (narrow) blood vessels, dilate the bronchioles (breathing tubes), increase blood sugar, and generally prepare the body for emergency. These effects can be beneficial. The effects on the lungs can actually improve the symptoms of asthma. Furthermore, fat is broken down to help mobilize energy, and this effect may contribute to the weight loss these drugs can cause. However, the effects on the heart can be so excessive that they may result in a disordered heartbeat or, eventually, failure of the cardiovascular system.

Most of the stimulants also increase body temperature, which presents a real problem when amphetamines are used in situations involving exercise. At the same time, amphetamines and cocaine seem to increase the capacity for muscular work. Whether this represents a real improvement in muscle function, a better delivery of sugar to fuel muscular work, or simply the perception of greater energy, these drugs have been popular with some endurance athletes, like cyclists, and with those attending all-night rave dance parties to permit dancing all night. Extreme physical exertion increases body temperature even without the amphetamine, and with amphetamine added, the increase in body temperature can become fatal.

EFFECTS ON MOTHER AND FETUS

No drug-associated problem has been the subject of more public scrutiny and more public outcry than "crack babies," the infants of women who abuse crack or other locomotor stimulants during pregnancy. Alarming statistics state that anywhere from 10 to 30 percent of the women who give birth in some inner-city hospitals have used cocaine during their pregnancy. Are the minds and bodies of these infants destroyed by their prenatal exposure to the drug? The answer is very hard to know, partly because almost no person abuses only one drug. The women who abuse cocaine almost invariably smoke cigarettes and abuse alcohol as well. Furthermore, they tend to have poor access to health care and as a result often do not receive adequate prenatal care. It is very difficult to distinguish the role of cocaine itself in any problems the infants experience.

Many cocaine-exposed babies are born prematurely and with low birth weight, and a few have experienced catastrophic events, like strokes, before they were born. Cocaine use is also associated with premature separation of the placenta from the uterus, a condition that can cut off the baby's blood supply and result in brain damage or death. However, if babies are carried to term, the consequences for many may not be drastic. Many cocaine-exposed infants are extremely irritable and overly sensitive to any form of sensory stimulus at birth. However, this condition usually resolves, and the infants develop fairly normally. What is most surprising is that many of the effects at birth (low birth weight, increased frequency of prematurity) are not unique to cocaine, but are also seen in babies whose mothers smoked tobacco during pregnancy. Nicotine and cocaine have something in common that explains this: both powerfully constrict blood vessels that supply blood to the fetus during pregnancy and deny the infant vital nutrients.

Does exposing children to drugs in utero increase the likelihood that children will abuse drugs as adults? Although this is a topic of intense research and controversy, we don't have a clear answer. Many people speculate that prenatal experience with the drugs will affect how they respond to drugs as adults, but the results of research are mixed: some find increased sensitivity to drugs in adulthood, and others find decreased response. Furthermore, biology is not destiny: many factors go into the development of drug use—not just brain biochemistry. In this regard, these children are at a disadvantage because they may well grow up in drug-using homes.

EPHEDRINE: HERBAL CURE OR DANGEROUS AMPHETAMINE SUBSTITUTE?

Ephedrine in various herbal preparations has become popular as a "safe and natural" stimulant and diet aid. Resourceful marketing targets a population that has become increasingly wary of artificial drugs and willing to endorse herbal cures. However, it is also a classic case of false advertising. Ephedrine enters the brain poorly compared to cocaine and amphetamine. Therefore, it has fairly weak amphetamine-like stimulant properties, and is not a particularly good appetite suppressant. However, ephedrine possesses all the other effects amphetamine has on the body, and at excessive doses can cause amphetamine-like excitation. At therapeutic doses, ephedrine has been used as a safe and effective drug for treating asthma for thousands of years, but it also causes an increase in heart rate and blood pressure that has been responsible for cardiovascular problems and deaths from excessive doses, mainly of unregulated herbal ephedrine preparations. Toxic effects of ephedrine can occur at doses just two or three times above the recommended doses. Unfortunately, many commercial vendors of ephedrine recommend taking three or four doses to get maximal effect! We have seen sales conducted at rock concerts where just that advice was given. (This drug is discussed in more detail in the "Herbal Drugs" chapter).

DESIGNER STIMULANTS

Methylphenidate, perhaps cathinone, and some new designer stimulants have the opposite profile of action from ephedrine. They seem to have only weak effects on the body, so effects on blood pressure and heart rate are minimal. In this sense they lack many of the dangerous short-term side effects of amphetamine. This is why methylphenidate is a relatively safe drug for treating attention deficit disorder. However, these drugs cause intense activation in the brain, and have euphoria-producing qualities. If used inappropriately, these drugs can be addicting, although appropriate medical use of methylphenidate is certainly possible and indeed commonplace.

HOW STIMULANTS WORK

What do euphoria, blood pressure, appetite, and attention have in common that causes them all to be affected by stimulants? These behaviors/bodily functions are all regulated by a related group of neurotransmitters—the biogenic amines, or monoamine, neurotransmitters. Norepinephrine, epinephrine, dopamine, and serotonin are the monoamine neurotransmitters. They are related in structure, but each is a neurotransmitter in its own right that regulates a particular set of behaviors. Locomotor stimulants increase the amount of all of the monoamine neurotransmitters in the synapse. So, the effects of stimulants mimic what would happen if every one of the neurons that released a monoamine fired at once. It's no wonder that the effects of stimulants are so complicated.

Norepinephrine was introduced earlier as the chemical transmitter of the sympathetic nervous system. Epinephrine (or adrenaline) is the transmitter of the adrenal medulla, a special part of the sympathetic nervous system that is particularly important in flight-or-fight responses. Norepinephrine also exists in certain neurons in the brain. Norepinephrine neurons are involved in the behavioral part of the flight-or-fight response. They prepare the body and mind for emergency. This entails paying attention to your environment (not doing simple body maintenance things, like eating) and deciding whether the risk is so great that physical action is needed. In addition, it involves preparing the body for physical activity: making the heart beat faster, bringing glucose and oxygen to muscles, and widening the breathing tubes to facilitate breathing. Dopamine neurons do a very different job. These neurons are responsible for reinforcement, or reward—the sense of pleasure—as we discuss in the "Addiction" chapter. In addition, these neurons control purposeful movement and influence release of some hormones. The loss of dopamine neurons in Parkinson's disease causes the gradual loss of voluntary movement that is so incapacitating. Serotonin is involved in regulation of sleep and mood, and also in controlling appetite, body temperature, and more "vegetative" functions, as they are strangely called (since when did a carrot control its body temperature?).

Imagine what happens when a person takes amphetamine: her body prepares for flight-or-fight both physically, by increasing heart rate and blood pressure, and mentally, by becoming hyperalert (via norepinephrine); she explores her environment, moves around (perhaps purposefully, perhaps not), and feels euphoric (courtesy of dopamine); she stops eating, raises her body temperature, and releases most of her body's hormones (through serotonin). Some of these actions seem to conflict with each other. For example, in preparing for physical activity, it would be better if your body were attempting to lose excess heat instead of gaining temperature. This is why the excessive use of stimulants can be so dangerous physically.

STIMULANTS PREVENT MONOAMINE "RECAPTURE"

Stimulants work by interfering with an ingenious mechanism that monoamine neurons have for stopping neurotransmission and "recycling" their products. Normally, monoamine neurons fire impulses and release their neurotransmitters, which go across the synapse and act on their receptors. Then the monoamine neurons recapture them, by "pumping" them back into the neuron. This process eliminates the monoamines from the synapse and is the main way that these neurons turn "off" neurotransmission once it is started by the release of neurotransmitter. The stimulants like cocaine and amphetamines prevent this process from working properly. The result is that the norepinephrine, dopamine, and serotonin all stay in the synapse much longer once they are released. The end result is that all the effects of these neurotransmitters combined last much longer.

HOW EACH NEUROTRANSMITTER CONTRIBUTES TO THE EFFECTS OF STIMULANTS

Norepinephrine	Blood pressure and heart rate increase Relaxation of bronchioles Activation of fat breakdown Arousing effects Appetite effects
Serotonin	Body temperature increase Appetite effects
Dopamine	Locomotor activation Euphoria: addiction Effects on attention

---

IS AMPHETAMINE REALLY DIFFERENT FROM RITALIN OR EPHEDRINE?

Amphetamine does not affect behavior exactly the way ephedrine or methylphenidate do. What determines the differences in effects of the stimulant drugs? First of all, drugs that don't get into the brain affect only the peripheral nervous system. Ephedrine is a good example of this. However, amphetamine, cocaine, and methylphenidate all enter the brain, but they do not cause exactly the same effect. Cocaine and amphetamine cause *all* the possible actions of stimulants; they increase attention and alertness and cause the pleasurable effects that become addicting. These drugs also mimic activation of the sympathetic nervous system, causing increased breathing, heart rate, and blood pressure because they increase levels of all the monoamines. In contrast, methylphenidate affects only dopamine, so it doesn't have the prominent effects on heart rate and breathing that the other stimulants have. Amphetamine actually does a particularly good job of increasing levels of norepinephrine and dopamine, and those of its effects that are mediated by monoamines, like suppressing the appetite and increasing blood pressure, are even greater than for cocaine.

COCAINE CAN CAUSE SEIZURES

Finally, cocaine has a unique effect all its own. Remember the initial use of cocaine by Freud's friend? It was first used for its ability to cause local anesthesia—to block the transmission of pain stimuli. Cocaine is used only rarely for this purpose today because drugs that have this effect but lack cocaine's addicting properties have been invented. However, the local anesthetic effects of cocaine may account for a toxicity that is unique to cocaine. At doses not much greater than those that cause maximal effects on mood, cocaine causes seizures. Other stimulants don't do this at all, or only do it rarely, and at extremely high doses. Since other local anesthetics also can cause seizures, we think that this effect of cocaine is a result of its anesthetic action.

Drugs with large effects on all monoamines	Cocaine, amphetamine, methamphetamine
Drugs with effects mainly on dopamine	Methylphenidate
Drugs with effects mainly on norepinephrine	Ephedrine

ADDICTION, TOLERANCE, DEPENDENCE, AND WITHDRAWAL

Cocaine addiction could be viewed as a problem created by successful science (and not the only one in our society, that's for sure). Cocaine addiction is basically unknown in the South American cultures, where cocaine has been used for millennia to increase endurance and the ability to work. Chewed with an alkaline substance and delivered to the stomach and then absorbed slowly, coca leaves provide only a mild stimulant effect. The rush doesn't happen, and the drug is used with relative safety.

The situation is quite different with the cocaine and amphetamine formulations available today. When purified cocaine is provided directly by injection, smoking, or application to mucous membranes, the euphoria is much more intense and the rate of addiction much higher. There are animal experiments that point out how uniquely compelling cocaine can be. If animals (rats or monkeys) are trained to press a lever to deliver an intravenous dose of cocaine, they will do so up to three hundred times for a single injection, and if they are given free access to cocaine, these animals simply keep taking it until they have seizures. Once the scientific establishment realized how powerfully reinforcing cocaine was in this form, these experiments were dramatically cut back out of concern for animal welfare. While most animals will not voluntarily ingest dangerous amounts of alcohol, nicotine, or heroin, they will take cocaine until they kill themselves. In part, this is because there are not enough unpleasant side effects at effective doses to offset the pleasurable effects. The side effects probably considerably limit the addictiveness of alcohol and nicotine. Recovering cocaine addicts tell a similar story. Usually the only thing that stops a serious addict during a binge is running out of cocaine. One user described it like this: "If I had been in a room full of cocaine, I would have kept using it until it was all gone, and I still would have wanted more."

Part of the addictiveness of cocaine may have much to do with how it is delivered to the body. The extremely fast rise in blood levels may be the important factor. Just as cigarettes deliver nicotine to the bloodstream rapidly, smoked cocaine (crack) delivers cocaine rapidly to the brain. The recent explosion of addiction to ice, the smokable form of methamphetamine, lends credence to this notion.

Does this mean that everyone who uses stimulants becomes addicted? There are thousands of people, ranging from children with attention deficit disorder to truck drivers, who regularly use stimulants but never develop a compulsive pattern of use. For the medical uses of stimulants, the reason is usually good prescribing practice by the physician, who should never give unlimited access to these drugs, but instead prescribe only a given amount for a particular period of time. Also, taking the drug according to a rigid schedule, instead of "as needed," helps to avoid a pattern of self-medication that can become compulsive. Similar differences have been observed in the laboratory. When monkeys have free access to cocaine, their intake increases to toxic levels, but if access is restricted to a few hours a day, their intake can remain stable for months. For truck drivers and students, the answer may be a little different. Usually, truck drivers and college students use stimulants only while engaged in a particular task in a particular environment (i.e., when on the road or pulling an all-nighter). When placed in a different environment, without all the typical stimuli associated with drug use, it is easier for them to abstain.

There is no question that locomotor stimulants are addictive. As described in the "Addiction" chapter, the dopamine neurons on which they act play a primary role in addiction, and taking amphetamine or cocaine can be viewed as simply substituting drugs for natural reinforcers, such as food and sex. No other drugs in this book act so directly on reward systems, or are so commonly addicting. Can some individuals use stimulants recreationally without addiction? Probably so, and yet we know that the drive to use cocaine or amphetamines is considerably stronger than that for any of the other addictive drugs.

Tolerance develops to some stimulant effects, such as the suppression of appetite, and develops more easily with continuous use than with irregular use. This is one reason why amphetamine isn't very useful as a diet pill. Tolerance also develops during a single run, so that the high becomes harder and harder to reach, which is why people keep taking more frequent injections ("chasing the high"). However, this rapidly developed tolerance also reverses rapidly, so a few days of abstaining can restore sensitivity to much greater levels. Some effects actually become progressively greater over time. The locomotor stimulation is one of the behavioral patterns that become more and more exaggerated. While people rarely show intense stereotyped behavior the first time they take amphetamine, it is a common behavioral effect on the long-time user. Do stimulants become more addictive over time? We really don't know the answer for sure, although the pattern of use probably plays an important role.

Is stimulant withdrawal dangerous? Although there are definite symptoms of stimulant withdrawal, it is not life-threatening. At the end of a long run, when people stop using they crash. There is a period of exhaustion, with excessive sleep, often depressive symptoms, and a rebound in appetite that probably results from a prolonged period of inadequate food intake. During this period, the craving for drug is very strong. One particularly difficult symptom is the inability to feel pleasure (anhedonia). This is not a big surprise if a person has been artificially and intensely stimulating their pleasure center with a drug. When the drug is removed, so is its artificial stimulus of the brain's pleasure center. There seems to be a suppression in dopamine neuron activity during the first few days after withdrawal. No one ever died from a few days without pleasure, but in the absence of any positive feelings, the temptation to use the drug to feel better becomes stronger and stronger. Anhedonia is thought to be a major reason why people start using stimulants after a period of attempted abstinence. We don't know for sure how long these symptoms last, but in very longtime users the craving for drug can last for months.

DIET PILLS

Amphetamine got its start, in part, as a diet pill. This use was based on the very real ability of amphetamine and drugs like it to suppress appetite. Unfortunately, it was impossible to separate the appetite-suppressing qualities from the addictive potential. The search for an effective nonaddicting diet pill fueled millions of dollars' worth of pharmaceutical company research, resulting in a new understanding of the neural mechanisms regulating appetite and the discovery of medications like dexfenfluramine, which suppress appetite without producing addiction. The appetite-inhibiting effects of amphetamine probably result from the release of norepinephrine, and its addictive qualities from the release of dopamine. Amphetamine also releases serotonin, the other monoamine involved in suppressing appetite, but drugs that release *only* serotonin can effectively suppress appetite without producing addiction, and this is the basis of many of the drugs used for this purpose today. Unfortunately, the serotonin-specific releasing drugs, like fenfluramine and its derivative dexfenfluramine (as well as some others used mainly in research), have proved potentially dangerous to the heart and blood vessels, and have been pulled off the market recently.

All effective drugs that suppress appetite require a prescription. However, there are many over-the-counter drugs marketed as effective that really have minimal or no effectiveness. Chromium is the favorite of health-food stores today for its supposed ability to burn fat—a claim based on a little shaky research about its slight ability to increase the actions of insulin. However, these effects are slight at best. There is little research to support them, and the safety of long-term use has not been established.

Ephedrine is another favorite, for both its ability to both suppress appetite and its thermogenic properties. There is a little more truth to this, but not much. If ephedrine is taken in safe amounts, it does not get into the brain and cannot suppress appetite.

STIMULANT TOXICITIES AND OVERDOSES

Locomotor stimulants can cause three kinds of severe health problems. The first are the single-dose toxicities that can cause death through overdose. The second are the consequences of repeated, chronic use of escalating doses. Finally, there are a myriad of health problems associated with long-term use that are not specifically caused by the drug, but result from the stimulant-using lifestyle.

All of these drugs can kill at doses people take recreationally. A single clinically appropriate dose of amphetamine, methamphetamine, cocaine, methylphenidate, or ephedrine would rarely cause death unless an individual had an underlying health problem (aneurysm, coronary artery disease, etc.). Yet people using bootleg drug sources rarely know the dose they are taking. Also, blood levels can gradually accumulate to toxic levels during the runs of repeated drug injections or inhalations at fairly closely spaced intervals, which are a common pattern of stimulant administration. It is commonplace for people to keep taking cocaine or amphetamine until they experience unpleasant side effects, but such warning signals may come too late if the drug accumulates in the body too rapidly. Finally, as we mentioned above, the marketers of "herbal" ephedrine products often recommend that their customers take excessive and potentially toxic doses of this drug.

What happens as blood levels rise to toxic levels? The first effects are simply exaggerations of the typical drug response: energy and alertness become jitteriness or even paranoia and hostility, and increased movement becomes repetitive aimless activities, such as drawing closely spaced lines, taking watches apart and putting them back together, or talking constantly without listening. A mild increase in heart rate becomes palpitations or chest pains as the heart rhythm is disturbed, and the skin becomes flushed as body temperature rises. Headaches are common, often from effects on blood vessels. Nausea and vomiting can accompany these changes. These toxic levels can also result in strokes, heart attacks, or fatal elevations in body temperature. For cocaine, the pattern is a little different. Elevated body temperature is relatively rare, but seizures are commonplace—so much so that an adolescent or young adult arriving at an emergency room with a seizure without a previous history is almost always screened for cocaine use. It was once argued that repeated use of cocaine led to increased sensitivity to seizures, but this theory has not held up in continued study. Seizures can happen at any time during a cocaine-using "career," either the first, twentieth, or hundredth time. However, it is true that many long-time users eventually have a seizure. Rather than some permanent change in the brain, the reason may be the escalating pattern of use that leads to higher and higher blood levels of drug.

Like alcohol, in the words of Shakespeare, "desire it provokith and unprovokith." Stimulants, especially cocaine, can increase interest in sex, but sexual activity can become more difficult. Stimulants constrict blood vessels in the penis in a way that makes it difficult to maintain an erection and can delay ejaculation. In fact, this latter characteristic of cocaine is occasionally exploited by local application of cocaine to the head of the penis to prolong sexual activity!

There are also more serious social consequences. The increasing hostility, paranoia, and belligerence associated with higher blood levels of stimulants result in more overt violence. Many high-dose stimulant users become increasingly convinced that people are "out to get them," while they also become more agitated and inclined toward action. In a country with fairly liberal gun laws, this combination can be lethal, and often is. The incidence of death by homicide is substantial for stimulant users.

Different problems develop with chronic use. As use escalates into more and more frequent runs, the bizarre, repetitive stereotyped movements become more extreme. They can take the form of very self-directed behaviors, like picking at imaginary insects under the skin or assembling and taking apart equipment, or more social forms, like repetitive, stereotyped sexual or conversational activity, such as saying the same thing over and over. The picking behavior leads people eventually to create large wounds in the skin that often become infected. When paranoid and hostile behavior takes over, a person in the midst of extreme chronic amphetamine intoxication often cannot be distinguished from a paranoid schizophrenic patient. Unlike some of the effects of chronic hallucinogen use, these symptoms mostly go away when the drug is metabolized, so after a few days of hospitalization the person generally returns tô normal.

What are the effects of long-term amphetamine use on major body functions? Part of the answer depends on how the drug is administered. Cocaine and the amphetamines are powerful vasoconstrictors, and so they cut off the blood supply to the area where drug is delivered. If cocaine is snorted, then the lining of the nose can develop ulcers from inadequate blood supply, while smoked cocaine or amphetamine can cause bleeding in the lungs as small blood vessels burst, and stomach ulcers or damage to the intestines can occur with long-term oral or even intranasal use. Heart problems are also fairly common. Long-term stimulant use seems to accelerate the development of atherosclerosis (development of fatty plaques that block blood vessels) and may cause direct damage to the heart muscle from lack of oxygen.

Long-time stimulant use is also associated with many problems not caused directly by the drug. Since these drugs suppress appetite, stimulant users are often undernourished and experience all the ill effects of that condition. The incidence of hepatitis, HIV, and other infectious diseases is high in users who share dirty needles or engage in sex to obtain money for drugs.

Finally, research in animals points to the possibility of long-term neurotoxic damage by chronic use of methamphetamine and perhaps cathinone. High-dose methamphetamine causes permanent damage to the nerve endings of serotonin and dopamine neurons. The nerves do not die, but the nerve endings are "pruned," or cut back, leaving a permanent deficit in the density of nerve terminals and the amount of dopamine and serotonin available for use. What is the functional implication of this loss? Right after the loss, the system probably can compensate enough that no behavior problems are obvious.

However, as people age and experience the normal aging-related loss of dopamine and serotonin neurons, this deficit could potentially be revealed in movement or mood disorders. As with Ecstasy, we don't know the answer yet, but, unfortunately, people are conducting the experiment on themselves now. This damage is produced reliably in every experimental animal species in which it has been studied, from rodents to nonhuman primates, so it is plausible that it could also happen in humans.

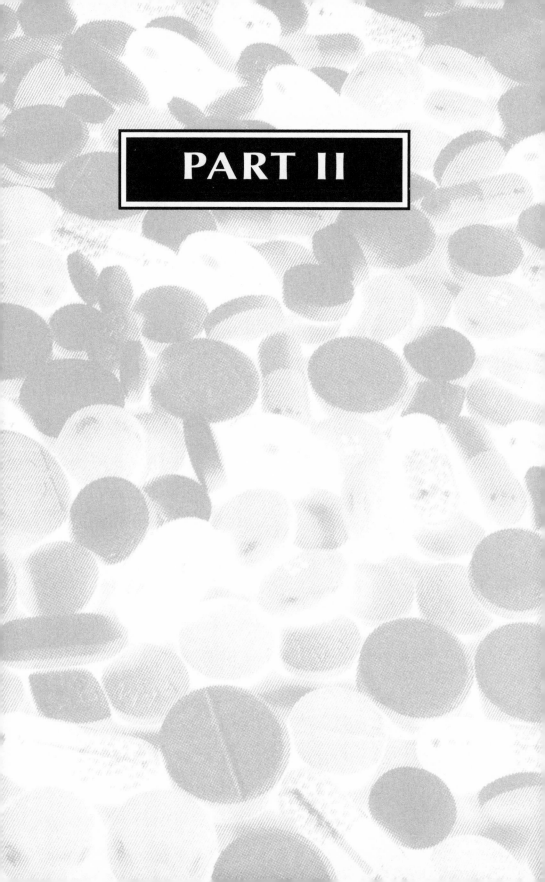

PART II

13

![square graphic]

Brain Basics

Nothing changes the way we feel or the way we perceive the world unless it interacts with our central nervous system (CNS). Whether we take a sip of wine, snort a line of cocaine, or see an attractive person, our CNS is the place where the action occurs. To understand how any drug works, we need to understand some very basic principles governing brain function.

THE PRINCIPLES

1. The brain is not only the organ that tells us who we are, what we are doing, and what we have done, but it also controls some very basic and critical body functions, such as heart rate, blood pressure, and breathing. Drugs can strongly affect these functions, which are critical to survival.

2. The brain is an extraordinarily complex structure, with thousands of different sites for drug action on thousands of different kinds of nerve cells. This complexity can cause different people to have very different experiences with the same drug.

3. The CNS, especially in children and young adults, has a remarkable capacity to change in response to experience, and this is called *plasticity*. We see it happen every day as learning and remembering, but the CNS, in response to a variety of influences, can undergo changes that occur without any awareness of them.

4. The ability of the CNS to undergo plasticity can be modified by chemicals, whether taken for medical benefit or for recreational purposes.

SINGLE NERVE CELLS

It is laughable to think that anyone completely understands how the brain functions. Every time neuroscientists make a discovery that explains some property of the nervous system, that discovery opens new doors and raises new questions. For example, no one knows exactly how the CNS stores memories, but we do know a lot about how to alter the storage process.

Often the brain is compared to a computer, and that analogy is overworked, but it's not such a bad one. Most people know how to use a computer, and they know that smashing the disks is a bad idea, but they do not know precisely how the circuits inside the computer do the job. However, not knowing just how the circuits work does not prevent the user from knowing where to insert the disk, how to turn on the monitor, and how to run a program. Likewise, there is a lot to know about the nervous system, and a little knowledge can help one keep his or hers healthy.

The first step is to appreciate what a miraculous structure the brain is. The real miracle is that such a complex structure can function so well even under some of the terribly difficult conditions that we impose on it. It has an ingenious balance of excitatory and inhibitory influences coursing through it. It's like a sports car moving along a winding country road with just the right amount of pressure on the accelerator (excitation) and the brakes (inhibition). In the brain, the brakes are the release of the inhibitory chemicals. They suppress the firing of nerve cells by opening channels in the cells membranes, letting ions flow in a direction that causes the cells' electrical potential to move away from the point at which it would fire a signal (an action potential). Without action potentials, there is no action, so we say that that cell or network of cells is inhibited. An inhibited network cannot carry out its function, so that function is lost. The lost function might be thinking, feeling anxiety, staying awake, having reflexes to pain, adjusting the circulatory system, or breathing. An overly excited network is like a pot of boiling water, or like that sports car out of control at high speed. There is a chaos of discharges that randomly fire in many parts of the brain, leading to all sorts of feelings and movements. It is a miracle that in most of us, for most of the time, the brain maintains the delicate balance that permits a normal life.

The first step to understanding that delicate balance, and how drugs disrupt it, is to understand the building blocks of the CNS—the nerve cells, or neurons. There are many other CNS cells that support the neurons, but the neurons are where the information is stored, where feelings are sensed, and where actions are initiated.

Neurons look a little like trees. Did you ever see a big tree uprooted? There's the trunk and the top with many branches and the leaves that receive the sunlight. Then there is the root system that is equally branched, with a large tap root going off into the earth. Under the microscope, many neurons look the same way. They have a "top" receiving area called the dendrites, where connections from other neurons make contact. Then they have a "trunk" area, where the body of the nerve cell is located, containing the genetic information for that cell. Finally, out of the cell body emerges the axon of the cell (like the root of a tree), which goes off and branches to make contact with other nerve cells or muscle cells and transmit signals to them.

Like all cells, a nerve cell is held together by its cell membrane, which is a mixture of lipids (fats) and proteins. Many nonneuronal cells (blood cells, muscle cells, etc.) have cell membranes that are more or less the same all over. The cell membranes of neurons, however, are vastly different in different parts of the cell. These differences allow a cell to receive different types of signals from many other cells, integrate these signals, and then send out signals of its own. Even a single neuron is a very complicated bit of biochemical machinery, but this complexity is what allows the enormous information storage and processing capacity of the human brain to exist in such a compact form.

CONNECTIONS BETWEEN NERVE CELLS

The dendritic, or receiving, area of neurons is where axons (transmitting fibers) from other nerve cells make contact. These points of contact are called synapses. A single synapse is, in itself, a complex structure, consisting of the presynaptic and the postsynaptic region. The presynaptic region is the termination point of the axon of the transmitting cell, and at that point the axon balloons from a very small fiber to a group of bulb-like endings called the presynaptic terminals. These terminals contain chemicals—neurotransmitters—which are released into the space between the presynaptic terminal and the dendrite of the postsynaptic (receiving) cell. The neurotransmitter molecules react with special receptors that are sensitive only to that neurotransmitter on the postsynaptic cell, and, in just thousandths of a second, these receptors cause electrical and/or biochemical signals within the receiving cell.

A single neuron can have millions of synapses on its dendrites, and it is the job of the neuron cell body to take in signals from all of those synapses and make a decision. That decision is whether to fire electrical signals itself down its transmitting fiber—its axon. The signals that are transmitted down the axon are called action potentials because they can cause action somewhere else. If they come from a nerve cell synapsing onto a muscle cell, they can cause the muscle cell to contract. If they come from a nerve cell connecting to another nerve cell, they can cause that follower nerve cell to either fire or stop firing, depending on what kind of signal it gets from the neurotransmitter molecules.

Thus, the input to a neuron is from synaptic connections from other neurons, while the output is a series of action potentials firing down its axon. The action potentials are all the same, just quick (about one thousandth of a second) discharges of electrical activity. The information is carried by the rate at which they occur. So, if a neuron fires lots of action potentials in a brief period (up to four hundred in one second), it can have a large influence on its follower cells, while slow firing would have less influence.

Some drugs may affect the generation and spread of action potentials down the axon, but that is not a common site of drug action. These drugs usually produce drastic and often toxic changes because they can completely stop a neuron from firing. One interesting toxin that does this is the chemical present in the ovaries of puffer fish, which are delicacies in Japan. This chemical, called tetrodotoxin, is so toxic that eating just part of a fish can paralyze the muscles responsible for breathing. Japanese restaurants have chefs who are specially trained and licensed to remove the ovaries before the fish is served. This same class of toxin is also thought to be used in Haitian voodoo rituals to induce zombie-like behavior.

Most drugs that don't make us zombies (and some that do!) act either at the presynaptic terminal, where the neurotransmitter is released, or at the postsynaptic membrane on the neurotransmitter receptor. The synapse is the primary site of action of the majority of drugs that affect human brain functions. To understand drugs, one must understand the synapse.

The presynaptic terminal is the place where neurotransmitters are synthesized, packaged, and released. When action potentials travel from the cell body of the transmitting neuron down to the terminal area, the electrical signals cause changes in the shape of protein molecules that reside in the terminal area. These molecules sense the electrical signals and, within thousandths of a second, reconfigure themselves to form pores, or channels, in the terminal membrane. Calcium ions flow into the terminal through these pores, and the calcium initiates a chain of biochemical reactions. The result of this biochemical sequence is that packets of neurotransmitter molecules break through the terminal membrane and move toward the postsynaptic area of the receiving cell.

What happens to the neurotransmitter molecules after they are released? After all, if they stayed around forever, the postsynaptic neuron, or muscle fiber, would constantly be under their influence and further signaling would be impossible. Removal of neurotransmitters is accomplished in three ways. First, the molecules just diffuse away into other areas where there are no receptors and are removed by the general circulation of fluids in the brain. Second, there can be specific chemicals that break the neurotransmitters into noneffective parts that are returned to the cells. Finally, there are specific sites on the presynaptic terminal that attach to the active neurotransmitter molecules and transport them back into the terminal for release again. These transport sites are often places where drugs act to prolong the presence of the transmitter in the postsynaptic area, therefore increasing its effect. Cocaine is an excellent example of such a drug, because it suppresses the uptake of the transmitter dopamine, which is important in the reward center of the brain.

This entire neurotransmitter release process can be controlled by chemicals active at the presynaptic terminal. In some cases there are receptors for the transmitter being released that serve to suppress further release of the transmitter, and thus limit the action at that synapse. In other cases there are receptors for different neurotransmitters that can regulate release. Any of these sites could be important places for drugs to act.

THE ROLE OF RECEPTORS

Next, consider the postsynaptic region of the cell, where the neurotransmitter receptors are located. The postsynaptic region contains the proteins bound in the lipid cell membrane that react with the neurotransmitter molecules. These proteins are, in themselves, very complex structures. They are three-dimensional molecules that have sites into which the neurotransmitter molecules can fit. In fact, this arrangement is just like a lock-and-key mechanism. The neurotransmitter molecules from the presynaptic cell are the keys and the postsynaptic receptors are the locks. When the key "enters" the lock by binding to the receptor molecule, the lock operates and the bioelectrical activity is initiated.

The lock-and-key analogy is good to a point, but certainly is too simplistic. Unlike a lock, which usually has only one action (to throw a bolt into a door), a receptor can have numerous actions, and each one of these steps can be changed by drugs. The first two actions that occur at a receptor are electrical and biochemical. The fastest signal is the electrical process.

Once the neurotransmitter binds, the receptor molecule can change its shape and open channels (pores) into the cell on which it is located. These channels allow the flow of charged molecules (ions) into or out of the cell, and this movement of electrical charge causes an electrical signal to develop across the cell membrane.

Normally neurons have an electrical charge so that the inside of the cell is negative (about .1 volt) compared to the outside. This is called the resting potential, and when a neuron is at rest, it fires no action potentials. When the inside of the cell at the point of the cell body becomes considerably less negative (about .04 volts), then action potentials begin to fire and the cell is then transmitting to its follower cells.

The electrical action at the synapse can thus control whether or not a cell will start to fire action potentials. For example, if a receptor opens a channel that lets in ions that make the cell less negative, then the electrical potential of the cell will move in the direction of firing action potentials. If the receptor opens a channel that causes the cell to become more negative inside, then the cell becomes less able to fire. Clearly, then, with millions of synapses, the cell must add all of this electrical activity together, and the sum of it determines whether or not a cell will fire. This addition of pro-and antifiring (excitatory and inhibitory) currents occurs in and around the cell body of the neuron, in a place where action potentials originate. Thus, all of the synaptic activity of the cell converges to the cell body, where the cell makes the decision to fire or not to fire, depending on the voltage across its cell membrane.

The two most common neurotransmitters in the CNS are the amino acids GABA (gamma-aminobutyric acid) and glutamate. These are referred to as inhibitory (GABA) and excitatory (glutamate) amino acid neurotransmitters. These neurotransmitters are responsible for much of the second-to-second processing in the CNS. If either of these is significantly blocked, the proper functioning of the CNS will be dramatically disrupted. There are many subtypes of these receptors, and each of these subtypes has different characteristics. Some of the most interesting drug effects come from activating just a particular subtype of a receptor rather than the whole class of receptors.

Receptors can initiate a cascade of biochemical events within neurons. Either by letting calcium ions into cells or by activating intracellular enzymes directly, activated receptors can profoundly change the biochemical environment of a cell. These biochemical signals can alter the numbers of receptors for different transmitters, change the degree to which they recognize their transmitters, or even change the systems that regulate the genetics of the cell—literally, thousands of different processes. It is no wonder that drugs that interact with receptors can be so specific and so powerful.

It is this diversity of receptors and biochemical signaling pathways that allows humans to devise drugs that have quite specific effects. Throughout this book there are references to actions of a drug at a specific receptor, receptor regulation site, or biochemical signaling pathway. Although we know much about the way these chemicals operate, it is important to remember the mantra of every pharmacologist: "Every drug has two effects—the one I know about and the one I don't know about."

COLLECTIONS OF NEURONS FORM SPECIALIZED BRAIN AREAS

While neurons are the basic components of the brain, the ways in which they are connected determine what functions will occur. An old cartoon shows a neurosurgeon in the operating room saying, "Well, there go the piano lessons." Like most humor, it's somewhat based in fact. The brain is organized into specialized areas that control speech, hearing, vision, fine movements, gross movements, learning, anger, fear, and much more.

It would be very useful to know which neurotransmitters and receptors carry the information for all of these functions, because then we could design specific drugs to modulate them with great precision. However, we are far from having that information, and even if we did have it, there is another complication—the pattern of connections between neurons. While neurochemistry is important, the patterns in which neurons connect is equally important. The connections are quite specific, and while we know a lot about the gross pathways connecting brain areas, we know little about how cells are connected *within* small brain areas.

Behaviors, even simple ones, are possible because neuronal connections are complicated. For example, even the simplest reaction, such as blinking when a dust particle gets in your eye, involves several nerves connected to each other. So, when a drug alters one process, the effect it has depends on how that process participates in the function of the network. Thus, our ignorance of nerve-cell connections accounts for some of the uncertainty in knowing the effects of drugs.

THE CENTRAL NERVOUS SYSTEM CONTROLS BASIC FUNCTIONS

In the section below we will talk about some of the most exciting parts of brain function, learning and memory. But it is crucial to understand that the central nervous system controls some very important body functions that sustain life. These are boring functions until they fail, and then they get attention right away. The three most vital functions that the CNS controls are the circulatory system (heart and blood vessels), the respiratory system (breathing), and the reflex system (which instantly, and without thinking, causes one to respond to a threat).

The circulatory system is maintained in a stable condition by its own built-in control system. However, the brain can easily modify this set point. For example, during periods of anger and frustration the heart will beat rapidly and blood pressure will rise. In this condition, the brain has decided that the "normal" status is incorrect and that the body needs to be prepared for *flight or fight*. In this condition, the CNS will also stimulate the respiratory system and cause breathing to increase. In contrast, when the mind is at peace, and perhaps meditative, the heart rate falls, blood pressure falls, and breathing is slowed.

The CNS reflex system is equally important, but often forgotten. People who think about drugs and safety often mention hearts and breathing, but they don't put as much emphasis on how reflexes keep us safe. Take, for example, how one jerks one's hand back from a hot surface. This is a pure reflex action that is signaled in the spinal cord. The sensing nerves in the fingers and hand send a powerful signal of distress to the spinal cord. This signal excites neurons that cause movement and, through a modestly complicated process, withdrawal of the hand. This all happens before the pain signals are even interpreted by the conscious brain.

A more important example is the reflex to clear the airway for breathing. Notice how fast and how strongly the body responds when something touches the airway in the back of the throat. This is a critical reflex to sustain life. If this reflex were suppressed by a drug, then something could easily occlude the airway (such as vomit) and it would not be cleared, and the person would die of asphyxiation. The list of basic body functions that can be impaired by drugs goes on and on. This is not a particularly glamorous or fascinating area of drug effects, but it is one that everyone must understand.

PLASTICITY IN THE CNS—LEARNING FROM EXPERIENCE

The third principle of this chapter stated that the CNS responds to experience by learning. That is, it reorganizes some of its neurochemistry and connections so that the experience is remembered. It is very important to understand that this plasticity is a broad concept. Not only does the CNS remember events that are consciously experienced but it also changes in response to all sorts of signals, such as the constant presence of drugs.

The most familiar plasticity in the CNS is the simple remembering of experiences—faces, smells, names, classroom lectures, and lots more. The neurobiological mechanisms through which this kind of learning happens are not completely understood, but we have some clues. One important site of learning appears to be the synapse.

As discussed above, synapses of nerve cells are quite complex and there is extensive biochemical machinery in both the presynaptic and the postsynaptic areas. We think memory is built one synapse at a time: some synapses that are stimulated repeatedly change how they function (learn) and maintain that change for a long time. There is an electrical manifestation of this learning that scientists call long-term potentiation (LTP). It is a long-lasting strengthening (potentiation) of the electrical signal between two neurons that occurs when the synapse between them is stimulated.

We're not sure how this happens, but it must be through some series of biochemical changes in how the first neuron releases its neurotransmitter, or in how the second neuron responds to it. On the presynaptic side, a synapse could be strengthened by increasing the number of presynaptic terminals by releasing more transmitter from the same number of terminals, or by a reduction in transmitter removal. On the postsynaptic side, strengthening could occur with an increase in the number of receptors, a change in the functional properties of the receptors, or a change in the biochemistry of the postsynaptic cell. There is scientific controversy about the true mechanisms of LTP, and the issue may not be clear for a number of years.

Almost every neuron can change many aspects of its function—by making more or less neurotransmitter, by changing the number of receptors on the surface of its cells, by changing the number of molecules responsible for the passage of the electrical stimulus down the axon, etc. If a neural circuit is being overstimulated, it can reduce the stimulation by removing some of the receptors for the neurotransmitter stimulating it. Therefore, even if it is being sent lots of signals, they don't get through. Alternatively, if a neural circuit is receiving much less stimulation than usual, it can adapt by becoming more sensitive to each stimulus. This is how the brain stays in balance.

This type of biochemical plasticity goes on all the time, and is part of normal brain function. However, these same changes can cause abnormal brain function. For example, we think that the tremendous mood changes in depression might result from changing numbers of neurotransmitter receptors following changing stimulation of specific neurons in the brain.

If neurons and synapses learn, do they also forget? The answer appears to be yes. We described above how stimulating a neural pathway in a certain way can cause it to "learn" to respond to stimulation differently. Stimulating it in another way (slowly, and for a long time) can cause a process called *depotentiation*, which appears to be the opposite of long-term potentiation. Why is this interesting? Depotentiation could be quite important because it may represent the synaptic equivalent of amnesia. Depotentiation can be produced by prolonged slow activity or by very strong high-frequency activity, like that which occurs in seizures. It may be a protective mechanism by which the CNS prevents a seizure or brain trauma from encoding new information into the circuits. Again, it is almost certainly under the control of cell signaling pathways, and thus could be manipulated by drugs.

This gradual change in the electrical strength of a connection seems subtle, but it makes intuitive sense that memories could form in this way. However, can the brain actually change physically? We used to think that once a person was mature, the brain didn't change anymore. However, more and more research shows that actual changes in the shapes of neurons also can happen in response to earlier experiences. We know that the shape of certain neurons in the brain change when different hormones become available. For example, at least in animals, treating them with hormones can stimulate the production of little protuberances, or "spines," on the dendrites of neurons. Other research has shown that synapses actually remodel themselves over time after different levels of activity. So, connections actually get lost or remade. It has been known for a long time that this happened in lower animals. For example, as songbirds learn new songs, the structure of certain parts of their brains change. It was once thought that the brains of mammals did not have this type of structural plasticity. However, more recent studies have shown similar changes in rats, and scientists think that they probably occur in all mammals.

Do All Parts of the Brain Learn?

The processes that we described above do not happen in just one part of the brain. There are indeed specialized neural networks, especially in a part of the brain called the hippocampus, where this process occurs and can create memories. We know this is important because people who have had damage to this part of the brain cannot learn new things, although they can remember things that happened before. However, most of these forms of plasticity can occur all over the brain and affect all brain function.

One final note about the changing brain. We are usually aware of memories, and the fact that the structure or biochemistry of the brain changes to create these memories makes a lot of sense. However, do our brains change without our awareness? The answer is a resounding yes. Many of the changes we described above happen without our knowing it.

For one to be able to function normally, all of these processes need to proceed unimpaired. All the neurotransmitter systems need to be working. Furthermore, one's brain needs to change with time to reflect previous experience, and needs to be able to restore balance if it is over- or understimulated. This means it needs to be able to make long-term changes that create and suppress memory, or restore biochemical balance to the brain.

THE DEVELOPING BRAIN

While the brains of adults change all the time, as we described above, what goes on in adults is trivial compared to the phenomenal changes that occur while the brain is developing. The brain assembles itself carefully through the process of neurons growing out, and through chemical signals around them, gradually finding their way to the correct destination, where they make the connections that they then maintain. During this time of life, the physical changes in the brain are dramatic. New synaptic connections are being made at a high rate every day. The growing brain also has its own way of "forgetting." Many of the neurons growing out never reach their destination, and die in the process. Others reshape their connections until they are correct. Through all of this furious growth, neurons must remain active or they can fail to make their appropriate connections. Therefore, changes in neuronal function that in an adult would simply shut down a pathway for a while, in a developing brain can have more drastic consequences.

Growing neurons are affected by processes that don't affect the neurons of adult brains. Exposure to substances that inhibit cell growth has some impact on an adult brain, but devastating impact on the developing brain. The neurotoxic element mercury provides a good example. Mercury affects the function of the adult brain, and can lead to serious, but largely reversible, disruption of brain function. However, exposure of the brain of the developing fetus to mercury disrupts brain development so totally that severe mental retardation results. For example, an industrial spill of mercury into the water near a small, coastal Japanese town called Minamata contaminated the fish that were the local food source. While many adults experienced diseases that eventually resolved, many children born during this time frame had terrible disruption of normal brain development and remained mentally retarded throughout their lives.

DRUGS AND PLASTICITY

Whatever the exact mechanisms are that underlie learning, there is strong evidence that supports the correlation between synaptic changes, neuroplasticity, and learning. The best of this evidence comes from drug studies. Chemicals that block the development of LTP tend to block other manifestations of neuroplasticity, and, in particular, can block learning.

For example, a drug called AP-5 (D-2-amino-5-phosphonopentanoate) blocks a certain subtype of the excitatory neurotransmitter glutamate. This particular subtype, the NMDA (the N-methyl-D-aspartate) receptor, has the very special property of letting calcium into the cell only when the cell is receiving excitatory signals through other synapses. The calcium causes LTP to occur at those synapses. Thus, the NMDA receptor is like a memory switch. When the cell is receiving a signal and the NMDA receptor is activated, the cell "remembers" the signal by strengthening that synapse.

It is wonderful that we have been lucky enough to find the NMDA receptor, because it appears to be one of the most important receptors for learning and other forms of neuroplasticity. It may teach us much about how memory occurs, and how some drugs disrupt it. For example, in laboratory experiments, if we chemically block the NMDA receptor so that glutamate cannot bind there, LTP does not occur, rats do not learn mazes, and the CNS does not reorganize its neuronal connections following injury. There is every reason to believe that learning and neuroplasticity are also suppressed in humans.

Alcohol in rats blocks NMDA receptors, suppresses LTP, and suppresses maze learning. So, now we may know why we forget what we did when we were drunk (see the "Alcohol" chapter for more information).

Many drugs affect the ability of the brain to learn—there is no question about it. But which drugs have which effects and for how long? One of the best stories about the effects of drugs on learning was told to one of us by a drug company representative during an airplane trip. It seems that some of the professional staff from his company were making a quick trip overseas to a meeting, and they needed to sleep during the plane ride over because their lectures were scheduled almost as soon as they were to arrive. So, this group had a few alcoholic drinks and then took one of their newly marketed sedatives to get to sleep. Everything went well, including the lectures, and the scientists returned home in a couple of days. The only problem was that when they returned they remembered nothing of the meeting—not their lectures or those of anyone else. They did not know that the drug they chose, in the dose they chose, would have powerful amnesiac effects, especially when mixed with alcohol.

This story is legend in the pharmaceutical industry, and whether or not it is exactly true does not make any difference. It illustrates the point that even the people who develop and manufacture drugs by the highest standards may not know every effect they can have, and how long these effects can last.

There are basically three ways in which drugs can affect memory. First, they can prevent learning by impairing the ability of the brain to store information (amnesia). Second, there is a glimmer of evidence that some chemicals can increase learning. Finally, they can cause distortions of reality that have such a powerful effect, they are stored and recalled as either good or bad experiences.

By far, the most common effect of drugs is to suppress learning, because this is the most complex process in the brain and is the first to go in response to almost any brain insult. Almost all of the drugs that have sedative or anxiety-reducing properties impair the retention of information. Although we do not know exactly how this happens, there are three mechanisms that have been proposed at the synaptic level.

The first of these is increased inhibition. We know that many sedative drugs increase GABA-mediated synaptic activity, which inhibits the firing of neurons. The experimental data suggest that this increase in inhibition can reduce the effects of the type of neuronal firing that is usually necessary for LTP, and thus prevent neuroplasticity.

The second of these mechanisms is reduced excitation. Some drugs, such as alcohol, not only increase GABA function (and thus inhibition) but also suppress the glutamate-mediated excitatory channels (the NMDA receptor-channels) that let calcium ions into the neurons. This reduction in calcium entry prevents the signaling mechanisms within the neurons that lead to long-term synaptic changes.

Finally, there are drugs, such as the THC in marijuana, that act through their own receptors to change cell biochemistry so that learning is impaired. As discussed in the "Marijuana" chapter, these THC receptors have just been identified, so not much is known about how they suppress learning. From what we know of their biochemistry, they may directly regulate the signal-processing pathways within the cell that govern the strength of synaptic activity, perhaps by suppressing the signals that mediate LTP or, alternatively, by enhancing the processes underlying LTD and/or depotentiation.

Now that we know about LTD and depotentiation, it is easy to imagine that there would be reasons for the CNS to reduce activity in some pathways and thus "forget" some neuroplastic changes. Therefore, it is completely reasonable that some drugs could enhance this type of signaling, reducing the ability to learn.

The opposite effect of learning suppression is enhancement of learning, and this is an area that neurobiology is just beginning to explore productively. As anyone can imagine, the pharmaceutical companies would just love to invent compounds that could make us smarter. The market would be huge. Many people suffer from Alzheimer's disease and other brain disorders that impair learning, and they desperately need help. Most of the rest of us would relish the ability to learn more or quicker. There are some tantalizing clues that this may be possible, but we are nowhere near success yet.

One of the most interesting clues about ways that we might enhance learning comes from an experience that almost all of us have had. It's the "Do you remember what were you doing when . . . ?" question. Every generation has at least one of these questions. For middle-aged people, it's what they were doing when they heard that Kennedy was shot. Younger people remember what they were doing when they heard that the space shuttle *Challenger* blew up. Think of an example: the first time you had a very important and emotional experience, either positive or negative.

Why is it that we remember some experiences so well, and not only the event but maybe what clothes we wore, what the room looked like, what we ate? A recent experiment sheds a lot of light on this phenomenon. Dr. Jim McGaugh (of the University of California at Irvine) took two similar groups of people and placed them in separate but similar rooms with all sorts of cues, or decorations, in the rooms. The goal was to subject the groups to an emotional story and to see how well they remembered the story and the environment (the room) in which they experienced the event.

What makes this experiment interesting is that one group was given a drug (propranolol) that blocks a particular subtype of adrenaline receptor — the beta-adrenaline receptor. This receptor is the one responsible for the increase in heart rate and blood pressure that occurs under physical or emotional stress, and the blocker, propranolol is used to control blood pressure and heart problems in some patients. So, one group was completely normal, while the other group had their excitatory adrenaline activity blocked.

The experimental subjects were then told a heartbreaking story about an injured child. After a period of time the two groups were removed from their rooms and then asked to recall the story and the details of their environment in the room. Both groups remembered the story. However, only the normal (undrugged) group remembered the details of the room. The treated group remembered very little of their environment.

What does this teach us? We all know that we tend to learn what interests us, and we know that we remember emotional events. Now we know why. The adrenergic system apparently delivers signals to the brain that facilitate learning and remembering the environment associated with an emotionally powerful event. This is probably a very important characteristic for both humans and other animals to have, because it tends to help us remember events and places that were either wonderful or threatening, and thus adjust our future behavior accordingly. So, now it is clear why a smell or a face or a place might make you feel good or bad, even if you cannot immediately recall why. It's the brain recalling an emotional experience.

This insight into learning is useful in several ways. First, it illustrates how important it is to be alert and interested in what one is trying to learn. A sleepy, depressed person is a poor learner, in part because his adrenergic system is not activated. If one really wants to learn or teach something, include an emotional component in it.

In addition, this experiment suggests that there may be ways to facilitate learning through manipulating brain chemistry. Neuroscientists already know that the adrenergic system is not the only modulator of learning. However, increasing the function of any of these systems has proven difficult to achieve without producing unacceptable side effects.

An important message for the audience of this book is the following: if anyone says that they have a drug that will improve learning, be very skeptical. Remember that the drug companies desperately want to find safe drugs that improve learning, and if the drug offered does not come from a pharmaceutical company, it is very likely ineffective or unsafe. Also, to improve learning, it is best to stay away from drugs that are depressants or that leave a person depressed after their use. Finally, and most important, study what is exciting (or get excited about what you must study!).

WHY SHOULD ANYONE CARE ABOUT ALL OF THIS?

We hope that this chapter offers some good reasons to develop a respect for the brain and the body that supports it, as well as some insight into why drugs do what they do. This is especially important for teenagers, because, as every teenager knows, they are different from adults.

What adults may not know is that the teenagers are right. For some time we have known that the very immature brain, as in babies, has a number of characteristics that are different from the adult brain. Now we are finding that the adolescent brain may be different also. It may respond differently to drugs and it may learn differently.

A psychologist at Duke University, Dr. David Rubin, has carried out a fascinating series of experiments showing just how different young people may be. The basic experiment was to take adults at various ages and ask them questions about events that occurred in every ten-year period of their lives, including a lot of trivia. Of course, recent events were remembered fairly well, but other than those, the events best recalled were those that occurred during young adulthood (from age eleven to age thirty). This means that a senior citizen recalled his life events and what was going on in the world during his adolescence even better than those events that had occurred just a few years earlier.

If our conclusions from this research are correct, then there is something very special about either our brain biochemistry or our psychological state during adolescence that enables us to store our experiences for life. Whatever the explanation, the implications are clear—the experiences, good or bad, that we have during our youth are very well stored in our memory systems and can be recalled for the rest of our lives. Thus, when teenagers say they are different, they are right, and when adults say that these are formative years, they too are right.

14

Drug Basics

Understanding drugs and their effects on our bodies begins with some very simple principles.

THE PRINCIPLES

1. A drug is any chemical put into the body that changes mental state or bodily function.

2. How a drug is taken can make a huge difference in its effects. Eating or swallowing a drug is usually the slowest route to the brain, and inhaling or intravenous injection is the fastest route. If a drug is potentially lethal, then rapid administration of the drug by inhaling it or injecting it is the most dangerous way to take it, and could result in almost immediate death.

3. The length of time a drug affects the central nervous system can vary tremendously. Some drugs are removed in only a few minutes, while others stay around for weeks. With any compound, it is crucial to know how long its effects will last—even those effects one does not notice.

4. The effects of drugs can change with time, as our bodies adapt to the drug. This is called tolerance. As a result, when drug use is stopped, these changes cause bodies to work abnormally once the drug is no longer present. This is called withdrawal.

CHAPTER CONTENTS

The term *drug* means one thing to politicians trying to get elected, another thing to high school students, and yet another to physicians. *A drug is any substance that changes mental state or bodily function.* This can mean megadoses of vitamins, herbal medications from health-food stores, birth control pills, over-the-counter cold remedies, aspirin, or beer. Psychoactive drugs are simply those that affect the brain. Psychoactive drugs can be found in foods or beverages (like coffee), are prescribed by doctors to treat illnesses of the brain (like epilepsy), and are taken for recreational purposes. There are thousands of compounds that fit this simple definition of drugs. Try to make a list of all the drugs you have ever taken. It will probably number at least twenty, even for those readers who "don't take drugs."

Some argue that certain foods are drugs (favorite culprits are sugar and chocolate), but this may be a stretch. While the analogy might be clear, as anyone who has ever had a chocolate binge will attest to, there simply isn't strong enough research to show that ingesting these substances changes behavior or physiology more than any other nutrient. Similarly, some addiction-treatment programs view behaviors such as compulsive sex, shopping, and gambling as similar to drugs. For the purpose of this book, we are going to assume that neither foods nor behaviors qualify as drugs.

A toxin, in distinction from a drug, is simply a substance that causes bodily harm. Pharmacologists joke that the only difference between a drug and a toxin is how much you take. There is a grain of truth in this. Many drugs produce good effects at some doses and bad effects at other doses. There is another difference between drugs and toxins. Drug taking is usually purposeful. This is not true of toxins. We are frequently exposed involuntarily to substances that are toxic, such as pesticide residues on our food, air pollutants, and vapors we inhale when we put gasoline in our cars. However, this last example shows how blurred these definitions can be. One of the substances present in gasoline in trace amounts (toluene) is the active ingredient in inhalants that some people sniff to get high. Is it a toxin or a drug? It is both, and it affects bodily function in a bad way, regardless of the intent of the drug user.

HOW DO DRUGS WORK: RECEPTORS

Drugs work by attaching to a particular molecule called a *receptor*. Many different molecules can be receptors for drugs. Proteins on the surface of a cell that normally respond to hormones circulating in the blood, enzymes that control the flow of energy in a cell, even structures like the microscopic tubes (microtubules) that give the cell its shape, can all be receptors. They can occur anywhere in the body: brain, heart, bone, skin. Almost any bodily function can be affected by a drug if it can bind to some element of the cell that is critical to that function.

When a drug binds to its receptor and activates it, the drug is called an *agonist*. Simply put, it means that the drug has an effect. Some drugs attach to a receptor but do not activate it. These drugs are *antagonists*. Antagonists keep other molecules from getting to the receptor, often the molecule that normally would be stimulating it. They act by preventing normal processes from happening. Many of the psychoactive drugs we will discuss in this book work by preventing the action of normal neurotransmitters.

The poisons used in poison darts provide a vivid example. One active compound in these poisons, curare, prevents the neurotransmitter acetylcholine from working on its receptor. Acetylcholine is necessary to transmit from brain to muscle the information that permits muscle contraction. When curare blocks the action of acetylcholine, the muscles are paralyzed and the dart's victim dies from paralysis of the muscles responsible for breathing.

HOW WELL DO DRUGS WORK: DOSE RESPONSE

How well a drug works depends on how much a user takes. The larger the dose, generally, the bigger the effect, until a maximum is reached. Usually this maximum is reached because all the available receptors become occupied by the drug. Taking more drug than this is pointless.

So, why do we take more of some drugs than others? Advertisements on TV are proud of bragging that one can take just one tiny pill of brand X instead of three pills of brand Y. Some drugs bind so tightly to their receptor that it takes very little to activate all the available receptors. Such a drug is very *po-*

tent. LSD is a good example of a very potent drug since only millionths of a gram can cause hallucinations. So, should you be happy to take brand X instead of brand Y? It depends on how much they cost. If brand X costs three times more and you take one-third as much, you have gained nothing!

What difference between brand X and brand Y could matter? Some drugs don't bind very well, but enough can activate all available receptors very well. Others bind very tightly but don't activate the receptor very well. *Efficacy* means how well a drug does what it does—how well it changes receptor function. It does matter if brand X has more efficacy than brand Y, because then the one pill would have more effect than three of brand Y. For example, both aspirin and a strong opiate like morphine diminish the sensation of pain. However, no matter how much aspirin one takes, one cannot come close to matching the pain relief from morphine, because aspirin has less efficacy for this particular action. So, why take aspirin instead of morphine? First of all, a morphine dose can kill you because the difference between an effective dose and a toxic overdose is not great. Second, morphine is addictive. For a garden-variety tension headache, the risks associated with using morphine are not worth the potential benefit. However, for very severe migraine headaches, sometimes the greater efficacy of opiate drugs is necessary.

HOW DRUGS GET INTO AND OUT OF THE BODY

GETTING IN

Drugs must get to their receptors to act. Even a skin cream like a cortisone ointment that relieves the itch of poison ivy must be able to pass through the fatty membrane that surrounds most cells to heal the cells that are irritated by poison ivy toxin.

Most drugs must go much farther than the skin to act. Drugs used to treat tumors deep inside the body must travel from where they are placed, through the bloodstream, to be delivered to distant organs. A few drugs dissolve so well in cells that when they are rubbed on the skin they travel through all the skin layers down to the layer of the skin where the smallest blood vessels (capillaries) are, through the capillary walls, and into the bloodstream. Nicotine is one, which is why the nicotine skin patch works. There is also a motion-sickness drug that is fat-soluble enough to travel through the skin to the brain. However, most drugs just don't dissolve well enough in these fatty membranes to travel all that distance.

Applying drugs to the mucous membranes is a more effective way of getting some drugs into the body because the mucous membrane surfaces of the body (as in the nose) are much thinner, and the capillaries are much closer to the surface. For these reasons, placing drugs in the nose, mouth, or rectum provides another pretty efficient route for administering some drugs. Cocaine and amphetamine are absorbed well from these sites, which is why they are often snorted by users. In contrast, one cannot take antibiotics nasally because they simply would not be well absorbed. Anyway, who would want to snort amoxicillin?

The most efficient way to get a drug into the bloodstream is to put it there directly. The invention of the hypodermic syringe provided the most direct means we have of getting drugs into the body: we inject them directly into a vein. The drug then goes to the heart and is distributed throughout the entire body. After intravenous injection, peak drug levels in the bloodstream are established within a minute or two. Then levels begin to fall as the drug crosses the capillaries and enters the tissues.

There are other places that drugs can be injected. Most immunizations are done by injecting the vaccine into the muscle (intramuscular). The drug is delivered a little more slowly this way, because it must leave the muscle and enter capillaries before it is distributed to the body. In the same way, drugs can be injected beneath the skin (subcutaneously, or skin-popping). This is a route used by many beginning heroin users who have not yet started injecting heroin intravenously.

Inhaling drugs into the lungs can deliver a drug to the circulation almost as quickly as intravenous injection if the drug is very fat-soluble. Anyone who smokes tobacco takes advantage of this characteristic to deliver nicotine to the brain. The drug simply has to dissolve through the air sacs of the lungs and into the capillaries. Since the surface area of the lungs is very large and drugs can move quickly across a large surface, and since the blood supply of the lungs goes directly to the heart and then out to the other tissues, smoking very fat-soluble compounds can deliver them to the tissues almost as quickly as intravenous injection.

The most common way that people get drugs into their system is to swallow them. Drugs that enter this way must pass through the walls of the stomach or intestine and then enter the capillaries. A large part of any drug that is swallowed never gets distributed to the rest of the body because it is removed by the liver and destroyed. The liver is placed cleverly to do this job. All the blood vessels that take nutrients from the intestine to the body must go through the liver first, where toxic substances can be removed. This protects the body from toxic substances in food. Swallowing may be the easiest way to deliver drugs, but it is the slowest way to deliver a drug to the body. So, the next time you take an ibuprofen for your headache, you should not wonder why the headache is not gone in five minutes.

To recapitulate, the way people take a drug (the route of administration), combined with the amount they take, determine the drug's effects. Injecting drugs intravenously or smoking them results in nearly instantaneous effects because the levels of drug in the blood rise very rapidly. This speed accounts for the lure of injecting heroin intravenously or smoking crack. The drug effect occurs much more rapidly than if the drug was snorted. Injecting a drug intravenously or smoking it also offers the greatest risk of overdose. Drugs like heroin can be lethal because they take effect so quickly after intravenous injection that the drug user can reach fatal drug levels before it would be possible to get help. The same dose of drug taken orally will never exert as great an effect because some of it will be lost to metabolism first and because the process of absorption is so gradual.

WHERE DO DRUGS GO IN THE BODY?

Once drugs are in the circulation, getting into most tissues is no challenge. There are big holes in most capillaries, and drugs are free to go into most tissues. The brain is an important exception because it has an especially tight defense—the blood brain barrier—that prevents the movement of many drugs into it. All of the drugs we discuss in this book are psychoactive, which means that they easily pass through this blood brain barrier because they dissolve easily in fat.

Although there are myths that drugs "hide" in specific places in the body (such as Ecstasy hiding in the spinal cord for months), they don't really. Since most psychoactive drugs are fat-soluble enough to enter the brain, they also accumulate in body fat. THC (the active component in marijuana) and PCP (phencyclidine, or angel dust) are particularly prone to accumulate in fat. As the drug eventually leaves the fat, it enters the bloodstream again and can enter the brain, but usually at levels low enough to produce only negligible effects.

There is a legal consequence to this storage in fat. Drugs like THC are so well stored in fat that they remain detectable in urine for weeks after the last time the drug was used. It is common in drug-treatment programs for people who have been testing "clean" to show drugs in their urine suddenly if they have been losing weight during their rehabilitation. The drug is simply driven out of the fat as the fat deposits shrink.

GETTING OUT

Most drugs do not leave the body the way they came in. Although a few drugs, like the inhalants, enter and leave through the lungs, most leave through the kidneys and the intestine. Many are changed in the liver to a form that is easily excreted in the urine. This process of metabolism and excretion in the urine determines how long the drug effect lasts. It is very difficult to change this rate, so once a dose of drug is ingested, there is no hurrying the recovery.

In extreme cases, there are emergency room procedures that can accelerate the removal of some drugs by the kidneys, but otherwise one must wait.

Some drugs, like cocaine, are removed by the body quickly. The combination of quick onset of action and rapid removal can lead to cycles of taking the drug repeatedly. Drug levels shoot up, then plummet, taking the user to an intense high followed by a "crash," which motivates the drug user to take another dose of drug. Some cocaine users get into "runs" of repeated doses and end up using grams of cocaine in a single sitting. This pattern often leads to overdosing—the user takes another dose as the drug effect wanes, but before the earlier dose has been completely eliminated. Drug levels in the brain gradually accumulate to dangerous levels.

Marijuana presents the opposite problem. THC, the active compound, is extremely fat-soluble (and thus accumulates in body fat) *and* its breakdown products are also active compounds. So, as the body tries to remove it, the metabolic products continue to have psychological effects. These two characteristics of marijuana mean that one can be under its influence for many hours after it is smoked.

THE EFFECTS OF DRUGS CHANGE OVER TIME

When people recall the first time they drank alcohol, most remember that they got drunker than they would now if they drank the same amount. This isn't all just fading memory. Many drugs cause much smaller reactions in the body after they have been taken for a while. This change is called *tolerance*. Usually the lesser reaction is due to previous experience with that drug or another similar drug, but even intense stress might change the reactions to some drugs.

Think about all the drugs we take that keep working even with many doses: our morning cup of coffee, an occasional aspirin for headache (imagine how much aspirin we all take over a lifetime!), an antacid to calm the stomach after a spicy meal. Why do these drugs keep working? The reason is that we usually take them only for a short time, or intermittently. *The more frequently one takes the drug, and the higher the dose, the more likely it is that tolerance will develop.* So, with just one aspirin once a week or even once a day, the body has plenty of time between doses to return to normal.

Coffee continues to provide that pleasant arousing effect that people associate with their morning cup of coffee or tea for years. However, bodies do adapt to the daily cup of coffee (see the "Caffeine" chapter), so that people who are regular coffee drinkers have smaller effects (show tolerance) to coffee compared to someone who never ingests caffeine. So, tolerance builds up, but the normal daily dose is not enough to cause the effect to go away entirely.

Tolerance to some drugs can be dramatic. For example, heroin addicts rapidly build up tolerance to opiate drugs. Longtime heroin addicts will take doses that would have killed them the first time they used the drug. This tolerance can last a long time (weeks or months). Some residual tolerance can last for years. Tolerance lasts this long because addicts typically take many doses a day, every day, sometimes for years.

What about antibiotics? Everyone probably remembers being exhorted to be sure to take every one of the two weeks' worth of pills, and tried (and perhaps failed) to be careful to take a dose every six or eight hours. Although no one bacterium survives the two weeks' worth of medication, and no one individual bacterium adapts to the drug, the population as a whole often does adapt. Since bacteria replicate between one and many times a day, new generations are constantly being born. When individual bacteria are born that happen to be resistant to the drug, this individual and its offspring survive, and the infection has now become *resistant*. With the rising use of antibiotics (antibiotics in beef, antibiotics for many childhood diseases, etc.), more and more humans are carrying resistant populations of bacteria in their body that are difficult to treat with currently available antibiotics. This is drug tolerance playing out at the population level rather than the individual level, and it is becoming more and more of a problem worldwide.

Some drugs actually become more effective over time. Cocaine is one such drug. Some of its effects become greater with each passing dose. There could be a beneficial side to this effect: drugs that gradually become more active could be delivered only occasionally and still be effective. This certainly would be cheaper! Some researchers have proposed that antidepressant drugs fit into this category, and that daily treatment may not be necessary.

In summary, tolerance develops to many drugs. Fortunately, many of the drugs we rely on to treat disease are given in doses that do not cause the development of tolerance, so they can continue working over a long period of time. This is especially important for drugs that are used to treat diseases like high blood pressure, which are lifelong conditions that require therapy for years.

HOW BODIES' RESPONSES TO DRUGS CHANGE

How do tolerance and sensitization happen? Bodies tend to adapt to the continuous presence of drugs, so bodily functions remain normal despite the presence of drugs. Of the many ways this happens, we will describe the three most important.

The first adaptation to long-term drug use happens in the liver, where drugs are inactivated by specific enzymes that change them into forms that can be excreted by the kidneys. The enzymes that inactivate drugs are not very specific. If they were, hundreds upon hundreds of them would be needed—one for each drug. Instead, humans have between twenty and thirty, which are responsible for metabolizing all drugs.

The activity of these enzymes changes with experience. When the body is exposed to frequent doses of a drug that one of the enzymes must inactivate, cellular machinery in the liver "tools up" to deal with the excess drug by making extra enzyme to get rid of the drug. As a result, the drug gets eliminated more quickly. This process causes tolerance in a simple way: less of the drug gets to the tissue where the receptors are. Smokers, who inhale many different substances each time they smoke cigarettes, typically metabolize many drugs much more quickly than nonsmokers because the constant presence of the substances in smoke results in increases in many drug-metabolizing enzymes. This can present problems when treating diseases in smokers. In the same way, the livers of heavy alcohol drinkers metabolize many drugs more quickly.

Nasal decongestants provide a great example of the second major tolerance process. The over-the-counter medications that people use to treat stuffy noses accomplish their effect by attaching to receptors on the blood vessels in the nose. These receptors are activated by the drug and cause the blood vessels to constrict. This decreases the volume of blood in the nose, and helps to reduce the inflammation and swelling. This works well for a while. However, the cells that have these receptors figure out that they are being overstimulated by these receptors. To reestablish balance, they simply remove some of the receptors from the surface of the cells. The result is that the nasal decongestant stops working! The warnings on the bottle about not using the drug for more than a few days are based on the reality that the drug will stop working anyway. This kind of change is a very common source of tolerance. The brain adapts in much the same way: overstimulation of receptors causes neurons simply to remove receptors and bring the level of stimulation back down to normal. Likewise, if the drug prevents receptors from working, the cell simply makes more.

Pavlov's dogs salivating when they heard a bell ringing to signal the arrival of dinner provides an example of the last tolerance mechanism. Our brains "learn" to expect the drug, and act accordingly. Sometimes this means activating processes that tend to oppose the effects of drugs. If people take drugs in a familiar environment (as do many people who take addictive drugs), they learn to associate the typical environment of drug taking with the experience of the drug. For example, a heroin addict might usually buy from the same dealer and take the drug to a "shooting gallery" to inject it. Soon, this environment becomes associated with the drug experience. When the heroin addict enters the shooting gallery, he or she will start breathing faster to offset the slowing that will happen once heroin is injected. This process is powerful. Often, when people OD after taking a dose of drug that they normally tolerate, it is because they took it in an unfamiliar place.

Unfortunately, this type of expectation can also work the opposite way. When heroin addicts have been in recovery and then return to their homes, many times simply being on the street where they used to take the drug will reawaken those same sensations and reawaken drug craving. This becomes a very strong urge, and is the reason why many treatment programs urge addicts to change their lifestyle in a dramatic way and avoid people and places that they associate with drug use.

WHAT HAPPENS WHEN WE STOP TAKING DRUGS?

When the drug is no longer present, all of these marvelous adaptations are counterproductive. Let's go back to the nose of the earlier example. Imagine that someone has been taking decongestants for two weeks. She probably is taking more and more to overcome the tolerance that is developing to the drug. What happens when she stops? The blood vessels of the nose don't have their normal number of receptors anymore. They are staying unstuffy only because the decongestant has been stimulating the few that are left like crazy. Once the drug is gone, the few receptors left are not enough to do the job, and there is a huge *rebound* in nasal congestion. So, the cure has become the disease.

This process is called *withdrawal*, and it is really the flip side of tolerance. She is not addicted to nose drops, but simply tolerant. This is one of the commonest misconceptions about withdrawal and addiction (more about this later, in the "Addiction" chapter). A person can go through withdrawal even from drugs that are not addicting, like nose drops.

All joking aside, *the consequences of withdrawal can be life-threatening*. For example, alcohol is a sedative drug that slows the firing of neurons. Imagine a neuron prevented from firing every day by alcohol. A logical response would be for it to do whatever it could to fire more often. Now imagine many cells in the brain affected in this way. They adapt by increasing receptors that stimulate neural firing and decreasing receptors that inhibit firing. Now imagine an alcoholic who enters treatment and stops drinking abruptly. All these neurons are very excitable, and result in tremendous overexcitation of the nervous system. This overexcitation can actually lead to seizures and death. Fortunately, there are medications which can be given to detoxifying alcoholics to keep these withdrawl symptoms at bay while the brain returns to normal.

Understanding how drugs work is not simply a matter of which drug does what, although that is the first thing to know. Everyone needs to understand how safe it is to take a drug in a particular way, how fast it gets in, how long it hangs around, and how it gets out; and we all need to understand the consequences of prolonged use of, and withdrawal from, anything we take.

15

Addiction

THE PRINCIPLES

1. Addiction is the repetitive, compulsive use of a substance that occurs despite negative consequences to the user.

2. Addictive drugs activate circuits in the brain that respond to normal pleasures, like food and sex. Every brain possesses these circuits, so every human could potentially become addicted to a drug.

3. Drug taking is maintained by many factors, including changes in the brain, the desire to experience pleasure from the drug, and the desire to avoid the discomfort of withdrawal.

4. Because addiction depends on many different factors in the life of an individual, such as family history, personality, mental health, and life experience, most people do not become addicted to drugs.

WHAT IS ADDICTION?

Addiction is the repetitive, compulsive use of a substance that occurs despite negative consequences to the user. Simply using cocaine or heroin may be illegal and health damaging, but it is not necessarily addiction. Addiction is often used to mean *psychological dependence*, to differentiate it from *physical dependence*. Simply undergoing changes when substance use is stopped (like the headache that many coffee users experience when they miss their morning cup of coffee) is physical dependence, but it is not necessarily addiction. Obviously, both psychological dependence and physical dependence coexist in people who are strongly addicted to some drugs.

This definition of addiction can be applied to the compulsive, repetitive use of alcohol, nicotine, opiate drugs like heroin, as well as cocaine and other stimulants. But what about activities like gambling, shopping, and sex? Some people obviously engage in these activities to the point that there are negative consequences for themselves (and their families). Some people clearly gamble away everything they have, or engage in promiscuous sex to the extent that they risk infection with HIV or other sexually transmitted diseases. These behaviors are clearly similar to drug-seeking behaviors in an addicted person. It is likely that the same neural circuits may be involved to some extent, but we don't really know.

THE BASIS OF ADDICTION: THE NEURAL CIRCUITS OF PLEASURE

What would lead someone to abandon his job, his family, and his life or to ignore the most basic, life-sustaining impulses to eat and reproduce? There must be something fundamentally different about "addicts" that leads them into such an extremely dysfunctional lifestyle. Addiction has often been attributed to personal characteristics, including a lack of "morals," having a different brain chemistry, or experiencing mental illness or extreme trauma.

While some of these factors may influence addiction, the neural mechanisms by which addictive drugs act are probably present in everyone. In fact, the reason why addiction is so powerful is that it mobilizes basic brain functions that are designed to guarantee the survival of the species. These mechanisms exist in the brains of all people, so potentially any human being could become a drug addict. The reason lies in a complicated neural circuit through which we appreciate the things that feel good. The job of this neural circuit, presumably, is to cause us to enjoy activities or substances that are life-sustaining. If it is successful, then it is more likely that we will engage in the activity again.

How does this "pleasure" circuit work? Let's use food as an example. If a person has a really great pastry at a bakery, it is more likely that he will go to this bakery again because the food tasted good. The good-tasting food is a *reinforcer* because it increases the likelihood that the person will engage in the same behavior (going to the bakery). Animals, including humans, will engage in all sorts of work to obtain access to food, water, sex, and the opportunity to explore an environment (perhaps to find food, water, or sex). These are the "natural reinforcers"—events or substances in the world that motivate behavior.

In a laboratory, an animal can learn to press a lever to obtain a food pellet. This is simply the laboratory equivalent of the bakery scenario. There is a critical neural circuit in the brain that must be intact for this to happen. If this circuit is damaged, even animals that are extremely hungry will not work to gain access to food. We think that this neural circuit is the pathway that causes the animal or person to experience the reinforcers as pleasurable. It is sometimes called the *reward* pathway. When this pathway is destroyed, an animal loses interest in food, in sex, and in exploring its environment. It is still *capable* of doing all these things; it is just not motivated. It can move around, have sex, and eat, but it simply doesn't seem to want to pursue reinforcers (or pleasure). If the reward pathway in an experimental animal is stimulated with a gentle electrical current, it will work very hard (pressing a bar or whatever) to turn on the current: the animal acts like it enjoys having the pathway stimulated electrically. This is called *self-stimulation*.

DRUGS AND THE PLEASURE CIRCUIT

To understand if this neural circuit has any relevance to addiction, first we need to know if addictive drugs are reinforcers. Here the experimental evidence is overwhelming and the answer is yes! The best evidence comes from studies in which animals could press a lever to obtain an injection of drug instead of food. Most experimental animals (pigeons, rats, monkeys) will press a lever to get an injection of cocaine, amphetamine, heroin, nicotine (sometimes), and alcohol. They will not press a lever for LSD, antihistamines, or many other drugs. This list of drugs for which experimental animals will work matches exactly the list of drugs that are viewed as clearly addictive in humans.

What is the evidence that this pathway has anything to do with drug addiction? There are two particularly convincing arguments. First, if this pathway is damaged in an animal, it will not work to gain access to drugs. Second, animals with an electrode placed in the reward pathway find smaller currents more "enjoyable" if the animal has received an injection of cocaine or heroin, for example. Some recent, very exciting studies in humans have provided evidence that this same system is activated in the brains of addicts. Cocaine addicts were shown pictures of cocaine or allowed to handle crack pipes while the activity of their brains was monitored. These activities sparked a craving for cocaine, and at the same time activated the reward pathway of the brain.

Drugs that are truly addictive (stimulants, opiates, alcohol, nicotine) can actually substitute for food, sex, or other primary reinforcers. This explains why rapid injection of cocaine or heroin produces a "rush" of pure pleasure that most users compare to the pleasure of orgasm. This isn't only true for certain people who lack willpower, or who are willing to engage in a deviant lifestyle. It is true for everyone who has a brain. It automatically becomes easier to understand why addiction is such a common problem across cultures.

Although the news media has certainly overdone the "what is the most addictive drug?" contest, it is also clear that animals will work much harder to get cocaine than to get most other drugs. Rats will press a bar up to two to three hundred times for one injection of cocaine. However, some drugs, like alcohol and nicotine, might be administered more if they didn't have other effects on the body that animals found unpleasant. Humans seem to be particularly good at ignoring unpleasant side effects in order to obtain reinforcement from drugs. If you judged the most addictive drug by the largest number of people who have trouble stopping their use of it, then nicotine would be the clear leader.

THE SPECIAL ROLE OF DOPAMINE

The neurotransmitter dopamine seems to play an important role in the normal process of reinforcement, and in the actions of most addictive drugs. One group of dopamine neurons runs directly through the reward circuit described above. If the dopamine neurons in this circuit are destroyed, then animals will not work for either food, sex, water, or addictive drugs. Furthermore, both natural reinforcers and most addictive drugs increase the release of dopamine from these neurons. Our favorite experiment was conducted by a scientist in Canada who measured the release of dopamine in the brain of a male rat before and after providing it with a female partner. Not surprisingly, access to a sexually receptive partner caused a large rise in dopamine levels in this part of the brain.

If this same experiment is done with drugs instead of natural reinforcers, much the same results are obtained. Animals given an injection of cocaine, morphine, nicotine, or alcohol will show large increases in dopamine in the same area of the brain in which sex causes a similar rise. Most neuroscientists think that addictive drugs affect neurons that connect, one way or another, with this critical dopamine circuit to stimulate its activity.

The experiments described above have been criticized because the animals in most of them have been given the drug involuntarily, a condition that does not match that of human addicts. Furthermore, dopamine neurons are not "the end of the line" for detecting pleasure, but clearly connect with other neurons. We are just beginning to understand how these other areas of the brain play a role.

THE DARK SIDE: PAIN, NOT PLEASURE

Enjoying the rush of pleasure when the drug is taken is only part of addiction. For established addicts, there is an opposing force, a yang for the yin. Once physical dependence is established, a daily cycle of drug taking, pleasure, gradual waning of drug effect, and the onset of withdrawal symptoms emerges. Withdrawal symptoms are different for each drug, and minimal for some (much of this is covered in detail in the chapters on individual drugs). For example, the waning of opiate effects is accompanied by an ill feeling similar to the onset of the flu. The drug user has chills and sweats, a runny nose, and a generally achy feeling. An alcoholic will feel restless and anxious. For *all* drugs, one part of withdrawal is a craving for more drug. Avoiding the unpleasant feelings of withdrawal and satisfying the desire for more drug can be strong motives for drug taking.

CUCUMBERS AND PICKLES: CHANGES IN THE BRAIN

If cocaine is enjoyable with the first experience, does that mean that a user is addicted after the first experience? The answer is no. Let's go back to the bakery. The first time our person went to the bakery, he simply liked the pastry. The pastry was not even a reinforcer until the person went back. And no one would describe an occasional trip to a favorite bakery as an addiction. But what if our pastry lover started going to the bakery two, three, four, five times a day.

Or what if he started waiting at the bakery door until opening time each day, neglecting his job or forgetting his children at school? It is this sort of compulsive, repetitive involvement in drug taking despite negative consequences that most experts view as addiction.

Use of addictive drugs can be viewed in a similar way. Many people drink alcohol occasionally, or even sometimes use cocaine at parties. However, for some people, the first social experiences with drugs gradually evolve into more continual use. Alcohol use provides an example. While 50 percent of the adult population of the United States drink alcohol occasionally, of these about 10 percent drink heavily, and some are engaged in addictive patterns of drinking.

Clearly, something happens in addicts that makes the need to consume drugs so great that they will go to extreme lengths to obtain the drug. What changes in the brain explain this? We have heard recovered addicts compare the change in their behavior and lives to the change from a cucumber to a pickle. Once a cucumber is turned into a pickle, it cannot be turned back. Is this a real analogy? If so, then the Alcoholics Anonymous approach of lifetime abstinence from drugs becomes a convincing solution to alcoholism.

Most scientists think that changes gradually occur in the reward circuit of the brain as it adapts to the continuous presence of the drug, although there are many complicated arguments about whether it becomes more sensitive to the drug or less so. At least in some circumstances, animals become more sensitive to cocaine when they are exposed to it repeatedly. When drug use ceases, the chemical stimulus stops and the reward system is shut down. Imagine the powerful cycle this could establish if it happens in people: with every drug-taking episode it would feel better and better, and with the absence of drug it would feel worse and worse!

This *sensitization* is not universal. For example, recovering heroin addicts often report that every time they inject heroin, they are trying to recapture the feeling of their early experience with the drug, which gave a pleasure that they never quite reached again. People who are in a stimulant "binge," taking hits every few hours, can have the same experience. They respond by "chasing the high," taking the drug every hour or so to recapture the first rush. Only when they stop taking the drug for a while does their initial sensitivity return.

Regardless of whether the pleasure circuit becomes more or less sensitive to the particular addictive drug, there are changes once a user stops taking drugs. Experiments with cocaine indicate that when an animal stops using cocaine, neurons in this part of the brain are less active, leading to a state in which the animal's reward pathways do not respond to food or sex.

Likewise, some recovering cocaine addicts say that they do not feel pleasure in anything for a while. Imagine how difficult it must be to stop using a drug that gives incredible pleasure, when even things that are usually enjoyable give no pleasure during withdrawal. This lack of ability to feel pleasure may be one of the powerful reasons why people have great difficulty giving up cocaine. If there is a substance at an addict's fingertips that can make him feel better immediately, clearly the impulse to take it can become overwhelming.

Many changes occur in the brain of a person who uses addictive drugs repeatedly, and not all of them are directly caused by the drugs themselves. For example, he will also learn to associate particular environments with the good feeling of being high. Let's go back to our bakery one more time. As our imaginary muffin addict approaches the store each day, he certainly remembers the route and looks forward to the smell of newly baked muffins wafting down the street. Pretty soon, the smell of the bakery alone can cause an intense longing for the pastries before he gets there. What happens when our muffin addict decides that the daily search for muffins is taking too long, or that the bakery raises prices so much that he won't pay? If he goes "cold turkey" and quits muffins altogether, he had better find another way to go to work, because he will find that the route to the bakery, the smell of the muffins, and many of the experiences associated with going to the bakery will cause an intense longing for a muffin. This type of longing has ruined many a diet, and this type of learning plays an important role in human addicts as well. Simply showing a former cocaine user a photograph of a crack pipe will trigger a strong craving for the drug, and recent studies of brain activity show that areas of the brain involved in memory are activated while he looks at these pictures.

We know less about the physical process of addiction than we do about the psychological process. For example, are the changes in the pleasure circuit the same with all addictive drugs? Do the brains of smokers, alcoholics, and cocaine users all adapt in the same way? Are these changes truly permanent, or do they gradually wane?

IS THERE A DEFICIENT BRAIN CHEMISTRY IN ADDICTS?

If everyone with a brain can become an addict, why are there relatively so few addicts? Could there be a unique group of people whose pleasure circuits are abnormal in some way, so that these drugs feel particularly good? Or could there be a group of people whose pleasure circuits don't work very well, so that they are inclined to drink alcohol, smoke, or take cocaine to feel normal? In studying many of these questions in human addicts, there is a real "chicken and egg" problem. If brain function is abnormal, it is impossible to know whether the abnormality was caused by years of substance abuse or was present before. Some scientists have tried to solve this problem by studying the children of alcoholics. There are certain EEG (brain wave) changes that have been noted in some alcoholics and in their sons. However, we don't really understand the significance of this EEG anomaly yet.

Are these differences due to a deficient gene that could simply be repaired? A few studies have analyzed specific genes: for example, the gene for one of the dopamine receptors. While a few subtle differences have been noted in the brains of alcoholics, other studies have not confirmed these findings. Studies in animals that voluntarily drink large amounts of alcohol have shown that there are definite genetic differences in these animals, and some of these differences are in how their pleasure circuits respond to alcohol. However, there are many types of mice that drink more alcohol, each of which probably has its own reason for excessive drinking. So, there probably won't be *one* gene for alcoholism, but twenty or thirty or one hundred such genes. Furthermore, even if an alcoholism gene associated with the pleasure circuit could be identified, this circuit is vital for normal brain function: without it, sex, food, drink, and many aspects of daily life would not be enjoyable. Eliminating the damaged gene could damage the reward system.

Finally, it is important to realize that biology is not destiny. People are more than bags of genes that produce behavior. They clearly are influenced by their environment, and can control their behavior voluntarily. Simply possessing a particular gene that has been found in the brains of some alcoholics does not mean that an individual will become an alcoholic. If he or she abstains from alcohol, for one thing, there will never be a problem. Maybe these slightly abnormal genes provide some benefit to the person that we don't fully understand.

PERSONALITY AND DRUG ADDICTION

How many people reading this book have worried about the possibility that they or a loved one may have an "addictive personality"? Although this concept is a favorite of some drug-abuse treatment professionals, psychology classes, and self-help books, there seems to be little agreement about what this is. Furthermore, the personality type prone to substance abuse changes with the times. In years gone by, the obsessive-compulsive personality was described as prone to drug abuse. Today, there is concern that risk-taking and impulsive people are more likely to develop substance-use problems. Many of these theories probably have a grain of truth to them. For example, if a person is uninhibited about trying new experiences, including those that are risky, he may be more likely to take drugs the first time. So, the risk of addiction in these people might rise from the greater likelihood that they will experiment with drugs. As with genetic arguments, it is important to remember that such traits do not condemn a person to drug addiction. Many risk takers channel their energies into daring sports like bungee jumping.

LIFE EXPERIENCE AND DRUG ADDICTION

Unfortunately, life experience can contribute to addiction as well as protect potential addicts. The life histories of people who have entered drug-treatment facilities show that certain characteristics are found more frequently in the substance users than in people without substance-use problems.

Two kinds of experience are found more frequently in the lives of substance abusers. First, they are more likely to have grown up in a family with a substance-using parent. Alcoholism can be passed on by the experience of living with an alcoholic parent (although almost as often this experience will motivate a life of abstinence). A substantial percentage of alcoholics grew up in a household with an alcoholic adult.

Do people growing up in an alcoholic household simply learn to respond to stress with alcohol? This can happen, but it is not necessarily the reason. Children of alcoholics also are more likely to have experienced physical and emotional abuse at the hands of their parents, and a past history of physical and emotional abuse is another characteristic of many substance abusers. This is particularly true among women. In studies of hospitalized alcoholics, 50 to 60 percent typically report having experienced childhood abuse.

Why should bad early experience lead to adult substance use? There are nearly as many explanations as there are scientists. One group of theories suggests a psychological origin for the substance use. However, recently a biological theory was developed from experimental work done on monkeys. Scientists at the National Institute of Health and elsewhere have shown that when infant monkeys are neglected or abused by their mothers, they have a number of behavioral problems as they grow up. As adults, they tend to get into fights, and if given the chance to drink alcohol, they drink to excess. This is not just a genetic tendency, because infants from perfectly normal mothers will show these tendencies if they are raised by neglectful mothers. None of this is surprising. However, the surprising part is that these behavioral problems are accompanied by changes in the brain. The alcohol-drinking monkeys show lower levels of the neurotransmitter serotonin in their brains. So, it appears that this early life experience may produce long-lasting changes in the brain that contribute to these behaviors.

A person's early experiences can influence his later use of drugs. We know that associating with drug-using peers increases the chances that a person will choose to try drugs. Also, early use of cigarettes, alcohol, or marijuana is associated with later use of other drugs. This association has lead to the popular "gateway theory" of drug addiction. This theory is based on evidence that most people who use illegal addictive drugs first used drugs like alcohol, tobacco, or marijuana. These drugs are viewed as a gateway to use of more dangerous drugs. However, the vast majority of people using cigarettes, alcohol, and marijuana never use "harder" drugs. Although the statistics are correct, this situation reminds us of our favorite statistics teacher, who is fond of saying that statistics don't prove how things happen. It is possible that people who are risk takers, or mentally ill, or living in chaotic families, are more likely to experiment with many deviant behaviors, including drug use. The drug use could just as likely be a symptom as a disease.

MENTAL ILLNESS AND DRUG ADDICTION

Depression and some other mental illnesses also occur more frequently in substance users. Did the drugs cause the problem, or did the problem cause the drug use? Once someone's life has become complicated by substance addiction, the turmoil that has been created can certainly contribute to the development of depression. This fact makes it very difficult to understand the complicated relationship between mental illness and drug addiction. However, some recovering addicts will describe an opposite cycle: that their anxious or depressed mood led them to drink or to use other substances in order to deal with feelings of inadequacy or despair. Then, as time passed and substance use became more frequent, the substance use became the dominant problem. This "self-medication" process probably contributes to addiction in many people.

THE BOTTOM LINE ON ADDICTION

The bottom line on addiction is that *anyone with a brain can get addicted to drugs*. However, most people don't, and there are a plethora of reasons. First and foremost, if a person does not experiment with addictive drugs, then he or she won't get addicted. Second, if a person is mentally healthy, has a stable family and work life, including supportive peers, and has no family history of substance abuse, she lacks some important risk factors and is less vulnerable. However, she still has a brain, and she is not immune to addiction. During the seventies' and eighties' cocaine craze, plenty of constructive, highly educated, well-employed professionals became addicted to cocaine despite these positive factors in their lives.

Finally, there may be some people for whom the pleasurable experience of these drugs is exceptionally high, and the drive to use the drugs is thus more compelling than for others. If these people do not try drugs, this underlying quality will not present a problem. However, if they have access to them, and if they do choose to use them, they are at significant risk. It is no accident that the rate of drug addiction among professionals in the United States is highest among medical personnel, who have easy access to such drugs.

16

■

Legal Issues

It is said that your life can change forever in a matter of seconds. When a person mixes drugs and the legal system, the combination can easily become life-changing. For a variety of reasons, the lawmaking bodies of most countries, especially the United States, have decided to suppress drug use by making drug laws harsh and certain. All who deal with drugs in an illegal manner are thus at risk for penalties that can disrupt their own lives and those of their families.

The use of almost all the drugs discussed in this book could involve violations of the law, depending on the circumstances. Many of these drugs are illegal in all circumstances—manufacturing, distribution, and possession. Others are legal when prescribed, but not for recreational use. Still others, such as alcohol, can be legal, but their use is prohibited for activities such as driving a car or operating a boat.

This chapter is written to inform readers about very basic laws and principles that come into play around drug issues. It is not intended to give advice about dealing with the law-enforcement community or the judicial system. If you feel that you need that advice, find a good lawyer and ask her all of your questions before you become legally involved.

THE PRINCIPLES

1. Everyone wants to know about the laws regarding the rights of a law officer to search one's car or one's home. This is a very complicated issue that is

often decided in the courts in individual cases. Generally one has the greatest "expectation of privacy" in one's home. There is less expectation of privacy in a car, and the least when one is out in public.

2. If a law-enforcement officer suspects you of a crime and really wants to search you or your car, you will be searched, whether or not you give permission. If you give your permission, the search will almost certainly be considered legal. If you refuse permission, the search may or may not be legal, but it may happen anyway. The debate over whether the search was permitted and legal will begin in the court system. The easiest way to avoid trouble is to avoid situations in which a random and unexpected search will yield anything illegal.

3. A person who is innocent of any crime, but is with someone arrested for possessing drugs, may become involved with the legal system until her innocence is proven. By that time, she may have hired an expensive lawyer, terrified her family, and spent some time under arrest.

4. The penalties for drug-related activities can be horrendous, especially in the United States federal judicial system, and particularly for selling drugs. Many casual drug users do not realize that simple possession of a modest amount of a drug can automatically be considered "intent to distribute," whether or not one actually plans to sell the drug.

5. One does not have to be on government property to be in violation of federal law. The federal drug laws apply everywhere in the United States at all times.

6. State and federal laws can be extremely strict about the use of guns in the commission of crimes. The possession of a gun—even having one just in the vicinity of a crime—can add many years onto the sentence for the original crime.

7. Many people believe that they are "safe" from serious legal consequences because they know the local officials, or because they believe the penalties are not serious. They are wrong. First, an arrest by a state or local officer can easily be referred to federal prosecutors not subject to local political influence. Second, in many states and in the federal system there is no parole. Even worse, "guideline" or "structured" sentencing laws give the judges practically no leeway for reduced sentences.

8. Finally, remember that while one may have and know one's rights as a citizen, those rights do not apply in foreign countries, and the legal consequences of drug-law violations in some places can literally mean death.

GETTING SEARCHED

There's this joke about a very large canary: "Where does an eight-hundred pound canary sit?" "Anywhere he wants to!" Likewise, a law-enforcement officer will search just about anywhere if he really wants to do it. Eventually the courts could decide whether the search was legal, but if an officer has reason to believe that a crime is being committed, he may well initiate the search process and let the lawyers settle the issue later.

Laws in the United States on the subject of a search are extremely complicated, in part because the legal rights of individuals have been defined over the years by many different court cases. However, there are a few general principles that govern when someone can legally be detained and searched.

First is the "expectation of privacy." The expression "A man's home is his castle" applies here. To search a residence usually requires more stringent legal prerequisites than searching elsewhere. Often a search warrant signed by a judge is required, unless there is evidence of a major and immediate threat to public safety.

Next is the automobile. This is the place where most individuals confront the law. An officer will see a traffic violation in progress, stop the vehicle, and then come to suspect that illegal drug activity is being carried out. If an officer reasonably believes that a crime is being committed, then he probably has the right to detain the occupants of the car until a legally proper investigation can be carried out. Remember, this officer can stop and hold someone if he *believes* that a crime is being committed, *even if he is wrong!*

A court official explains an extreme example: Say a murder has been committed in the course of a bank robbery and the killer is driving away in a 1994 blue four-door sedan. In the heat of the moment, an incompetent 911 operator becomes confused and broadcasts that the killer is leaving the scene in a 1987 red pickup truck. An officer down the road sees a 1987 red pickup truck and stops it, removes the occupants, and searches the truck for weapons. He finds illegal substances. Was the search legal? Probably, because the officer had reason to suspect that the occupants were criminals. He was wrong, but with good reason, and the occupants may well be convicted for whatever offense they committed.

There are equally odd outcomes in which convictions are not possible because the officer was found to have no reason to search a vehicle. That is why most officers ask permission to search a car and obtain written permission before doing so. That permission probably makes the search legal and any evidence is thus legally obtained. If permission is not given, then the officer may choose to detain the individuals further and call for a search warrant or a "drug dog" to examine the outside of the vehicle. This issue then gets very complicated.

The practical side of all this is that a law officer has quite a lot of power to detain and arrest, because the lawmakers have decided it is in the public good to be able to detain potential criminals, and, to some extent, to ask questions later. Even if an officer is eventually found in court to be wrong, the suspected individuals would have suffered loss of time and perhaps arrest, legal bills, and considerable life discomfort.

Finally, there is the situation when a person is out in public and walking about. This is the least "private" act, and so there is the least expectation of privacy. In this case a law officer has much more leeway in searching a person, for the protection of the officer herself and for that of the general public. For example, imagine that an officer sees a person walking down the street in and out of traffic, in an erratic manner. She has the right to stop and talk to that person to ensure that he and the driving public are safe. If, in the process of that stop, the officer feels that the individual may be carrying a weapon, she could search him and find no weapon, but find an illicit drug. Can the person be convicted of a drug-law violation? It is very likely that he can because the search was legal.

The same rules might apply at a concert. Two students are obviously intoxicated and fighting. An officer moves to stop the fight, the students resist, they are searched for weapons, and illicit substances are discovered. If the officer chooses to charge them, there is a good probability that the charges will stick.

Do law-enforcement officers have a pathological agenda to harass drivers and students at a concert, looking for drugs everywhere? Rarely. Most law officers see their work as a job, not a mission. Think of all the traffic laws that are broken every day and how seldom stops occur. Think of how seldom someone who is innocent of any law violation is stopped in a car or interdicted at a concert. By and large, the legal community just does its job.

ILLEGAL ACTS

The drug laws are complicated, and the states differ from each other and from the federal system. So, there is no easy way to explain them in detail. However, there are a few very powerful and relatively unknown aspects of the law that should be explained to everyone.

First is the difference between a felony and a misdemeanor. A misdemeanor is a minor crime that might result in a fine, a public service, or a short prison sentence. A felony is considered such a serious crime that convicted individuals lose many rights that ordinary citizens enjoy. This includes the right to hold many kinds of highly paid jobs. A felony conviction is truly a life-changing event. Understanding this is important for drug users because possession of some amounts of some drugs can be considered a misdemeanor, while larger amounts are always felonies.

The law always sets the level of punishment based on the amount of a drug that one possesses or distributes, and in this case size counts a lot. For example, there is a current public controversy because the federal laws are terribly tough for possession of even a few grams of crack cocaine, but one would have to possess much more powdered cocaine to receive the same punishment. Anyone who contemplates drug usage should understand the severity of the penalties that various levels of drug possession invoke.

Most people know that conviction for selling drugs (distribution) results in stiffer penalties than for possession. What they don't know is that simply possessing certain amounts of a drug can be considered "intent to distribute," and thus may subject the person to the much stiffer distribution penalties. Moreover, money may not have to change hands for distribution to take place from a legal perspective. Simply handing a package of a drug from one person to another can be considered distribution.

Another obscure criminal area is conspiracy. In drug cases, there are many convictions for conspiracy to commit a crime because very often a drug deal involves much more than the simple transfer of money and drugs. The conspiracy laws are broad and powerful, and even people peripheral to the planning of a crime, who may not have participated in the crime itself, are often charged under these laws, sometimes in the hope that they will cooperate with the court officials to convict others. Anyone hanging around individuals involved in drug possession and distribution should be aware of the risk of being charged with conspiracy for seemingly innocent acts, such as lending a boyfriend a car, cashing a check, or allowing a friend who is a dealer to use a telephone. From the standpoint of law enforcement, drug dealing is considered a business (although it is illegal), and, just as in a legal business, different people play different roles and have different levels of importance. In general, being around drug dealing is legally very risky.

Finally, there is the issue of confiscation of property. Most of us have heard about auctions where the property of drug dealers are sold. This happens because of forfeiture laws that allow property used in drug dealing to be confiscated and sold by the government. The particularly devastating aspect of this is that property of a more or less innocent individual might be confiscated because it was being used in violation of drug laws. Imagine, for example, a student distributing cocaine from his father's home and car. Suppose the father knew something about this and told the student to stop it. If the prosecutor could prove that the father knew something and allowed it to continue, it is possible that both the home and the car could be confiscated as part of the criminal prosecution.

We cannot stress enough the seriousness with which the lawmaking bodies are taking drug issues. The drug penalties get more severe every day. The situation has, in some cases, reached the point of near hysteria. As this is written, there have been news reports of two children in different parts of the United States being thrown out of school for giving a completely legal over-the-counter painkiller to a classmate. In one case it was a common preparation for premenstrual pain, and in the other, an ibuprofen tablet. In both cases the children were punished for breaking the rules against distributing any substance. In this kind of environment it is critical that everyone be extraordinarily thoughtful about involvement with drugs.

GETTING CAUGHT

Most people believe that it will not happen to them. Teenagers, in particular, have the feeling that they are "beyond the law." But it does happen. It happens to grandmothers, teenagers, lawyers, doctors, and the most ordinary people on the face of the earth.

Many drug arrests come from the most random events imaginable. In Virginia, an officer stopped a car for having something hanging off the rearview mirror. He became suspicious, legally searched the car, and found major quantities of cocaine. Another drug transporter thought he had the perfect scheme, and filled fruit juice cans with cocaine, then resealed them. It is a regular practice for tourists to bring back food from vacation in the Caribbean, and he expected to walk right through customs. What he did not realize was that customs officials knew there was no reason to bring canned fruit juice from the Caribbean, where it is expensive, to the United States, where it is cheap. He was arrested and convicted for transporting millions of dollars' worth of cocaine.

Even grandmothers are not immune to arrest. A pair of Drug Enforcement Administration agents working a bus station in North Carolina noticed an elderly woman behaving oddly. When they approached her, she moved away and they became suspicious. They conducted a legal search and found a large quantity of cocaine in her luggage.

A college student came back to her dorm room to find the place crawling with campus and city police. While she had absolutely no role in any illegal activity, a friend of her roommate had come to town from another college with a shipment of drugs. Another student, obeying the honor code, had called the campus police. Fortunately, the innocent student was not arrested because the roommate cleared her, but it was a very close call.

The law-enforcement community is actually quite sophisticated in its drug-enforcement efforts. Drug Enforcement Administration agents work all over the world trying to prevent the transport of drugs into the United States. They have agents working major and minor airports, and even the bus stations. The highway patrols of most states have drug interdiction units looking for suspicious vehicles. This is not a trivial effort, and it results in so many convictions that both the state and federal prison populations have grown dramatically in the last fifteen years.

Yet everyone realizes that most countries are overrun with drugs. It is usually easy to buy the most common illegal drugs in many areas of cities and on college campuses. So why is the legal interdiction effort perceived as failing? It is not exactly failing, but rather it is being overwhelmed. Many, many people are caught in the legal system, but there is always someone else to replace each person caught. Routine usage of cocaine, crack, or heroin can be a very expensive habit, and the only way that most people can maintain such expensive behavior is to turn to dealing. As we say elsewhere in this book, cocaine and opiates can be extremely reinforcing, and they are also expensive in the quantities that habitual users consume. The combination of dependence and expense often leads users to become dealers until they are stopped by medical intervention, arrest, or death.

What does this have to do with the average reader of this book? Anyone who can read this book no doubt has the ability to do honest and legal work and have a successful life. Such a reader might feel that she is above being caught, or just not in the right "circle of friends" to be caught. This might be the most dangerous attitude of all, because, like most jobs, illegal drug dealing depends on knowledge, skills, and having a network of people. Most casual dealers do not have the knowledge or, fortunately, are not willing to do what is necessary to involve themselves fully in the drug culture. Thus, they approach the whole issue as amateurs, and, like many amateurs in anything, they fail miserably. Only in this case, the stakes are much higher. They can get caught, lose a lot of money, become victims of criminal violence, or become heavily dependent on the substance they are dealing.

As we all know, some people think they have few opportunities and only a short time to live. They will deal drugs no matter what anyone says. In their lives they see jail time as just the cost of doing business. However, a district attorney who has prosecuted thousands of drug cases had just one bit of advice: people with families, an opportunity for education, and a supportive network of friends have so much to lose from being on the wrong side of the legal system that they should never become involved with it. A felony conviction can strip a person of so many opportunities in this society, and can cost families so much in pain, suffering, and financial loss, that no amount of money or drug experience is worth the risk.

GETTING CONVICTED: THE PENALTY BOX

The penalty laws of most states and countries are built on a series of legislative acts that happened over a long period of time, and thus they are complicated and not easily summarized. Possession of modest amounts of marijuana can result in a slap on the wrist in some places and serious jail time in others. The same is true for other drugs, although they are usually taken more seriously, even in very small amounts. Often the prosecuting attorney has some leeway about the level of crime with which to charge an individual. The problem is that it is difficult to be sure of: (1) the latest changes in the law that probably made them stricter; (2) the attitude that the prosecutor is taking toward drug crimes; and (3) whether one will be charged under state or federal statutes. Thus, conviction for the possession of a small, recreational amount of heroin or cocaine could result in either a modest sentence or a huge fine and a long prison term, depending on the exact circumstances and the mood of the legal officials overseeing the case, or even on the social status of the accused.

It is important to recall that in some states and in the federal system there is structured, or guideline, sentencing. That means that once an individual is convicted of some drug crimes, the sentence is fixed by law and cannot be altered by the judge, no matter what the circumstances. Coupled with the fact that there is no parole in the federal system (and increasingly in the state systems), a conviction can mean long prison time, even if the prosecutor and judge wish it were otherwise.

The increasing severity of the drug laws and their enforcement is a result of a near panic by prosecutors and lawmakers over the drug issue. Unfortunately, the casual user can easily be caught up in this and the consequences may be awful. This happened in 1995 in Raleigh, North Carolina, after a 1994 study indicated that drug usage was up in local high schools, and Raleigh education and law-enforcement officials decided to respond with Operation Checkup, a three-month-long undercover investigation in which police officers and criminal justice students posed as students. In December 1996, the highly respected *Raleigh News and Observer* published an investigative report examining the consequences of the operation one year later.

The undercover agents had infiltrated suspected groups of students and attempted to buy drugs, mostly marijuana. According to the newspaper report, parents said that their children were repeatedly "pestered" by the agents until the students agreed to sell them some marijuana. Here's a particularly sad story from the article (with the names of the parties omitted):

[A student] said he agreed to sell a quarter-ounce of marijuana after repeated requests from [an] agent. Enrolled as a senior, [the agent] often gave [the student] rides home in his pickup truck.

"He'd see me two, three times a day, and every time he'd ask if I could get him some," [the student] said.

After several days, he sold the marijuana for $45 when [the agent] came to his home. That deal was the one charge against [the student].

The operation ended on December 1, 1995, with the arrest of eighty-five young people—seventy-five high school students and ten nonstudents. The district attorney made it clear from the beginning that there would be no plea bargaining, so felony charges would not be reduced to misdemeanors (as is commonly done), regardless of the amount of drug involved.

Thus, there were severe consequences for those arrested. First, the students were suspended from the school system for the rest of the year. Because the district attorney was unwilling to plea bargain for these cases, many of the students received felony convictions—some for selling less than a gram of marijuana. Only one of these students had a prior drug conviction.

The *News and Observer* checked the history of marijuana prosecutions in that county and found that prosecution for felony "sell and deliver" marijuana charges were very low except in the years that high school undercover operations were conducted. When high schools were targeted, they went up almost to five times the normal amount.

This illustrates perfectly the point that drug law enforcement can be capricious. During "normal" years, Raleigh officials apparently go to very little trouble to enforce the marijuana laws. Then, on some occasions (four times since 1979), they decide that it is time to crack down and they prosecute high school students to the limit of the law.

This level of inconsistency in enforcement can deliver the wrong message. In the years between crackdowns, people begin to believe that a community is "safe" for minor drug usage, then they are caught in the sting.

In the Raleigh case, the newspaper article reviewed a conversation with the police chief, who indicated that officers regularly stationed at the schools reported that the on-campus drug trade was increasing just a year after the sting. Clearly, police officers stationed at schools can be aware of drug dealing and yet nothing happens. Perhaps this is because it is more difficult to prove something than to know something is happening. But this can lead students to believe that the school is, by its lack of action, giving permission for minor drug usage. It is usually easy to buy marijuana, heroin, crack, and other drugs, and even a modest street-level enforcement effort would bring in hundreds of users and dealers. The fact is that Raleigh and other cities do very little about minor dealing and usage until someone decides to crack down. Then a lot of people get into serious trouble.

The newspaper also interviewed students who said that the sting changed nothing. Drugs are still in the schools, and a few unlucky students have had their lives wrecked by a capricious system.

The truth is that one can never assume that one is safe from severe consequences for drug-law violations, as seen in Raleigh schools. No matter what message a community or college or high school sends by lack of enforcement, the law-enforcement community can always reach out to inflict the most severe penalties allowed.

WHERE DO WE GO FROM HERE?

As this is written, there is a raging debate in the United States about legalization or decriminalization of drugs by society. California and Arizona have passed laws allowing the use of marijuana for medical purposes, but these laws are being challenged by antidrug groups, and there is the additional problem that these state laws may be in conflict with federal laws, so no one knows what the outcome will be.

A number of prominent Americans—including the conservative writer William F. Buckley—have concluded that the current drug policy of strong interdiction and enforcement efforts, coupled with stiff punishment, is expensive and not working. In an article entitled "The War on Drugs is Lost" (*National Review*, February 12, 1996), Buckley says, ". . . but the data here cited instruct us that the cost of the drug war is many times more painful, in all its manifestations, than would be the licensing of drugs combined with intensive education of non-users and intensive education designed to warn those who experiment with drugs."

On the other side, many people honestly have believed that any effort to reduce the pressure on drug users and dealers will result in a flood of illegal substances that, in their worst nightmares, will become readily available to children. Unfortunately, drugs are already readily available to anyone, including children from all economic levels. So, that nightmare is here right now, as the U.S. government has recognized. The 1997 National Drug Control Strategy includes as a goal, "Explicit recognition that demand reduction must be the centerpiece of the national anti-drug effort."

To reduce demand, we need to increase education. As we have said elsewhere in this book, effective drug education is not just a matter of exhortations to refuse all drugs, because many individuals believe that the drugs they use are harmless. It is a matter of teaching the basic science that can help us appreciate what complex and delicate organisms our brains are, how body chemistry may vary from person to person, and how little we know about the many ways, both positive and negative, short-term and long-term, that the powerful chemicals we call "drugs" can affect us. Good education is expensive, but we would be healthier, and as a society, we would save the enormous costs of lost wages, law enforcement, and prisons that drugs have brought us.

Further Reading

DOING YOUR OWN RESEARCH

If reading this book has raised your level of interest and you want more specific information, or you want the straight story about a new development, there is no substitute for doing your own research.

Reading both scholarly review articles and original research papers is much easier than most people believe. In fact, one of the first steps in writing this book was gathering such research. Much of the library work was done by two college students, neither of whom had any previous experience using a medical library. Should you decide to investigate for yourself, here are some suggestions about where to begin.

Public libraries are not likely to have the sorts of journals and books you will need. Because there is such a vast amount of medical literature published, most universities with a medical school have a separate library just to house all this information. Find a medical library at a nearby medical school. If, for some reason, you cannot get to a medical school, check to see if there is a college or university biology department nearby and use the library they use.

Next, go to the library and make friends with the reference librarian, because you will need his or her help until you are familiar with the library and the search mechanisms. The most efficient way of searching the literature is to use MEDLINE. Once you get to MEDLINE the fun begins! This is a database of the National Library of Medicine, a U.S. government institution that allows you to search almost all the published medical literature on any subject you can think of related to health. You can search by author, title, subject, keyword, institution, and many other descriptors.

In most cases you will find far more information than you need. A good place to start is with reviews. Reviews are documents that consolidate and summarize the research and literature available in a given area and they are usually written in less technical language. Reading several recent reviews about the topic you are researching will help you form a base of knowledge about the subject. Practice using MEDLINE by starting out with simple concepts; for example, search for marijuana articles. There are hundreds of them, and many of the titles will be so technical that they might seem indecipherable. So ask the computer to select for marijuana and review articles. This will reduce the number markedly.

If you have read *Buzzed*, then you know that one of the active ingredients in marijuana is THC. Try searching for THC and you will get more articles. Reduce the number by asking for reviews and you will get different articles than you did when you searched for marijuana. Play with the database and have fun. Search for all kinds of combinations of key words, like THC and learning, or THC and adolescent. You will soon have an idea of the enormous amount of information about just this chemical. Understand, though, that no one study tells the whole story.

As a final note, we caution you not to accept everything you read as directly applicable to the human condition. Often scientists employ very high levels of a chemical to test for toxic effects in animals, and sometimes the chemical levels they use in/on animals are hundreds or thousands of times higher than a human would ever use, taking into account the weight of the human compared to the animal. Consequently, some of the toxic effects seen in animals may not apply to humans. On the other hand, animal experiments cannot reveal many subtle effects of chemicals, particularly psychological ones, and thus animal studies almost certainly miss some important effects that humans will experience. So, as you read a scientific paper, remember that it is just a small part of the literature about a drug, and, while the data may be true, it is important to understand that data in the context of everything else known about the drug.

GENERAL REFERENCES

Cooper, J. R., F. E. Bloom, and R. H. Roth. *The Biochemical Basis of Neuropharmacology.* New York: Oxford University Press, 1996.

Hardman, J. G., L. E. Limbird, P. B. Molinoff, and R. W. Ruddon, eds. *Goodman and Gilman's the Pharmacological Basis for Therapeutics.* New York: McGraw Hill, 1996.

Karch, S. B. *The Pathology of Drug Abuse.* Boca Raton: CRC Press, 1996.

Musto, D. F. "Opium, Cocaine and Marijuana in American History." *Scientific American* 265 (1991): 40–47.

Ray, O., and C. Ksir. *Drugs, Society, and Behavior* (7th ed.). St. Louis: Mosby Press, 1996.

Schivelbusch, W. *Tastes of Paradise.* Trans. D. Jacobson. New York: Random House, 1992.

Snyder, S. *Drugs and the Brain.* New York: W. H. Freeman, 1995.

Trends in Pharmacological Sciences 13(5). Elsevier Science Publishers, May 1992.

ALCOHOL

Diamond, I., and A. S. Gordon. "Cellular and Molecular Neuroscience of Alcoholism." *Physiological Reviews* 77 (1997): 1–20.

Herz, A. "Endogenous Opioid Systems and Alcohol Addiction [review]." *Psychopharmacology* 129 (1997): 99–111.

Hobbs, W., T. Rall, and T. Verdoorn. "Hypnotics and Sedatives; Ethanol." This is Chapter 17 in *Goodman and Gilman's the Pharmacological Basis of Therapeutics* listed in the general references above.

Koperafrye, K., S. Dehaene, and A. P. Streissguth. "Impairments of Number Processing Induced by Prenatal Alcohol Exposure." *Neuropsychologia* 34 (1996): 1187–1196.

Musto, D. F. "Alcohol in American History." *Scientific American* 274 (1996): 78–83.

Streissguth, A., P. Sampson, H. Olson, F. Bookstein, H. Barr, M. Scott, J. Feldman, and A. Mirsky. "Maternal drinking during pregnancy: Attention and short-term memory in 14-year-old offspring—a longitudinal prospective study." Alcoholism: *Clinical and Experimental Research* 18 (1994): 202–218.

The National Clearinghouse for Alcohol and Drug Information (www.health.org/index.htm) is a national resource sponsored by the U.S. government. For users of the Internet it has the advantage of providing searchable databases (www.health.org/dbases.htm) which allow the user to search for references to research papers on any topic related to alcohol actions or use.

U.S. Dept. of Health and Human Services. *Eighth Special Report to the U.S. Congress on Alcohol and Health.* Alexandria, Va.: EEI, September 1993.

CAFFEINE

Edwards, B. *America's Favorite Drug: Coffee and Your Health.* Berkeley, Calif.: Odonian Press, 1992.

Jurich, N. *Espresso: From Bean to Cup.* Seattle: Missing Link Press, 1991.

Lamarine, R. J. "Selected Health and Behavioral Effects Related to the Use of Caffeine." *Community Health* 19 (1994): 449–466.

Thompson, W. G. "Coffee: Brew or Bane?" *American Journal of the Medical Sciences* 308 (1994): 49–57.

COCAINE

Hammer, R. P., ed. *The Neurobiology of Cocaine.* Boca Raton Fla.: CRC Press, 1995.

"Neurobiology of cocaine abuse." *Trends in Pharmacological Sciences* 13 (1992): 193–200.

ENACTOGENS

Demirkiran, M., J. Jankovic, and J. M. Dean. "Ecstasy Intoxication: An Overlap Between Serotonin Syndrome and Neuroleptic Malignant Syndrome." *Clinical Neuropharmacology* 19 (1996): 157–164.

McCann, U. D., A. Ridenour, Y. Shaham, and G. A. Ricaurte. "Serotonin neurotoxicity after (±) 3,4-methylenedioxymethamphetamine (MDMA; 'Ecstasy'): a controlled study in humans." *Neuropsychopharmacology* 10 (1994): 129–138.

Ricaurte, G. A., A. L. Martello, J. L. Katz, and M. B. Martello. "Lasting effects of (±) 3,4-methylenedioxymethamphetamine (MDMA) on central serotonergic neurons in nonhuman primates: neurochemical observations." *Pharmacology and Experimental Therapeutics* 261 (1992): 616–622.

Rudnick, G., and S. C. Wall. "The molecular mechanism of 'ecstasy' [3,4-methylenedioxymethamphetamine (MDMA)]: serotonin transporters are targets for MDMA-induced serotonin release." *Proceedings of the National Academy of Sciences* 89 (1992): 1817–1821.

Steele, T. D., E. D. McCan, and G. A. Ricaurte. "3,4-Methylenedioxymethamphetmiane (MDMA, 'Ecstasy'): pharmacology and toxicology in animals and humans." *Addiction* 89 (1994): 539–551.

HALLUCINOGENS

Abraham, H. D., A. M. Aldridge, and P. Gogai. "The Psychopharmacology of Hallucinogens." *Neuropsychopharmacology* 14 (1996): 285–298.

Holmstedt, B., and N. Kline., eds. "Ethnopharmacologic Search for Psychoactive Drugs." Public Health Service Publication no. 1645 (1967).

Jacobs, B. L. "How hallucinogenic drugs work." *American Scientist* 75 (1987): 386–392.

Schultes, R. E. *The Botany and Chemistry of Hallucinogens.* Thomas Press. New York: Thomas Press, 1980.

Schultes, R. E., and A. Hoffman. *Plants of the Gods.* Rochester, Vt.: Healing Arts Press, 1992.

INHALANTS

Dinwiddie, S. H. "Abuse of inhalants: a review." *Addiction.* 89 (1994): 925–939.

Meadows, R., and A. Verghese. "Medical complications of glue sniffing." *Southern Medical Journal* 89 (1996): 455–462.

Sharp, C. W., F. Beauvais, and R. Spence, eds. National Institute of Drug Abuse Research Monograph 129 (1992). This can be obtained from the National Institute on Drug Abuse at 5600 Fishers Lane, Rockville, MD 20857.

Nitrites and volatile anesthetic gasses are well described in *Goodman and Gilman's the Pharmacological Basis of Therapeutics* listed in the general references above. This book contains numerous references to the research literature.

MARIJUANA

Abood, M., and B. Martin. "Neurobiology of marijuana abuse." *Trends in Pharmacological Sciences* 13 (1992): 201–206.

Adams, I. B., and B. R. Martin. "Cannabis: Pharmacology and toxicology in animals and humans." *Addiction* 91 (1996): 1585–1614.

Clarke, R. C. *Marijuana Botany.* Berkeley, Calif.: And/Or Press, 1981.

Devane, W. "New dawn of cannabinoid pharmacology." *Trends in Pharmacological Sciences* 15 (1994): 40–41.

Grinspoon, L., and J. Bakalar. "Marijuana as Medicine." *Journal of the American Medical Association* 273 (1995): 1875–1876. See also the replies to this article in volume 274 (1995): 1837–1838.

Hollister, L. "Health aspects of cannabis." *Pharmacological Reviews* 38 (1986): 1–20.

Lichtman, A. H., and B. R. Martin. "Delta (9)-Tetrahydrocannabinol Impairs Spatial Memory Through a Cannabinoid Receptor Mechanism." *Psychopharmacology* 126 (1996): 125–131.

Pollan, M. "How pot has grown." *The New York Times Magazine,* 19 February 1995.

NICOTINE

Julien, R. M. *A Primer of Drug Action.* San Francisco: W. H. Freeman, 1995.

Porchet, H. "Pharmacokinetics and pharmacodynamics of nicotine: Implications for tobacco addiction apprehension." In *Drugs of Abuse and Neurobiology,* R. R. Watson, ed. Boca Raton, Fla.: CRC Press, 1992.

OPIATES

R. P. Hammer. *The Neurobiology of Opiates.* Boca Raton, Fla.: CRC Press.

"The Neurobiology of Opiates." *Trends in Pharmacological Sciences* 13 (1992): 185–193.

SEDATIVES

All legal sedatives are well described in *Goodman and Gilman's the Pharmacological Basis of Therapeutics* listed in the general references above. This book contains numerous references to the research literature.

For GHB reading we recommend:

Galloway, G. P., S. L. Frederick, F. E. Staggers Jr, S. Gonzales, and D. E. Smith. "-Gamma-hydroxybutyrate: an emerging drug of abuse that causes physical dependence." *Addiction* 92 no. 1 (1997): 89–96.

Maitre, Michel. "The Gamma-hydroxybutyrate signalling system in brain: organization and functional implications." *Progress in Neurobiology* 51 (1997): 337–361.

STIMULANTS

Hatsukami, D. K., and M. W. Fischman. "Crack Cocaine and Cocaine Hydrochloride—Are the Differences Myth or Reality?" *Journal of the American Medical Association* 276 (1996): 1580–1588.

Kuhar, M. J., and N. S. Pilotte. "Neurochemical Changes in Cocaine Withdrawal." *Trends in Pharmacological Science* 17 (1996): 260–264.

Lakoski, Joan M., Matthew P. Galloway, and Francis J. White, eds. *Cocaine: Pharmacology, Physiology, and Clinical Strategies.* Boca Raton, Fla.: CRC Press, 1992.

Van Dyke, C., and R. Byck "Cocaine." *Scientific American.* 246 no. 3 (1982): 128–141.

Williams, R. G., K. M. Kavanagh, and K. K. Teo. "Pathophysiology and Treatment of Cocaine Toxicity: Implications for the Heart and Cardiovascular System." *Canadian Journal of Cardiology* 12 (1996): 1295–1301.

ADDICTION

Di Chiara, G., and A. Imperato. "Drugs abused by humans preferentially increase synaptic dopamine concentrations in the mesolimbic system of freely moving rats." *Proceedings of the National Academy of Science* 85 (1988): 5274–5278.

Goldstein, A. *Addiction: From Biology to Drug Policy.* New York: W. H. Freeman, 1994.

Kiyatkin, E. A. "Functional Significance of Mesolimbic Dopamine." *Neuroscience & Biobehavioral Reviews* 19 (1995): 573–598.

Koob, G. F., and F. E. Bloom. "Cellular and Molecular Mechanism of Drug Dependence." *Science* 242 (1988): 715–723.

Robinson, T. E., and M. K. C. Berridge. "The neural basis of drug craving: an incentive-sensitization theory of addiction." *Brain Research Reviews* 18 (1993): 247–291.

White, N. M. "Addictive Drugs as Reinforcers: multiple partial actions on memory systems." *Addiction* 91 (1996): 921–949.

Wise, R. A. "The role of reward pathways in the development of drug dependence." *Pharmacology and Therapeutics* 35 (1987): 227–263.

LEGAL ISSUES

We do not recommend that anyone act on any legal information obtained from any source without first speaking with a legal expert. The laws of each state and the federal system are different from one another and extremely complicated. What may be legal in one place may be a felony in another.

For general reading on search, seizure, and privacy, we recommend the following book:

McWhirter, Darien A. *Search, Seizure and Privacy.* Exploring the Constitution Series, Darien A. McWhirter, Series Editor. Phoenix, Ariz.: Oryx Press, 1994.

For information on U.S. government laws, drug scheduling, and penalties, we recommend obtaining a free copy of *Drugs of Abuse* by the U.S. Department of Justice, Drug Enforcement Administration, Arlington, Virginia 22202.

WEB SITE

Check http://www.buzzed.org for more information from the authors.

Glossary of Drug-Related Street Terms/Slang Words

The following list of drug terms is based on a list published on the Internet by David Brocato at the Addictions and Life Page: http://www.addictions.com. It is reproduced with his permission. The authors caution that the drug world is full of rapidly changing terminology and that this list should be viewed as incomplete and, in some cases, outdated.

A

A Bean—MDMA
Abe—$5 worth of drugs
Abe's cabe—$5 bill
Abolic—veterinary steroid
Aborts—Absolut vodka and port, mixed together
Acapulco gold—marijuana from southwest Mexico
Acapulco red—marijuana
Ace—marijuana; PCP
Acid—LSD
Acid head—LSD user
AD—PCP
Adam—MDMA
African black—marijuana
African bush—marijuana
African woodbine—marijuana cigarette
Agonies—withdrawal symptoms

Ah-pen-yen—opium
AIP—heroin from Afghanistan, Iran, and Pakistan
Air blast—inhalant
Airhead—marijuana user
Airplane—marijuana
Alamout black hash—hash; belladona (small amount)
Alice—LSD; mushrooms
Alice B. Toklas—marijuana brownie
Alien sex fiend—very strong powdered PCP mixed with heroin
All lit up—under the influence of drugs
All-American drug—cocaine
All-star—user of multiple drugs
Alpha-ET—alpha-ethyltyptamine
Ames—amyl nitrite
Amidone—methadone
Amies—amphetamine; amyl nitrite
Amoeba—PCP

Amp—amphetamine

Amp joint—marijuana cigarette laced with some form of narcotic

Amped and queer—to be high on coke or crystal

Amped-out—fatigue after using amphetamines

Amping—accelerated heartbeat

AMT—dimethyltryptamine

Amys—amyl nitrite

Anadrol—oral steroid

Anatrofin—injectable steroid

Anavar—oral steroid

Angel—PCP

Angel dust—PCP

Angel hair—PCP

Angel mist—PCP

Angel poke—PCP

Angel tears—liquid LSD

Angels in a sky—LSD

Angie—cocaine

Angola—marijuana

Animal—LSD

Animal trank—PCP

Animal tranquilizer—PCP

Antifreeze—heroin

Anything going on?—Do you have drugs for sale?

Apache—fentanyl

Apple jacks—crack

Aries—heroin

Aroma of men—isobutyl nitrite

Artillery—equipment for injecting drugs

Ashes—marijuana

Ate up—someone who's always wasted

Atom bomb—marijuana and heroin

Atshitshi—marijuana

Aunt Hazel—heroin

Aunt Mary—marijuana

Aunt Nora—cocaine

Aunti—opium

Aunti Emma—opium

Aurora borealis—PCP

B

B—amount of marijuana to fill a matchbox

Babe—drug used for detoxification

Baby—marijuana

Baby bhang—marijuana

Baby habit—occasional use of drugs

Baby slits—MDMA

Baby T—crack

Babysit—guide someone through a first drug experience

Back door—residue left in a pipe

Backbreakers—LSD and strychnine

Backjack—to inject opium

Back-to-back—smoking crack after injecting heroin or heroin used after smoking crack

Backtrack—to allow blood to flow back into a needle during injection

Backup—to prepare a vein for injection

Backwards—depressant

Bad—crack

Bad bundle—inferior-quality heroin

Bad go—bad reaction to a drug

Bad seed—peyote; heroin; marijuana

Bad trip—bad acid trip

Bag—container for drugs

Bag bride—crack-smoking prostitute

Bag man—person who transports money

Bagboy—someone who sells dope for someone else

Bagging—using inhalant

Bale—marijuana

Ball—crack

Baller—one who sells a variety of drugs

Balling—vaginally implanted cocaine

Balloon—heroin supplier

Ballot—heroin

Bam—depressant; amphetamine

Bambalacha—marijuana

Bambs—depressant

Bammer—term given to weak marijuana

Bang—to inject a drug; inhalant

Bank bandit pills—depressant

Bar—marijuana

Barb—depressant

Barbara Jean—pot

Barbies—depressant

Barbs—cocaine

Barrels—LSD

Bart Simpsons—LSD
Base—cocaine; crack
Base crazies—searching on hands and knees for crack
Base head—person who bases
Baseball—crack
Bash—marijuana
Basuco—cocaine; coca paste residue sprinkled on marijuana or regular cigarette
Bat—marijuana pipe, easily disguised as a cigarette
Bathtub speed—methcathinone
Batt—IV needle
Battery acid—LSD
Batu—smokable methamphetamine
Bazooka—cocaine; crack
Bazulco—cocaine
BC Budd—very high-grade marijuana from British Columbia
Beam me up, Scottie—crack dipped in PCP
Beamer—crack user
Beaners—drugs
Beans—amphetamine; depressant; mescaline
Beast—LSD
Beat artist—person selling bogus drugs
Beat vials—vials containing sham crack to cheat buyers
Beautiful boulders—crack
Bebe—crack
Bedbugs—fellow addicts
Bee—bong hit
Beemers—crack
Behind the scale—to weigh and sell cocaine
Beiging—chemicals altering cocaine to make it appear a higher purity
Belladonna—belladonna
Belt—effects of drugs
Belushi—cocaine and heroin
Belyando spruce—marijuana
Bender—drug party
Bennie—amphetamine
Benz—amphetamine
Bernice—cocaine
Bernie—cocaine

Bernie's flakes—cocaine
Bernie's gold dust—cocaine
B-40—cigar laced with marijuana and dipped in malt liquor
Bhang—marijuana (Indian term)
Big bag—heroin
Big bloke—cocaine
Big C—cocaine
Big D—LSD
Big 8—⅛ kilogram of crack
Big flake—cocaine
Big H—heroin
Big Harry—heroin
Big man—drug supplier
Big O—opium
Big rush—cocaine
Bill Blass—crack
Billie hoke—cocaine
Bindle—small packet of drug powder; heroin
Bing—enough of a drug for one injection
Binger—bong hit
Bingers—crack addicts
Bingo—to inject a drug
Bings—crack
Binky—marijuana cigarette
Birdie powder—heroin; cocaine
Biscuit—50 rocks of crack
Bite one's lips—to smoke marijuana
Biz—bag or portion of drugs
B.J.'s—crack
Black—opium; marijuana
Black acid—LSD; LSD and PCP
Black and white—amphetamine
Black bart—marijuana
Black beauties—amphetamine
Black birds—amphetamine
Black bombers—amphetamine
Black button—dried button of peyote
Black ganja—marijuana resin
Black gold—high-potency marijuana
Black gungi—marijuana from India
Black gunion—marijuana
Black hash—opium and hashish
Black maria—highly potent marijuana
Black mo/black moat—highly potent marijuana
Black mollies—amphetamine

Black mote—marijuana mixed with honey

Black pearl—heroin

Black pill—opium pill

Black powder—black hash ground into powder

Black rock—crack

Black Russian—hashish mixed with opium

Black star—LSD

Black stuff—heroin

Black sunshine—LSD

Black tabs—LSD

Black tar—heroin

Black whack—PCP

Blacks—amphetamine

Blanco—heroin

Blanket—marijuana cigarette

Blanks—low-quality drugs

Blast—to smoke marijuana; to smoke crack

Blast a joint—to smoke marijuana

Blast a roach—to smoke marijuana

Blast a stick—to smoke marijuana

Blasted—under the influence of drugs

Blind squid—ketamine; belladona; LSD

Blitzed—under the influence of drugs

Blizzard—white cloud in a pipe used to smoke cocaine

Block—marijuana

Block busters—depressant

Blonde—marijuana

Blotter—LSD; cocaine

Blotter acid—LSD

Blotter cube—LSD

Blow—cocaine; to inhale cocaine; to smoke marijuana

Blow a fix—injection misses the vein and is wasted in the skin

Blow a shot—injection misses the vein and is wasted in the skin

Blow a stick—to smoke marijuana

Blow blue—to inhale cocaine

Blow coke—to inhale cocaine

Blow one's roof—to smoke marijuana

Blow smoke—to inhale cocaine

Blow the vein—injection misses the vein and is wasted in the skin

Blowcaine—crack diluted with cocaine

Blowing smoke—marijuana

Blue—depressant; crack

Blue acid—LSD

Blue angels—depressant

Blue barrels—LSD

Blue birds—depressant

Blue boy—amphetamine

Blue bullets—depressant

Blue caps—mescaline

Blue chairs—LSD

Blue cheers—LSD

Blue de hue—marijuana from Vietnam

Blue devil—depressant

Blue dolls—depressant

Blue fly—New York City LSD

Blue heaven—LSD

Blue heavens—depressant

Blue madman—PCP

Blue microdot—LSD

Blue mist—LSD

Blue moons—LSD

Blue sage—marijuana

Blue sky blond—high-potency marijuana from Columbia

Blue star—LSD; PCP

Blue tips—depressant

Blue vials—LSD

Blunt—marijuana inside a cigar

Blunted out—smoked many blunts of marijuana

Boat—PCP

Bob—marijuana cigarette

Bo-bo—marijuana

Bobo—crack

Bobo bush—marijuana

Body packer—person who ingests crack or cocaine to transport it

Body stuffer—person who ingests crack vials to avoid prosecution

Bogart a joint—salivate on a marijuana cigarette; refuse to share

Bohd—marijuana; PCP

Bolasterone—injectable steroid

Bolivian marching powder—cocaine

Bolo—crack

Bolt—isobutyl nitrite

Bomb—crack; heroin; large marijuana cigarette; high-potency heroin

Bomb squad—crack-selling crew

Bomber—marijuana cigarette

Bombido—injectable amphetamine; heroin; depressant

Bombita—amphetamine; heroin; depressant

Bombs away—heroin

Bone—marijuana; $50 piece of crack

Bonecrusher—crack

Bones—crack

Bong—pipe used to smoke marijuana

Bonita—heroin

Boo—marijuana

Booger—cocaine (in the Florida Keys)

Boogered up—high on cocaine (in the Florida Keys)

Boom—marijuana

Boomers—psilocybin/psilocin

Boost—to inject a drug; to steal

Boost and shoot—steal to support a habit

Booster—to inhale cocaine

Boot—to inject a drug

Boot the gong—to smoke marijuana

Booted—under the influence of drugs

Booty juice—MDMA dissolved in liquid

Boppers—amyl nitrite

Botray—crack

Bottles—crack vials; amphetamine

Boubou—crack

Boulder—crack; $20 worth of crack

Boulya—crack

Bouncing powder—cocaine

Bowl—between ⅟₃₂ and ⅟₁₆ ounce of marijuana

Boxed—in jail

Boy—heroin

Bozo—heroin

Brain ticklers—amphetamine

Break night—staying up all night until day break

Breakdowns—$40 crack rock sold for $20

Breakfast of champions—crack

Brewery—place where drugs are made

Brick—1 kilogram of marijuana; crack

Brick gum—heroin

Bridge up or bring up—ready a vein for injection

Britton—peyote

Broccoli—marijuana

Broker—go-between in a drug deal

Brome/Bromage—dextromethorphane hydrobromide (active ingredient in Robitussin DM), popular in clinical powder form in some cities as a street drug

Brown—heroin; marijuana

Brown bombers—LSD

Brown crystal—heroin

Brown dots—LSD

Brown rhine—heroin

Brown sugar—heroin

Brownies—amphetamine

Browns—amphetamine

Buck—to shoot someone in the head

Bud—marijuana

Buda—a high-grade marijuana joint filled with crack

Budda—marijuana

Buffer—crack smoker; a woman who exchanges oral sex for crack

Buger sugar—powdered cocaine

Bugged—annoyed; to be covered with sores and abscesses from repeated use of unsterile needles

Bull—narcotics agent or police officer

Bullet—isobutyl nitrite

Bullet bolt—inhalant

Bullia capital—crack

Bullion—crack

Bullyon—marijuana

Bumblebees—amphetamine

Bummer trip—unsettling and threatening experience from PCP intoxication

Bump—crack; fake crack; to boost a high; small dose of crystal meth

Bundle—heroin

Bunk—fake cocaine

Burese—cocaine

Burn one—to smoke marijuana

Burn the main line—to inject a drug

Burned—purchased fake drugs

Burned out—collapse of veins from repeated injections; permanent impairment from drug abuse

Burnie—marijuana

Burning logs—smoking marijuana cigarettes

Burnout—heavy abuser of drugs
Burnt—smoked too much weed
Bush—cocaine; marijuana
Businessman's LSD—dimethyltryptamine
Businessman's special—dimethyltryptamine
Businessman's trip—dimethyltryptamine
Busted—arrested
Busters—depressant
Busy bee—PCP
Butt naked—PCP
Butter—marijuana; crack
Butter flower—marijuana
Buttons—mescaline
Butu—heroin
Buzz—under the influence of drugs
Buzz bomb—nitrous oxide

C

C—cocaine
C & M—cocaine and morphine
C joint—place where cocaine is sold
Caballo—heroin
Cabello—cocaine
Caca—heroin
Cacti joint—a joint of dried and ground up peyote
Cactus—mescaline
Cactus buttons—mescaline
Cactus head—mescaline
Cad/Cadillac—1 ounce
Cadillac—PCP
Cadillac express—methcathinone
Caine—cocaine; crack
Cakes—round disks of crack
California cornflakes—cocaine
California sunshine—LSD
Cam trip—high-potency marijuana
Cambodian red/Cam red—marijuana from Cambodia
Came—cocaine
Can—marijuana; 1 ounce
Canadian black—marijuana
Canamo—marijuana
Canappa—marijuana
Canceled stick—marijuana cigarette

Candy—cocaine; crack; depressant; amphetamine
Candy C—cocaine
Candy flip—1 hit Ecstasy per 3 hits LSD
Cannabinol—PCP
Cannabis indica—marijuana that is very strong and causes hallucinations
Cannabis sativa—marijuana that is milder than indica and does not cause hallucinations
Cannabis tea—marijuana
Cannon—huge joint
Canoe—when a joint gets a hole in the side or looks like a canoe
Cap—crack; LSD
Cap up—transfer bulk-form drugs to capsules
Capital H—heroin
Caps—crack; heroin; psilocybin/psilocin
Carburetor—crack stem attachment
Carga—heroin
Carmabis—marijuana
Carne—heroin
Carnie—cocaine
Carpet patrol—crack smokers searching the floor for crack
Carrie—cocaine
Carrie Nation—cocaine
Cartucho—package of marijuana cigarettes
Cartwheels—amphetamine
Cashed—bowl is finished/empty
Casper the ghost—crack
Cat—methcathinone
Cat valium—ketamine
Catnip—marijuana cigarette
Caviar—crack
Cavite all-star—marijuana
C-dust—cocaine
Cereal—marijuana being smoked in a bowl
Cecil—cocaine
Cess—marijuana
C-game—cocaine
Chalk—methamphetamine; amphetamine
Chalked up—under the influence of cocaine

Chalking—chemically altering the color of cocaine so that it looks white

Chamber—pipe used for marijuana

Chandoo/chandu—opium

Channel—vein into which a drug is injected

Channel swimmer—one who injects heroin

Charas—marijuana from India

Charge—marijuana

Charged up—under the influence of drugs

Charley—heroin

Charlie—cocaine

Chase—to smoke cocaine; to smoke marijuana

Chaser—compulsive crack user

Chasing the dragon—crack and heroin

Chasing the tiger—to smoke heroin

Chaze—to christen a new bowl or pipe

Cheap basing—crack

Check—personal supply of drugs

Cheeba—marijuana

Cheeo—marijuana

Chemical—crack

Chestbonz—the one who takes the biggest bong hit

Chewies—crack; marijuana cigar with powdered cocaine inside

Chiba chiba—high-potency marijuana from Columbia

Chicago black—marijuana (term from Chicago)

Chicago green—marijuana (term from Chicago)

Chicken powder—amphetamine

Chicken scratch—searching on hands and knees for crack

Chicle—heroin

Chief—LSD; mescaline

Chieva—heroin

Chillie Willies—snorting vodka or gin out of a bottle cap

Chillun—pipe used to smoke hashish

China—opium

China cat—high-potency heroin

China girl—fentanyl

China town—fentanyl

China white—fentanyl

Chinese dragons—LSD

Chinese molasses—opium

Chinese red—heroin

Chinese tobacco—opium

Chinese-eyed—when the eyes become slanted from the influence of marijuana

Chip—heroin

Chipper—occasional Hispanic user

Chippie—marijuana

Chipping—using drugs occasionally

Chippy—cocaine

Chira—marijuana

Chocolate—opium; amphetamine

Chocolate chips—MDMA

Chocolate ecstasy—crack made brown by adding chocolate-milk powder during processing

Chocolate rocket—crack made brown by adding chocolate-milk powder during processing

Chocolate Thi—marijuana

Choker—large or powerful hit of crack cocaine

Cholly—cocaine

Chorals—depressant

Christina—amphetamine

Christine—crystal methamphetamine

Christmas rolls—depressant

Christmas tree—marijuana; depressant; amphetamine

Chronic—marijuana; marijuana mixed with crack

Chucks—hunger following withdrawal from heroin

Church—LSD paper with a cross on it

Churus—marijuana

Cid—LSD

Cigarette paper—packet of heroin

Cigarrode cristal—PCP

Citrol—high-potency marijuana from Nepal

CJ—PCP

Clarity—MDMA

Clear up—stop drug use

Clicker—crack and PCP

Cliffhanger—PCP

Climax—crack; isobutyl nitrite; heroin

Climb—marijuana cigarette

Clips — rows of vials heat-sealed together

Clocking paper — profits from selling drugs

Closet baser — user of crack who prefers anonymity

Cloud — crack; huge hit from ice pipe

Cloud nine — crack

Cluck — crack smoker

Coasting — under the influence of drugs

Coasts to coasts — amphetamine

Coca — cocaine

Cocaine blues — depression after extended cocaine use

Cochornis — marijuana

Cocktail — cigarette laced with cocaine or crack; partially smoked marijuana cigarette inserted into regular cigarette

Cocoa puff — to smoke cocaine and marijuana

Coco rocks — crack made dark brown by adding chocolate pudding during production

Coco snow — benzocaine used as cutting agent for crack

Coconut — cocaine

Cod — large amount of money

Coffee — LSD

Coke — cocaine; crack

Coke bar — bar where cocaine is openly used

Cola — cocaine

Cold turkey — sudden withdrawal from drugs

Coli — marijuana

Coliflor tostao — marijuana

Colorado — cocaine

Colorado cocktail — marijuana

Columbian — marijuana

Columbo — PCP

Columbus black — marijuana

Come home — end a trip from LSD

Comeback — benzocaine and mannitol used to adulterate cocaine for conversion to crack

Conductor — LSD

Connect — to purchase drugs; supplier of illegal drugs

Contact lens — LSD

Cook — to mix heroin with water; heating heroin to prepare it for injection

Cook down — process in which users liquefy heroin in order to inhale it

Cooker — to inject a drug

Cookies — crack

Cool — someone who uses drugs

Cooler — cigarette laced with a drug

Coolie — cigarette laced with cocaine

Cop — to obtain drugs

Co-pilot — amphetamine

Copping zones — specific areas where buyers can purchase drugs

Coral — depressant

Coriander seeds — cash

Cork the air — to inhale cocaine

Corn-stalker — marijuana cigarette rolled in the shuck of a corn cob sealed with honey

Corrinne — cocaine

Cosa — marijuana

Cotics — heroin

Cotton — currency

Cotton brothers — cocaine, heroin, and morphine

Courage pills — heroin; depressant

Course note — bill larger than $2

Cozmo's — PCP

Crack — cocaine

Crack attack — craving for crack

Crack back — crack and marijuana

Crack cooler — crack soaked in wine cooler

Crack gallery — place where crack is bought and sold

Crack head — someone who uses crack cocaine

Crack spot — area where people can purchase crack

Crack star — someone who uses crack cocaine

Crack weed — marijuana laced with crack

Cracker jacks — crack smokers

Crackers — LSD

Crank — methamphetamine; amphetamine; methcathinone

Cranking up — to inject a drug

Crankster—someone on crank
Crap/crop—low-quality heroin
Crash—to sleep off effects of drugs
Crazy coke—PCP
Crazy Eddie—PCP
Crazy weed—marijuana
Credit card—crack stem
Creeperbud—marijuana that creeps up on you
Crib—crack
Crill—marijuana cigarette laced with cocaine
Crimmie—cigarette laced with crack
Crink—methamphetamine
Crip—meth
Cripple—marijuana cigarette
Cris—methamphetamine
Crisco—crystal methamphetamine
Crisscross—amphetamine
Crissy—crystal methamphetamine
Cristina—methamphetamine
Cristy—smokable methamphetamine
Croak—crack and methamphetamine
Cross tops—amphetamine
Crossroads—amphetamine
Crown crap—heroin
Crumbs—tiny pieces of crack
Crumbsnatcher—a junkie who steals tiny pieces of crack
Crunch & Munch—crack
Crusty treats—cocaine
Cruz—opium from Veracruz, Mexico
Crying weed—marijuana
Crypto—methamphetamine
Crystal—methamphetamine; PCP; amphetamine; cocaine
Crystal joint—PCP
Crystal meth—methamphetamine
Crystal pop—cocaine and PCP
Crystal T—PCP
Crystal tea—LSD
Cube—1 ounce; LSD
Cubes—marijuana tablets
Culican—high-potency marijuana from Mexico
Cupcakes—LSD
Cura—heroin
Cushion—vein into which a drug is injected

Cut—adulterate drugs
Cut-deck—heroin mixed with powdered milk
Cycline—PCP
Cyclones—PCP

D

D—LSD; PCP
Dabble—use drugs occasionally
Daddy—marijuana joint
Dagga—marijuana
Dama blanca—cocaine
Dance fever—fentanyl
Dank—marijuana
Dawamesk—marijuana
Dead on arrival—heroin
Dealer—one who sells drugs
Deca-duabolin—injectable steroid
Decadence—MDMA
Deck—1–15 grams of heroin, also known as a bag; packet of drugs
Deeda—LSD
Delatestryl—injectable steroid
Demo—crack stem; a sample-size quantity of crack
Demolish—crack
Dental floss—LSD
Dep-testosterone—injectable steroid
DET—dimethyltryptamine
Detroit pink—PCP
Deuce—$2 worth of drugs; heroin
Devil's dandruff—crack
Devil's dick—crack pipe
Devilsmoke—crack
Dew—marijuana
Dews—$10 worth of drugs
Dexies—amphetamine
Diablo—LSD paper with a devil on it
Diambista—marijuana
Dianabol—veterinary steroid
Diesel—heroin
Diet pills—amphetamine
Diggidy—good marijuana
Digie—refers to scales used to weigh drugs
Dihydrolone—injectable steroid
Dimba—marijuana from western Africa

Dime—crack; $10 worth of crack; $\frac{1}{16}$ ounce of marijuana

Dime bag—$10 worth of drugs

Dime's worth—amount of heroin to cause death

Ding—marijuana

Dinkie dow—marijuana

Dinosaurs—LSD

Dip—crack

Dipper—PCP

Dipping out—crack runners taking a portion of crack from vials

Dirge—PCP

Dirt—heroin

Dirt grass—inferior-quality marijuana

Dirty basing—crack

Disco biscuits—depressant

Disease—drug of choice

Ditch—marijuana

Ditch weed—inferior-quality marijuana from Mexico

Divider—sharing a joint with someone

Dizz—marijuana

Djamba—marijuana

D.L. spot—safe place to buy and use drugs

DMT—dimethyltryptamine

Do a joint—to smoke marijuana

Do a line—to inhale cocaine

Do it, Jack—PCP

DOA—PCP; crack

Doctor—MDMA

Dog—good friend

Dog food—heroin

Dogie—heroin

Doja—strong marijuana

Dollar—$100 worth of drugs

Dolls—depressant

Domes—LSD

Domestic—locally grown marijuana

Domex—PCP and MDMA

Dominoes—amphetamine

Don jem—marijuana

Dona Juana—marijuana

Dona Juanita—marijuana

Doobie/dubbe/duby—marijuana

Doogie/doojee/dugie—heroin

Dooley—heroin

Dope—heroin; marijuana; any other drug

Dope fiend—crack or marijuana addict

Dope smoke—to smoke marijuana

Dopium—opium

Doradilla—marijuana

Dose/Doses—LSD

Dots—LSD or mescaline

Doub—$20 rock of crack

Double bubble—cocaine

Double cross—amphetamine

Double dome—LSD

Double rock—crack diluted with procaine

Double trouble—depressant

Double ups—a $20 rock that can be broken into 2 $20 rocks

Double yoke—crack

Dove—$35 piece of crack

Dover's powder—opium

Downer—depressant

Downie—depressant

Downtown—heroin

Draf weed—marijuana

Drag weed—marijuana

Draw up—to inject a drug

Dream—cocaine

Dream gum—opium

Dream stick—opium

Dreamer—morphine

Dreams—opium

Dreck—heroin

Drink—PCP

Dropper—to inject a drug

Drowsy high—depressant

Drug deal—the exchange of money for drugs

Dry high—marijuana

DT—heroin

Dub sack—$20 worth of drugs (marijuana)

Duct—cocaine

Due—residue of oils trapped in a pipe after smoking crack

Dugout—pipe used for marijuana

Duji—heroin

Dummy dust—PCP

Durabolin—injectable steroid

Durog—marijuana
Duros—marijuana
Dust—heroin; cocaine; PCP; marijuana mixed with various chemicals
Dust joint—PCP
Dust of angels—PCP
Dusted—high on PCP
Dusted parsley—PCP
Dusting—adding PCP, heroin, or another drug to marijuana
Dynamite—heroin and cocaine
Dyno—heroin
Dyno-pure—heroin

E

E—MDMA
Earth—marijuana cigarette
Easing powder—opium
Eastside player—crack
Easy score—obtaining drugs easily
Eat—to take acid or mushrooms
Eater—someone who eats marijuana
Eating—taking a drug orally
Ecstasy—MDMA
Egg—crack
Eight ball—⅛ ounce of drugs
Eightball—crack and heroin
Eighth—heroin or marijuana
El Cid—LSD
El diablito—marijuana, cocaine, heroin, and PCP
El diablo—marijuana, cocaine, and heroin
El Gato Diablo—crystal methamphetamine
Elaine—Ecstasy
Electric Kool-Aid—LSD
Elephant—PCP
Elephant tranquilizer—PCP
Elle Momo—marijuana laced with PCP
Ellis Day—LSD
Embalming fluid—PCP
Emergency gun—instrument used to inject other than a syringe
Emsel—morphine
Endo—marijuana

Energizer—PCP
Enoltestovis—injectable steroid
Ephedrone—methcathinone
Equipose—veterinary steroid
Erth—PCP
Esra—marijuana
Essence—MDMA
Estuffa—heroin
ET—alpha-ethyltyptamine
Euphoria—MDMA, mescaline, and crystal methamphetamine
Eve—MDEA
Explorers' club—group of LSD users
Eye opener—crack; amphetamine

F

Fachiva—heroin
Factory—place where drugs are packaged, diluted, or manufactured
Fake STP—PCP
Fall—arrested
Fallbrook redhair—marijuana (term from Fallbrook, CA)
Famous dimes—crack
Fantasia—dimethyltryptamine
Fat bags—crack
Fat pappy—fat marijuana cigarette or cigar
Fatty—marijuana cigarette
Feed bag—container for marijuana
Ferry dust—heroin
Fi-do-nie—opium
Fields—LSD
Fiend—someone who smokes marijuana alone
Fifteen cents—$15 worth of drugs
Fifty-one—crack
Finajet/finaject—veterinary steroid
Fine stuff—marijuana
Finger—marijuana cigarette
Fir—marijuana
Fire—to inject a drug; crack and methamphetamine
Fire it up—to smoke marijuana
First line—morphine
Fish scales—crack

Five C note—$500 bill

Five-cent bag—$5 worth of drugs

Five-dollar bag—$50 worth of drugs

Fives—amphetamine

Fix—to inject a drug

Fizzies—methadone

Flag—appearance of blood around the vein

Flake—cocaine

Flakes—PCP

Flame cooking—smoking cocaine base by putting the pipe over a stove flame

Flamethrower—cigarette laced with cocaine and heroin

Flash—LSD

Flashers—LSD that is very hallucinogenic

Flat blues—LSD

Flat chunks—crack cut with benzocaine

Flea powder—low-purity heroin

Florida snow—cocaine

Flower—marijuana

Flower tops—marijuana

Fly Mexican airlines—to smoke marijuana

Flying—under the influence of drugs

Following that cloud—searching for drugs

Foo foo stuff—heroin; cocaine

Foo-foo dust—cocaine

Foolish powder—heroin; cocaine

Footballs—amphetamine

Forty-five-minute psychosis—dimethyltryptamine

Forwards—amphetamine

420—marijuana

Fraho/frajo—marijuana

Freebase—to smoke cocaine; crack

Freeze—cocaine; to renege on a drug deal

French blue—amphetamine

French fries—crack

Fresh—PCP

Friend—fentanyl

Fries—crack

Frios—marijuana laced with PCP

Frisco special—cocaine, heroin, and LSD

Frisco speedball—cocaine, heroin, and LSD

Friskie powder—cocaine

Fry—crack or marijuana laced with embalming fluid

Fry daddy—crack and marijuana; cigarette laced with crack

Fu—marijuana

Fucked up—high on drugs

Fuel—marijuana mixed with insecticides; PCP

Fuete—hypodermic needle

Fuma D'Angola—marijuana (Portuguese term)

Future—crystal methamphetamine

G

G—$1,000; 1 gram of drugs; term for an unfamiliar male

G spot tornado—equal parts of rum and NyQuil

Gaffel—fake cocaine

Gaffus—hypodermic needle

Gage/gauge—marijuana

Gagers—methcathinone

Gaggers—methcathinone

Gak—line of methamphetamine or cocaine

Galloping horse—heroin

Gamot—heroin

Gange—marijuana

Gangster—marijuana

Gangster pills—depressant

Ganja—marijuana from Jamaica

Gank—fake crack

Gar—marijuana rolled in cigar paper

Garbage—inferior-quality drugs

Garbage heads—users who buy crack from street dealers instead of cooking it themselves

Garbage rock—crack

Garr—large joint of marijuana

Gash—marijuana

Gasper—marijuana cigarette

Gasper stick—marijuana cigarette

Gato—heroin

Gauge butt—marijuana

G.B.—depressant

Gee—opium

Geek—crack and marijuana
Geeker—crack user
Geeze—to inhale cocaine
Geezer—to inject a drug
Geezin a bit of dee gee—injecting a drug
George smack—heroin
Get a gage up—to smoke marijuana
Get a gift—to obtain drugs
Get down—to inject a drug
Get high—to smoke marijuana
Get lifted—under the influence of drugs
Get off—to inject a drug; to get high
Get the wind—to smoke marijuana
Get through—to obtain drugs
Ghana—marijuana
GHB—gamma-hydroxybuterate
Ghost—LSD
Ghost busting—smoking cocaine;
    searching for white particles in the
    belief that they are crack
Gick monster—crack smoker
Gift-of-the-sun—cocaine
Giggle smoke—marijuana
Gimmick—drug-injection equipment
Gimmie—crack and marijuana
Gin—cocaine
Girl—cocaine; crack; heroin
Girlfriend—cocaine
Give wings—to inject someone or teach
    someone how to inject heroin
Glacines—heroin
Glad stuff—cocaine
Glading—using inhalant
Glass—hypodermic needle;
    amphetamine
Glass gun—hypodermic needle
Glo—crack
Gluey—person who sniffs glue
Go into a sewer—to inject a drug
Go loco—to smoke marijuana
Go on a sleigh ride—to inhale cocaine
Godfather—marijuana cigarette laced
    with cocaine; cigar filled with
    marijuana or other type of drug
God's drug—morphine
God's flesh—psilocybin/psilocin
God's medicine—opium
Go-fast—methcathinone
Going 90 mph—the peak of a trip

Going to the dentist—nitrous oxide
Gold—marijuana; crack
Gold dust—cocaine
Gold star—marijuana
Golden dragon—LSD
Golden girl—heroin
Golden leaf—very high-quality marijuana
Golf ball—crack
Golf balls—depressant; LSD
Golpe—heroin
Goma—opium; black tar heroin
Gondola—opium
Gong—marijuana; opium
Gong ringer—a fat marijuana cigarette
Goob—methcathinone
Good—PCP
Good and plenty—heroin
Good butt—marijuana cigarette
Good giggles—marijuana
Good go—proper amount of drugs for
    the money paid
Good H—heroin
Good lick—good drugs
Goodfellas—fentanyl
Goof butt—marijuana cigarette
Goofball—cocaine and heroin;
    depressant
Goofers—depressant
Goofy's—LSD
Goon—PCP
Goon dust—PCP
Gopher—person paid to pick up drugs
Goric—opium
Gorilla biscuits—PCP
Gorilla pills—depressant
Gorilla tab—PCP
Got it going on—fast sale of drugs
Graduate—to completely stop using
    drugs; to progress to stronger drugs
Gram—hashish
Grape parfait—LSD
Grass—marijuana
Grass brownies—brownies made with
    marijuana
Grata—marijuana
Gravel—crack
Gravy—to inject a drug; heroin
Grease—currency
Great bear—fentanyl

Great tobacco—opium
Green—inferior-quality marijuana; PCP; ketamine
Green button—fresh button of peyote
Green cigarette—marijuana cigarette
Green double domes—LSD
Green dragons—depressant
Green frog—depressant
Green goddess—marijuana
Green gold—cocaine
Green goods—paper currency
Green leaves—PCP
Green single domes—LSD
Green tea—PCP
Green wedge—LSD
Greens/green stuff—paper currency
Greeter—marijuana
Greta—marijuana
Gray shields—LSD
Griefo—marijuana
Griff—marijuana
Griffa—marijuana
Griffo—marijuana
Grit—crack
Groceries—crack
G-rock—1 gram of rock cocaine
Grogged—really stoned or burned out on marijuana
Ground control—guide or caretaker during a hallucinogenic experience
G-shot—small dose of drugs used to hold off withdrawal symptoms until full dose can be taken
Gum—opium
Guma—opium
Gun—to inject a drug; needle
Gungun—marijuana
Gunther—neighborhood marijuana dealer
Gutter—vein into which a drug is injected
Gutter junkie—addict who relies on others to obtain drugs
Gyve—marijuana cigarette

H

H—heroin
H & C—heroin and cocaine

H caps—heroin
Hache—heroin
Hail—crack
Hairy—heroin
Half—½ ounce
Half a football field—50 rocks of crack
Half G—$500
Half load—15 bags (decks) of heroin
Half moon—peyote
Half piece—½ ounce of heroin or cocaine
Half track—crack
Half-a-C—$50 bill
Hamburger helper—crack
Hand-to-hand—direct delivery and payment
Hand-to-hand man—a transient dealer who carries small amounts of crack
Hanhich—marijuana
Hanyak—smokable speed
Happy cigarette—marijuana cigarette
Happy dust—cocaine
Happy powder—cocaine
Happy trails—cocaine
Hard candy—heroin
Hard line—crack
Hard rock—crack
Hard stuff—opium; heroin
Hardcore—heavy drug user
Hardware—isobutyl nitrite
Harm reducer—marijuana
Harry—heroin
Hash—marijuana
Hats—LSD
Have a dust—cocaine
Haven dust—cocaine
Hawaiian—very high-potency marijuana
Hawaiian sunshine—LSD
Hawaii's finest—methamphetamine
Hawk—LSD
Hay—marijuana
Hay butt—marijuana cigarette
Haze—LSD
Hazel—heroin
HCP—PCP
Head drugs—amphetamine
Headlights—LSD
Heart-on—inhalant
Hearts—amphetamine

Heaven and hell—PCP
Heaven dust—heroin; cocaine
Heavenly blue—LSD
Heeled—having plenty of money
Helen—heroin
Hell dust—heroin
He-man—fentanyl
Hemp—marijuana
Henpicking—searching on hands and knees for crack
Henry—heroin
Henry VIII—cocaine
Her—cocaine
Herb—marijuana
Herb and Al—marijuana and alcohol
Herba—marijuana
Herms—PCP
Hero—heroin
Hero of the underworld—heroin
Heroina—heroin
Hessle—heroin
High—the effect drug users feel when using drugs
Highbeams—the wide eyes of a person on crack
Hikori—peyote
Hikuli—peyote
Hikuli—peyote
Him—heroin
Hinkley—PCP
Hippie crack—inhalant
Hiropon—smokable methamphetamine
Hit—crack; marijuana cigarette; to smoke marijuana
Hit the hay—to smoke marijuana
Hit the main line—to inject a drug
Hit the needle—to inject a drug
Hit the pit—to inject a drug
Hitch up the reindeers—to inhale cocaine
Hits—LSD
Hitter—little pipe designed for only one hit
Hitting up—injecting drugs
HO—½ ounce of marijuana
Hocus—opium; marijuana
Hog—PCP
Holding—possessing drugs
Holli—a marijuana cigarette stuck in a pipe and then smoked

Hombre—heroin
Hombrecitos—psilocybin
Homegrown—marijuana
Honey—currency
Honey blunts—marijuana cigars sealed with honey
Honey oil—ketamine; inhalant
Honeymoon—early stages of drug use before addiction or dependency develops
Hong-yen—heroin in pill form
Hooch—marijuana
Hoochie-mamma—a two-paper joint
Hooked—addicted
Hooter—cocaine; marijuana
Hop/hops—opium
Hopped up—under the influence of drugs
Horn—to inhale cocaine; crack pipe
Horning—heroin; to inhale cocaine
Horse—heroin
Horse heads—amphetamine
Horse tracks—PCP
Horse tranquilizer—PCP
Hot box—to fill up a closed area with secondhand marijuana smoke
Hot dope—heroin
Hot heroin—heroin that has been poisoned to give to a police informant
Hot ice—smokable methamphetamine
Hot load/hot shot—lethal injection of an opiate
Hot stick—marijuana cigarette
Hotcakes—crack
House fee—money paid to enter a crackhouse
House piece—crack given to the owner of a crackhouse or apartment where crack users congregate
How do you like me now?—crack
Hows—morphine
HRN—heroin
Hubba, I am back—crack
Hubba pigeon—crack user looking for rocks on the floor after a police raid
Hubbas—crack (term from northern CA)
Huff—inhalant
Huffer—inhalant abuser (gas, glue, Pam, etc.)

Hulling—using others to get drugs

Hunter—cocaine

Hustle—to attempt to obtain drug customers

Hyatari—peyote

Hydro—marijuana

Hydroponic—hydroponically grown marijuana

Hype—heroin addict; an addict

Hype stick—hypodermic needle

I

I am back—crack

Ice—cocaine; methamphetamine; smokable amphetamine; MDMA; PCP

Ice cream habit—occasional use of drugs

Ice cube—crack

Icing—cocaine

Idiot pills—depressant

In—connected with drug suppliers

Inbetweens—depressant; amphetamine

Inca message—cocaine

Incense—opium

Indian boy—marijuana

Indian hay—marijuana from India

Indica—species of cannabis found in hot climate that grows to 3.5 to 4 feet tall

Indo—marijuana (term from northern CA)

Indonesian bud—marijuana; opium

Infinity—LSD that lasts for a long period of time

Instant zen—LSD

Interplanetary mission—traveling from one crackhouse to another in search of crack

Isda—heroin

Issues—crack

IZM—marijuana

J

J/J's—marijuana cigarette(s)

Jab/job—to inject a drug

Jack—to steal someone else's drugs

Jackpot—fentanyl

Jack-up—to inject a drug

Jag—to keep a high going

Jam—amphetamine; cocaine

Jam cecil—amphetamine

Jamaican red—potent marijuana from Jamaica

Jane—marijuana

Jay—marijuana cigarette

Jay smoke—marijuana

Jee gee—heroin

Jefferson airplane—used match cut in half to hold a partially smoked marijuana cigarette

Jellies—depressant

Jelly—cocaine

Jelly baby—amphetamine

Jelly bean—amphetamine; depressant

Jelly beans—crack

Jesus Christ acid—especially potent LSD

Jet—ketamine

Jet fuel—PCP

Jim Jones—marijuana laced with cocaine and PCP

Jive—heroin; marijuana; drugs

Jive doo jee—heroin

Jive stick—marijuana

Johnny go fast—speed

Johnson—crack

Joint—marijuana cigarette

Jojee—heroin

Jolly bean—amphetamine

Jolly green—marijuana

Jolly pop—casual user of heroin

Jolt—to inject a drug; strong reaction to drugs

Jones—heroin

Jonesing—need for drugs

Joy flakes—heroin

Joy juice—depressant

Joy plant—opium

Joy pop—to inject a drug

Joy popping—occasional use of drugs

Joy powder—heroin; cocaine

Joy smoke—marijuana

Joy stick—marijuana cigarette

Joyride—going out and getting high

Juan Valdez—marijuana

Juanita—marijuana
Juggle—to sell drugs to another addict to support a habit
Juggler—teenage street dealer
Jugs—amphetamine
Juice—steroids; PCP
Juice joint—marijuana cigarette sprinkled with crack
Ju-ju—marijuana cigarette
Jum—sealed plastic bag containing crack
Jumbos—large vials of crack sold on the streets
Junk—cocaine; heroin
Junkie—addict

K

K—ketamine
Kabayo—heroin
Kabuki—crack pipe made from a plastic rum bottle and a rubber sparkplug cover
Kaksonjae—smokable methamphetamine
Kaleidoscope—a type of LSD
Kali—marijuana
Kangaroo—crack
Kaps—PCP
Karachi—heroin
Kate bush—good marijuana, or "kind bud"
Kaya—marijuana
KB—potent marijuana
K-blast—PCP
Keesh—a fat bag
Keller—ketamine
Kelly's day—ketamine
Kentucky blue—marijuana
Keyed—high on drugs
KGB (killer green bud)—marijuana
K-hole—periods of ketamine-induced confusion
Kibbles & Bits—small crumbs of crack
Kick—to get off a drug habit; inhalant
Kick stick—marijuana cigarette
Kicked—to pass out or about to pass out
Kiddie dope—prescription drugs
Kiff—marijuana

Killer—marijuana; PCP
Killer weed (1960s)—marijuana
Killer weed (1980s)—marijuana and PCP
Kilo—2.2 pounds
Kilter—marijuana
Kind—marijuana
Kind bud—marijuana
King ivory—fentanyl
King Kong pills—depressant
King's habit—cocaine
Kit—equipment used to inject drugs
KJ—PCP
Kleenex—MDMA
Klingons—crack addicts
Knuckle samich—fat marijuana cigarette
Kokomo—crack
Koller joints—PCP
Kona gold—strong marijuana grown on the Big Island in Hawaii
Kools—PCP
Kram—to pack the bowl tightly
Krippies—moist marijuana to be smoked only out of a bowl or a bong
Kryptonite—crack
Krystal—PCP
Krystal joint—PCP
Kumba—marijuana
Kushempeng—marijuana
Kutchie—marijuana
KW—PCP

L

L—LSD
L.A.—long-acting amphetamine
L.A. glass—smokable methamphetamine
L.A. ice—smokable methamphetamine
Lace—cocaine and marijuana
Lady—cocaine
Lady caine—cocaine
Lady snow—cocaine
Lakbay diva—marijuana
Lamborghini—crack pipe made from a plastic rum bottle and a rubber sparkplug cover
Las mujercitas—psilocybin
Lason sa daga—LSD

Laugh and scratch—to inject a drug
Laughing gas—nitrous oxide
Laughing grass—marijuana
Laughing weed—marijuana
Lay back—depressant
Lay-out—equipment for taking drugs
LBJ—LSD; PCP; heroin
Leaf—marijuana; cocaine
Leaky bolla—PCP
Leaky leak—PCP
Leapers—amphetamine
Leaping—under the influence of drugs
Leary's—LSD
Lemonade—heroin; poor-quality drugs
Lenllo—joint
Lens—LSD
Lethal weapon—PCP
Lettuce—money
Lib (Librium)—depressant
Lid—1 ounce of marijuana
Lid proppers—amphetamine
Life Saver—heroin
Light stuff—marijuana
Lightning—amphetamine
Lima—marijuana
Lime acid—LSD
Line—cocaine
Linga—crank
Lipton Tea—inferior-quality drugs
Lit up—under the influence of drugs
Little bomb—amphetamine; heroin; depressant
Little bowl of Buddha—10-gram bowl of marijuana buds or hash
Little green friends—marijuana
Little ones—PCP
Little smoke—marijuana; psilocybin/psilocin
Live ones—PCP
L.L.—marijuana
Llesca—marijuana
Load—25 bags of heroin
Loaded—high
Loaf—marijuana
Lobo—marijuana
Locker room—isobutyl nitrite
Locoweed—marijuana
Log—PCP; marijuana cigarette
Logor—LSD

Loused—covered by sores and abscesses from repeated use of unsterile needles
Love—crack
Love affair—cocaine
Love boat—marijuana dipped in formaldehyde; PCP
Love doctor—MDMA
Love drug—MDMA; depressant
Love nuggets—marijuana
Love pearls—alpha-ethyltyptamine
Love pills—alpha-ethyltyptamine
Love potion #9—MDMA
Love trip—MDMA and mescaline
Love weed—marijuana
Lovelies—marijuana laced with PCP
Lovely—PCP
LSD—lysergic acid diethylamide
Lubage—marijuana
Luch head—alcoholic
Lucky Charmz—Ecstacy
Lucy in the sky with diamonds—LSD
Ludes—depressant
Luding out—high on a depressant
Luds—depressant
Lunchbox—kids who do drugs

M

M—marijuana; morphine
M&M—depressant
Machinery—marijuana
Macon—marijuana
Mad dog—PCP
Mad scientist—someone who makes crank
Madman—PCP
Magic—PCP
Magic dust—PCP
Magic mushroom—psilocybin/psilocin
Magic smoke—marijuana
Main line—to inject a drug
Mainliner—person who injects into the vein
Make up—need to find more drugs
Mama coca—cocaine
Manhattan silver—marijuana
Manteca—Puerto Rican slang for heroin

Marathons—amphetamine
Mari—marijuana cigarette
Marimba—marijuana
Marshmallow reds—depressant
Mary—marijuana
Mary and Johnny—marijuana
Mary Ann—marijuana
Mary Jane—marijuana
Mary Jonas—marijuana
Mary Warner—marijuana
Mary Weaver—marijuana
Maserati—crack pipe made from a
   plastic rum bottle and a rubber
   sparkplug cover
Matchbox—1/4 ounce of marijuana or 6
   marijuana cigarettes
Matsakow—heroin
Maui waui—marijuana from Hawaii
Max—gamma-hydroxybuterate
   dissolved in water and mixed with
   amphetamines
Maxibolin—oral steroid
Mayo—cocaine; heroin
MDM—MDMA
MDMA—
   methylenedioxymethamphetamine
Mean green—PCP
Meg—marijuana
Megg—marijuana cigarette
Meggie—marijuana
Mellow yellow—LSD
Merchandise—drugs
Merk—cocaine
Mesc—mescaline
Mescal—mescaline
Mescap—capsule of mescaline
Mescy—peyote
Mese—mescaline
Messorole—marijuana
Meth—methamphetamine
Meth head—regular user of
   methamphetamine
Meth monster—person who has a
   violent reaction to
   methamphetamine
Method—marijuana
Methyltestosterone—oral steroid
Mexican brown—heroin; marijuana
Mexican horse—heroin

Mexican mud—heroin
Mexican mushroom—
   psilocybin/psilocin
Mexican red—marijuana
Mexican reds—depressant
Mezc—mescaline
Mickey Finn—depressant
Mickey's—depressant
Microdot—LSD
Midnight oil—opium
Midnight toker—person who smokes
   marijuana before bed
Mighty Joe Young—depressant
Mighty mezz—marijuana cigarette
Mighty Mite—breed of marijuana plant
   with huge buds
Mighty Quinn—LSD
Mind detergent—LSD
Minglewood—cigar filled with good
   marijuana and hashish
Minibennie—amphetamine
Mint leaf—PCP
Mint weed—PCP
Mira—opium
Miss Emma—morphine
Missile basing—crack liquid and PCP
Mission—trip out of the crackhouse to
   obtain crack
Mist—PCP; crack smoke
Mister blue—morphine
M.J.—marijuana
M.O.—marijuana
Modams—marijuana
Mohasky—marijuana
Mojo—cocaine; heroin
Monkey—drug dependency; cigarette
   made from cocaine paste and tobacco
Monkey dust—PCP
Monkey tranquilizer—PCP
Monos—cigarette made from cocaine
   paste and tobacco
Monte—marijuana from South America
Mooca/moocah—marijuana
Moon—mescaline
Moonrock—crack and heroin
Mooster—marijuana
Moota/mutah—marijuana
Mooters—marijuana cigarette
Mootie—marijuana

Mootos—marijuana
Mor a grifa—marijuana
More—PCP
Morf—morphine
Morning wake-up—first blast of crack from the pipe
Morotgara—heroin
Mortal combat—high-potency heroin
Mosquitos—cocaine
Mota/moto—marijuana
Mother—marijuana
Mother of God—LSD paper with a naked woman on it
Mother's little helper—depressant; specifically, Valium
Mouth worker—one who takes drugs orally
Movie-star drug—cocaine
Mow the grass—to smoke marijuana
Mowing the lawn—smoking marijuana
M.S.—morphine
M.U.—marijuana
Mud—opium; heroin
Muerte—overdosing
Muggie—marijuana
Mujer—cocaine
Mule—carrier of drugs
Munchies—to get real hungry after smoking marijuana
Murder 8—fentanyl
Murder one—heroin and cocaine
Mushrooms—psilocybin/psilocin
Musk—psilocybin/psilocin
Mutha—marijuana
Muzzle—heroin

N

Nail—marijuana cigarette
Nailed—arrested
Nanoo—heroin
Nazi vitamins—crystal methamphetamine
Nebbies—depressant
Nemmies—depressant
New acid—PCP
New Jack Swing—heroin and morphine
New magic—PCP

Newspapers—LSD
Nice and easy—heroin
Nick—0.5 gram of marijuana (1/2 gram)
Nickel—0.5 gram of marijuana (1/2 gram)
Nickel bag—$5 worth of drugs; heroin
Nickel deck—heroin
Nickel note—$5 bill
Nickelonians—crack addicts
Niebla—PCP
Nimbies—depressant
Nitro—speed or nitrous oxide
Nitrous—nitrous oxide
Nix—stranger among the group
Nod—effects of heroin
Noise—heroin
Nontoucher—crack user who doesn't want affection during or after smoking crack
Northern lights—extremely high-grade marijuana
Nose—heroin
Nose candy—cocaine
Nose drops—liquefied heroin
Nose stuff—cocaine
Nose powder—cocaine
Nubs—peyote
Nugget—amphetamine
Nuggets—crack
Number—marijuana cigarette
Number 3—cocaine; heroin
Number 4—heroin
Number 8—heroin
Number 9—Ecstacy

O

O—opium; 1 ounce of marijuana
Oboy—marijuana
Octane—PCP laced with gasoline
Ogoy—heroin
Oil—heroin; PCP
O.J.—marijuana
Old Steve—heroin
On a mission—searching for crack
On a trip—under the influence of drugs
On ice—in jail
On the bricks—walking the streets

On the nod—under the influence of narcotics or depressant
One and one—to inhale cocaine
One box tissue—1 ounce of crack
One hitter quitter—marijuana that takes one hit to obtain a high
One way—LSD
One-fifty-one—crack
O.P.—opium
Ope—opium
O.P.P.—PCP
Optical illusions—LSD
Orange barrels—LSD
Orange crystal—PCP
Orange cubes—LSD
Orange haze—LSD
Orange micro—LSD
Orange wedges—LSD
Oranges—amphetamine
Oregano—hash
Outerlimits—crack and LSD
Outfit—heroin
Owl—marijuana
Owsley—LSD
Owsley's acid—LSD
Oz—inhalant; 1 ounce of marijuana or other drugs
Ozone—PCP
Ozzie—1 ounce of marijuana

P

P—peyote; PCP
Pack—heroin; marijuana
Pakalolo—marijuana
Pakistani black—marijuana
Panama cut—marijuana
Panama gold—marijuana
Panama red—marijuana
Panatella—large marijuana cigarette
Pancakes and syrup—combination of glutethimide and codeine cough syrup
Pane—LSD
Pangonadalot—heroin
Panic—drugs are not available
Paper acid—LSD
Paper bag—container for drugs

Paper blunts—marijuana within a paper casing rather than a tobacco-leaf casing
Paper boy—heroin peddler
Paps—rolling papers
Parabolin—veterinary steroid
Parachute—crack and PCP smoked; heroin
Paradise—cocaine
Paradise white—cocaine
Parlay—crack
Parsley—marijuana; PCP
Paste—crack
Pat—marijuana
Patico—crack (Spanish)
Paz—PCP
PCP—phencyclidine
PCPA—PCP
P-dope—20 to 30 percent pure heroin
Peace—LSD; PCP
Peace pill—PCP
Peace tablets—LSD
Peaches—amphetamine
Peanut—depressant
Peanut butter—PCP mixed with peanut butter; a type of methamphetamine that is brown in color
Pearl—cocaine
Pearls—amyl nitrite
Pearly gates—LSD; morning glory seeds
Pebbles—crack
Peddler—drug supplier
Pee wee—crack; $5 worth of crack
Peep—PCP
Peg—heroin
Pellets—LSD
Pen yan—opium
Pep pills—amphetamine
Pepsi habit—occasional use of drugs
Perfect high—heroin
Perico—cocaine
Permafried—high all the time
Perp—fake crack made of candle wax and baking soda
Peruvian—cocaine
Peruvian flake—cocaine
Peruvian lady—cocaine
Peter Pan—PCP
Peth—depressant

Peyote—mescaline
P-funk—heroin; crack and PCP
Phennies—depressant
Phenos—depressant
Pianoing—using the fingers to find lost crack
PID—possession with intent to distribute
Piece—1 ounce; cocaine; crack
Piedras—crack (Spanish)
Pig killer—PCP
Piles—crack
Pimp—cocaine
Pimp your pipe—lend or rent out your crack pipe
Pin—marijuana
Pin gon—opium
Pin yen—opium
Pine—marijuana
Ping-in-wing—to inject a drug
Pink blotters—LSD
Pink hearts—amphetamine
Pink ladies—depressant
Pink Panther—LSD
Pink robots—LSD
Pink wedge—LSD
Pink witches—LSD
Pinner—small joint of marijuana
Pipe—crack pipe; marijuana pipe; vein into which a drug is injected; to mix drugs with other substances
Pipero—crack user
Pit—PCP
Pixies—amphetamine
Piznacle—marijuana pipe
Pizza—marijuana; LSD
Pizza toppings—psilocybin/psilocin mushrooms
Plant—hiding place for drugs
Pocket rocket—marijuana
Pod—marijuana
Poison—heroin; fentanyl
Poke—marijuana
Polvo—heroin; PCP
Polvo blanco—cocaine
Polvo de angel—PCP
Polvo de estrellas—PCP
Pony—crack
Poof—smoking methamphetamine
Poor man's pot—inhalant

Pop—to inhale cocaine
Poppers—isobutyl nitrite; amyl nitrite
Poppy—heroin
Pot—marijuana
Potato—LSD
Potato chips—crack cut with benzocaine
Pothead—someone who smokes marijuana
Potten bush—marijuana
Powder—heroin; amphetamine
Powder diamonds—cocaine
Power puller—rubber piece attached to a crack stem
Pox—opium
P.R. (Panama red)—marijuana
Pregnant—when a joint has a lump in the middle
Prescription—marijuana cigarette
Press—cocaine; crack
Pretendica—marijuana
Pretendo—marijuana
Primo—crack; marijuana mixed with crack
Primobolan—injectable and oral steroid
Primos—cigarettes laced with cocaine and heroin
Proviron—oral steroid
Prudential—crack user
Pseudocaine—phenylpropanolamine (an adulterant for cutting cocaine)
Puff—to smoke marijuana
Puff the dragon—to smoke marijuana
Puffer—crack smoker
Puffy—PCP
Pulborn—heroin
Pull a will—vomiting from too much drug use
Pullers—crack users who pull at parts of their bodies excessively
Pumping—selling crack
Pure—heroin
Pure love—LSD
Purple—ketamine
Purple barrels—LSD
Purple flats—LSD
Purple haze—LSD
Purple hearts—LSD; amphetamine; depressant
Purple ozoline—LSD

Purple rain—PCP
Push—to sell drugs
Push shorts—to cheat or sell short amounts
Pusher—one who sells drugs; metal hanger or umbrella rod used to scrape residue in crack stems

Q

Q—depressant
Q.P.—¼ pound of marijuana
Quad—depressant
Quarter—¼ ounce, or $25 worth, of drugs
Quarter bag—$25 worth of drugs
Quarter moon—hashish
Quarter piece—¼ ounce
Quartz—smokable speed
Quas—depressant
Queen Anne's lace—marijuana
Queeted—when you get *way* too high off half a bowl
Quicksilver—isobutyl nitrite
Quill—methamphetamine; heroin; cocaine
Quinolone—injectable steroid

R

Racehorse charlie—cocaine; heroin
Ragweed—inferior-quality marijuana; heroin
Rail—large dose of crystal methamphetamine
Railroad weed—marijuana
Rainbows—depressant
Rainy day woman—marijuana
Rambo—heroin
Rane—cocaine; heroin
Rangood—marijuana grown wild
Rap—criminally charged; to talk with someone
Raspberry—female who trades sex for crack or for money to buy crack
Rasta weed—marijuana
Rat—someone who turns drug dealers in to the police

Rave—party designed to enhance a hallucinogenic experience through music and behavior
Raw—crack
Razed—under the influence of drugs
RB—resin bud (marijuana)
Ready rock—cocaine; crack; heroin
Recompress—to change the shape of cocaine flakes to resemble "rock"
Recycle—LSD
Red—under the influence of drugs
Red and blue—depressant
Red bullets—depressant
Red caps—crack
Red chicken—heroin
Red cross—marijuana
Red devil—depressant; PCP
Red dirt—marijuana
Red eagle—heroin
Red phosphorus—smokable speed
Reds—depressant
Reefer—marijuana
Register—to allow blood to flow back into the needle just prior to injecting heroin
Regular P—crack
Reindeer dust—heroin
Rhine—heroin
Rhythm—amphetamine
Riding the train—using cocaine
Riding the wave—under the influence of drugs
Rig—equipment used to inject drugs
Righteous bush—marijuana
Ringer—good hit of crack
Ripped—under the influence of drugs
Rippers—amphetamine
Roach—butt of a marijuana cigarette
Roach clip—instrument that holds a partially smoked marijuana cigarette
Road dope—amphetamine
Robo-ing—drinking Robitussin with codeine
Roca—crack (Spanish)
Roche—Rophynol (see "Roofies")
Rock(s)—cocaine; crack
Rock attack—crack
Rock house—place where crack is sold and smoked

Rock star—female who trades sex for crack or for money to buy crack

Rocket—marijuana cigarette

Rocket caps—dome-shaped caps on crack vials

Rocket fuel—PCP

Rockette—female who uses crack

Rocks of hell—crack

Rocky III—crack

Roid rage—aggressive behavior caused by excessive steroid use

Roll—MDMA

Roller—to inject a drug

Rollers—police

Rolling—MDMA

Roofies—Rohypnol (a sedative that makes users feel very drunk)

Rook—a person who can't handle his drugs

Rooster—crack

Root—marijuana

Rope—marijuana

Roples—Rohypnol (see "Roofies")

Rosa—amphetamine

Roses—amphetamine

Rox—crack

Roxanne—cocaine; crack

Royal blues—LSD

Royal Temple Ball—resin mixed with LSD, then rolled in to a ball

Roz—crack

Ruderalis—species of cannabis found in Russia that grows to 1 to 2.5 feet tall

Ruffles—Rophynol (see "Roofies")

Runners—people who sell drugs for others

Running—MDMA

Rupture—PCP

Rush—isobutyl nitrite

Rush snappers—isobutyl nitrite

Russian sickles—LSD

S

Sack—heroin

Sacrament—LSD

Sacre mushroom—psilocybin

Sak—bag of marijuana

Salt—heroin

Salt and pepper—marijuana

Sam—federal narcotics agent

San Pedro—mescaline

Sancocho—to steal (Spanish)

Sandoz—LSD

Sandwich—two layers of cocaine with a layer of heroin in the middle

Santa Marta—marijuana

Sasfras—marijuana

Satan's secret—inhalant

Satch—papers, letter, cards, clothing, etc., saturated with drug solution (used to smuggle drugs into prisons or hospitals)

Satch cotton—fabric used to filter a solution of narcotics before injection

Sativa—species of cannabis found in cool, damp climates that grows up to 18 feet tall

Scaffle—PCP

Scag—heroin

Scat—heroin

Scate—heroin

Schmeck—cocaine

Schoolboy—cocaine; codeine

Schoolcraft—crack

Scissors—marijuana

Score—to purchase drugs

Scorpion—cocaine

Scott—heroin

Scottie—cocaine

Scotty—cocaine; crack; the high from crack

Scramble—crack

Scratch—money

Scruples—crack

Scuffle—PCP

Seccy—depressant

Seeds—marijuana

Seggy—depressant

Sen—marijuana

Seni—peyote

Sernyl—PCP

Serpico 21—cocaine

Server—crack dealer

Sess—marijuana

Set—place where drugs are sold

Sevenup—cocaine; crack

Sewer—vein into which a drug is injected

Sezz—marijuana

Shabu—methamphetamine

Shake—marijuana

Shaker/baker/water—materials needed to freebase cocaine: shaker bottle, baking soda, water

Shaman—peyote

Sharps—needles

She—cocaine

Sheet rocking—crack and LSD

Sheets—PCP

Sherm—a cigarette that has been dipped into embalming fluid

Shermans—PCP or PCP-laced cigarettes

Sherms—PCP; crack

Shmagma—marijuana

Shmeck/schmeek—heroin

Shoot/shoot up—to inject a drug

Shoot the breeze—nitrous oxide

Shooting gallery—place where drugs are used

Shot—to inject a drug

Shot down—under the influence of drugs

Shotgun—someone puts the marijuana cigarette or cigar into his mouth backward and blows the smoke into someone else's mouth

Shrimp—marijuana

Shrooms—psilocybin/psilocin

Shwag—low-grade marijuana

Siddi—marijuana

Sightball—crack

Silly Putty—psilocybin/psilocin

Simple Simon—psilocybin/psilocin

Sinse—marijuana

Sinsemilla—potent variety of marijuana

Sixty-two—2½ ounces of crack

Skee—opium

Skeegers/skeezers—crack-smoking prostitute

Sketch—a bad reaction to LSD or marijuana

Sketching—coming down from a speed-induced high

Skid—heroin

Skied—under the influence of drugs

Skies—scales used to weigh drugs

Skin-popping—injecting drugs under the skin

Skuffle—PCP

Skunk—marijuana

Slab—crack

Slack—a bag that doesn't weigh out

Slam—to inject a drug

Slanging—selling drugs

Sleeper—heroin; depressant

Sleet—crack

Slick superspeed—methcathinone

Slime—heroin

Slinging—dealing drugs

Slits—MDMA

Smack—heroin

Smears—LSD

Smoke—heroin and crack; crack; marijuana

Smoke Canada—marijuana

Smoke you out—smoke marijuana with you

Smoke-out—under the influence of drugs

Smoking—PCP

Smoking gun—heroin and cocaine

smoochywoochypoochy—marijuana

Snap—amphetamine

Snappers—isobutyl nitrite

Sniff—to inhale cocaine; inhalant; methcathinone

Snite—lighter used to smoke drugs

Snop—marijuana

Snort—to inhale cocaine; to use inhalant

Snot—residue produced from smoking amphetamine

Snot balls—rubber cement rolled into balls and burned

Snow—cocaine; heroin; amphetamine

Snow bird—cocaine

Snow pallets—amphetamine

Snow seals—cocaine and amphetamine

Snow soke—crack

Snow white—cocaine

Snowball—cocaine and heroin

Snowcones—cocaine

Society high—cocaine

Soda—injectable cocaine used in Hispanic communities

Softballs—depressant

Soles—hashish

Soma—PCP

Sopers—depressant

Space base—crack dipped in PCP; hollowed-out cigar refilled with PCP and crack

Space cadet—crack dipped in PCP; someone who is high on drugs

Space dust—crack dipped in PCP

Spaced out—high on marijuana

Spaceship—glass pipe used to smoke crack

Spare time—possessing marijuana

Spark an owl—smoke a gigantic joint

Spark it up—to smoke marijuana

Sparking an owl—lighting a joint

Sparkle plenty—amphetamine

Sparklers—amphetamine

Special K—ketamine

Special la coke—ketamine

Speed—methamphetamine; amphetamine; crack

Speed boat—marijuana; PCP; crack

Speed for lovers—MDMA

Speed freak—habitual user of methamphetamine

Speedball—heroin and cocaine; amphetamine

Spider blue—heroin

Spike—to inject a drug; needle

Splaff—marijuana cigarette laced with acid

Splash—amphetamine

Spliff/Spliffy—marijuana cigarette

Splim—marijuana

Split—to leave

Splivins—amphetamine

Spoc—police officers (*cops* spelled backward)

Spoon—1/16 ounce of heroin; paraphernalia used to prepare heroin for injection

Spores—PCP

Sporting—to inhale cocaine

Spray—inhalant

Sprung—person just starting to use drugs

Square dancing tickets—LSD

Square mackerel—marijuana (term from Florida)

Square time Bob—crack

Squirrel—smoking cocaine, marijuana, and PCP; LSD

Stack—marijuana

Stacking—taking steroids with a prescription

Stackola—stack of money

Star—methcathinone

Stardust—cocaine; PCP

Star-spangled powder—cocaine

Stash—place to hide drugs

Stash areas—drug storage and distribution areas

Stat—methcathinone

Steamroller—pipe used to smoke marijuana

Steerer—person who directs customers to spots for buying crack

Stem—cylinder used to smoke crack

Stems—marijuana

Step on—dilute drugs

Stick—marijuana; PCP

Stimey—dime bag

Stink weed—marijuana

Stinky—pot

Stoned—under the influence of drugs

Stoner—someone who stays high on marijuana

Stones—crack

Stoppers—depressant

STP—PCP

Straw—marijuana cigarette

Strawberries—depressant

Strawberry—female who trades sex for crack or for money to buy crack

Strawberry fields—LSD

Strung out—heavily addicted to drugs

Stuff—heroin

Stumbler—depressant

Sugar—cocaine; LSD; heroin

Sugar block—crack

Sugar cubes—LSD

Sugar lumps—LSD

Sugar weed—marijuana

Sunshine—LSD

Super—PCP

Super acid—ketamine

Super C—ketamine
Super grass—PCP
Super ice—smokable methamphetamine
Super joint—PCP
Super kools—PCP
Super weed—PCP
Supergrass—marijuana
Super-jaded—blitzed off drugs; unable to think clearly
Surfer—PCP
Swag—poor-quality marijuana
Sweet Jesus—heroin
Sweet Lucy—marijuana
Sweet stuff—heroin; cocaine
Sweets—amphetamine
Swisher—cigar emptied and filled with marijuana
Synthetic cocaine—PCP

T

T—acid tabs; cocaine; marijuana
Tabs—LSD
Tail lights—LSD
Taima—marijuana
Taking a cruise—PCP
Takkouri—marijuana
Tampon—a fat joint
Tango & Cash—fentanyl
Tar—opium; heroin
Tardust—cocaine
Taste—heroin; small sample of drugs
Taxing—price paid to enter a crackhouse; charging more per vial depending on race of customer or if not a regular customer
T-buzz—PCP
Tea—marijuana; PCP
Tea party—to smoke marijuana
Teardrops—dosage units of crack packaged in the cut-off corners of plastic bags
Tecate—heroin
Tecatos—Hispanic heroin addicts
Teddy bears—LSD
Teenage—¹⁄₁₆ gram of methamphetamine
Teeth—cocaine; crack
Tension—crack

Texas pot—marijuana
Texas tea—marijuana
Tex-Mex—marijuana
Thai sticks—bundles of marijuana soaked in hash oil; marijuana buds bound on short sections of bamboo
THC—tetrahydrocannabinol
The beast—heroin
The C—methcathinone
The devil—crack
The great white hope—crack
The witch—heroin
Therobolin—injectable steroid
Thing—heroin; cocaine; main drug interest at the moment
Thirst monsters—heavy crack smokers
Thirteen—marijuana
Thoroughbred—drug dealer who sells pure narcotics
Thrust—isobutyl nitrite
Thrusters—amphetamine
Thumb—marijuana
Tic—PCP in powder form
Tic tac—PCP
Ticket—LSD
Tie—to inject a drug
Tin—container for marijuana; a marijuana pipe made out of tinfoil
Tish—PCP
Tissue—crack
Titch—PCP
Toilet water—inhalant
Toke—to inhale cocaine; to smoke marijuana
Toke up—to smoke marijuana
Toncho—octane booster that is inhaled
Tooles—depressant
Tools—equipment used for injecting drugs
Toot—cocaine; to inhale cocaine
Tootie—methamphetamine
Tooties—depressant
Tootsie roll—heroin
Top gun—crack
Topi—mescaline
Tops—peyote
Torch—marijuana
Torch cooking—smoking crack cocaine by using a propane or butane torch as the source of flame

Torch up—to smoke marijuana

Torpedo—crack and marijuana

Toss up—female who trades sex for crack or for money to buy crack

Totally spent—MDMA hangover

Toucher—user of crack who wants affection before, during, or after smoking crack

Tout—person who introduces buyers to sellers

Toxy—opium

Toys—opium

Tracers—visual effects of hallucinogens

Track—to inject a drug

Tracks—row of needle marks on a person

Tragic magic—crack dipped in PCP

Trails—LSD-induced perception that moving objects leave multiple images or trails behind them

Trank—PCP

Tranq—depressant

Trap—hiding place for drugs

Trash—heroin

Trashed—under the influence

Travel agent—LSD supplier

Trays—bunches of vials

Trees—marijuana

Trip—LSD; alpha-ethyltyptamine

Troop—crack

Trophobolene—injectable steroid

TR-6s—amphetamine

Truck drivers—amphetamine

TT1—PCP

TT2—PCP

TT3—PCP

Tubes—water pipes or bongs

Tuie—depressant

Turbo—crack and marijuana

Turf—place where drugs are sold

Turkey—cocaine; amphetamine; hashish

Turnabout—amphetamine

Turned on—introduced to drugs; under the influence

Tutti-frutti—flavored cocaine developed by a Brazilian gang

Tweak mission—on a mission to find crack

Tweaker—crack user looking for rocks on the floor after a police raid

Tweaking—drug-induced paranoia; peaking on speed

Tweeds—marijuana

Tweek—methamphetamine-like substance

Tweeker—methcathinone; person addicted to methamphetamines

Twenty—$20 rock of crack

Twenty-five—LSD

Twist—marijuana cigarette

Twistum—marijuana cigarette

Two for nine—2 $5 vials or bags of crack for $9

U

Ultimate—crack

Uncle—federal agents

Uncle Fester—glass pipe

Uncle Milty—depressant

Unkie—morphine

Up against the stem—addicted to smoking marijuana

Uppers—amphetamine

Uppies—amphetamine

Ups and downs—depressant

Utopiates—hallucinogens

Uzi—crack; crack pipe

V

V—the depressant Valium

Valley dolls—LSD

Vaporizer—vaporizes marijuana and leaves you with just the THC

Venom—PCP

Viper's weed—marijuana

Vodka acid—LSD

Volcano 5—red LSD paper

W

Wac—PCP mixed with marijuana

Wack—PCP

Wacky tobacky—marijuana

Wacky weed—marijuana

Waffles—hits of LSD

Wake ups—amphetamine
Water—methamphetamine; PCP
Wave—crack
Wedding bells—LSD
Wedge—LSD
Weed—marijuana; PCP
Weed out—weed for sale
Weed tea—marijuana
Weightless—high on crack
Weltschmerz—heroin withdrawal
Wet—PCP
Whack—PCP and heroin
Wheat—marijuana
When-shee—opium
Whippets—nitrous oxide
White—amphetamine
White ball—crack
White boy—heroin
White cloud—crack smoke
White cross—methamphetamine;
   amphetamine
White dust—LSD
White fluff—LSD
White ghost—crack
White girl—cocaine; heroin
White horizon—PCP
White horse—cocaine
White junk—heroin
White lady—cocaine; heroin
White lightning—LSD
White mosquito—cocaine
White nurse—heroin
White Owsley's—LSD
White powder—cocaine; PCP
White stuff—heroin
White sugar—crack
White tornado—crack
White-haired lady—marijuana
Whiteout—isobutyl nitrite
Whites—amphetamine
Whiz bang—cocaine and heroin
Wiggin—needing some drugs
Wild cat—methcathinone and cocaine
Window glass—LSD
Window pane—LSD
Wings—heroin; cocaine
Winstrol—oral steroid
Winstrol V—veterinary steroid
Witch—heroin; cocaine
Witch hazel—heroin

Wizard—1 ounce of marijuana
Wizard of Oz—1 ounce of marijuana
Wobble weed—PCP
Wolf—PCP
Wollie—rocks of crack rolled into a
   marijuana cigarette
Wonder star—methcathinone
Wooer—a marijuana cigarette
Woolah—a hollowed out cigar refilled
   with marijuana and crack
Woolas—cigarette laced with cocaine;
   marijuana cigarette sprinkled with
   crack
Woolies—marijuana and crack or PCP
Wooly—cocaine in a marijuana
   cigarette
Wooly blunts—crack or PCP in a
   marijuana cigar
Wooz—marijuana
Working—selling crack
Working half—crack rock weighing ½
   gram or more
Works—equipment for injecting drugs
Worm—PCP
Wrecking crew—crack
Wuwoo—marijuana and cocaine

X

X—marijuana; MDMA; amphetamine
X-ing—MDMA
XTC—MDMA

Y

Yahoo/yeaho—crack
Yale—crack
Yeh—marijuana
Yellow—LSD; depressant
Yellow bam—methamphetamine
Yellow bullets—depressant
Yellow dimples—LSD
Yellow fever—PCP
Yellow jackets—depressant
Yellow submarine—marijuana
Yellow sunshine—LSD
Yen pop—marijuana
Yen Shee Suey—opium wine

Yen sleep—restless, drowsy state after LSD use

Yerba—marijuana

Yerba mala—PCP and marijuana

Yesca—marijuana

Yesco—marijuana

Yeyo—cocaine (Spanish term)

Yimyom—crack

Ying—marijuana

Yuppie flu—the ongoing effects of a cocaine-snorting habit

Z

Z—1 ounce of heroin

Zacatecas purple—marijuana from Mexico

Zambi—marijuana

Zen—LSD

Zero—opium

Zig Zag man—LSD; marijuana; marijuana rolling papers

Zip—cocaine

Zips—1 ounce of any type of drug

Zoinked—intoxicated on drugs to the point of uselessness

Zol—marijuana cigarette

Zombie—PCP; heavy user of drugs

Zombie weed—PCP

Zooie—instrument that holds the butt of a marijuana cigarette

Zoom—PCP; marijuana laced with PCP

Zoomers—individuals who sell fake crack and then flee

Index

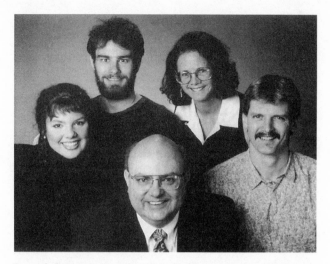

From left: Leigh Heather Wilson, Jeremy Foster, Wilkie Wilson, Cynthia Kuhn, and Scott Swartzwelder.
PHOTO BY JIM WALLACE.

CYNTHIA KUHN is a professor of pharmacology at Duke University Medical Center and heads the Pharmacological Sciences Training Program at Duke. She is married with two teenaged children.

SCOTT SWARTZWELDER is a professor of psychology at Duke University and a clinical professor of psychiatry at Duke University Medical Center. He is also a research career scientist and has served as the program specialist in alcoholism and drug dependence for the Department of Veterans Affairs. He is married with three young children.

WILKIE WILSON is a professor of pharmacology at the Duke University Medical Center. He is also a research career scientist and has served as neurobiology program specialist for the Department of Veterans Affairs. He is married with two daughters, one teenaged and one, college-aged, who also worked on this book.

LEIGH HEATHER WILSON is a junior at Hollins College, majoring in psychology.

JEREMY FOSTER is a senior at the University of North Carolina at Chapel Hill, majoring in journalism and mass communications.